THE WASHINGTON MANUAL™

Gastroenterology

Subspecialty Consult

FOURTH EDITION

Editor

C. Prakash Gyawali, MD, MRCP

Professor
Division of Gastroenterology
Washington University School of Medicine
St. Louis, Missouri

Executive Editors

Thomas Ciesielski, MD

Assistant Professor
Division of General Medicine
Washington University School of Medicine
St. Louis, Missouri

Thomas M. De Fer, MD, FACP

Professor of Medicine
Associate Dean for Medical Student
   Education
Department of Medicine
Washington University School of Medicine
St. Louis, Missouri

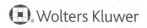 Wolters Kluwer

Philadelphia · Baltimore · New York · London
Buenos Aires · Hong Kong · Sydney · Tokyo

Executive Editor: Sharon Zinner
Development Editor: Thomas Celona
Editorial Coordinator: Tim Rinehart
Marketing Manager: Phyllis Hitner
Senior Production Project Manager: Alicia Jackson
Manager, Graphic Arts & Design: Stephen Druding
Senior Manufacturing Coordinator: Beth Welsh
Prepress Vendor: Aptara, Inc.

4th edition

Library of Congress Cataloging-in-Publication Data

Names: Gyawali, C. Prakash, editor. | Ciesielski, Thomas, editor. |
    Washington University (Saint Louis, Mo.). School of Medicine, sponsoring body.
Title: The Washington manual gastroenterology subspecialty consult /
    editor, C. Prakash Gyawali ; executive editor, Thomas Ciesielski.
Other titles: Gastroenterology subspecialty consult | Washington manual
    subspecialty consult series.
Description: Fourth edition. | Philadelphia : Wolters Kluwer, [2021] | Series: Washington manual subspecialty consult series | Includes bibliographical references and index. | Summary: "Advances in the field of gastroenterology since the last edition of this manual have been incorporated into the chapters in this edition. The manual continues to provide succinct, precise recommendations on the evaluation and management of common gastrointestinal symptoms and disorders. Each chapter has been thoroughly revised, and some chapters have been rewritten, to update content to modern concepts and guidelines. The chapters were written predominantly by Washington University subspecialty fellows, with support and guidance from their faculty mentors. Similar to previous editions, the fourth edition of the manual is targeted to medical students, novice and advanced trainees, physician extenders, nurse practitioners, other health care providers, and physicians, and will provide easy access to clinically relevant recommendations for diagnosis and management of gastrointestinal disorders"– Provided by publisher.
Identifiers: LCCN 2020022589 | ISBN 9781975113308 (paperback)
Subjects: MESH: Digestive System Diseases–diagnosis | Digestive System
    Diseases–therapy | Handbook
Classification: LCC RC801 | NLM WI 39 | DDC 616.3–dc23
LC record available at https://lccn.loc.gov/2020022589

MPP0722

Contributing Authors

Bader A. Alajlan, MD
Fellow
Division of Gastroenterology
Washington University School of Medicine
St. Louis, Missouri

Saad Alghamdi, MD
Fellow
Division of Gastroenterology
Washington University School of Medicine
St. Louis, Missouri

Ghadah Al Ismail, MD
Adjunct Associate Professor
Division of Gastroenterology
Washington University School of Medicine
St. Louis, Missouri

Osama Altayar, MD
Instructor
Division of Gastroenterology
Washington University School of Medicine
St. Louis, Missouri

Surachai Amornsawadwattana, MD
Instructor
Division of Gastroenterology
Washington University School of Medicine
St. Louis, Missouri

Motaz H. Ashkar, MD
Fellow
Division of Gastroenterology
Washington University School of Medicine
St. Louis, Missouri

Ricardo Badillo, MD
Fellow
Division of Gastroenterology
Washington University School of Medicine
St. Louis, Missouri

Michael C. Bennett, MD
Assistant Professor
Division of Gastroenterology
Washington University School of Medicine
St. Louis, Missouri

Jason G. Bill, MD
Fellow
Division of Gastroenterology
Washington University School of Medicine
St. Louis, Missouri

Elizabeth J. Blaney, MD
Assistant Professor
Division of Gastroenterology
Washington University School of Medicine
St. Louis, Missouri

Jeffrey W. Brown, MD
Instructor
Division of Gastroenterology
Washington University School of Medicine
St. Louis, Missouri

Chien-Huan Chen, MD, PhD
Professor
Division of Gastroenterology
Washington University School of Medicine
St. Louis, Missouri

Adeeti J. Chiplunker, MD
Fellow
Division of Gastroenterology
Washington University School of Medicine
St. Louis, Missouri

George P. Christophi, MD
Fellow
Division of Gastroenterology
Washington University School of Medicine
St. Louis, Missouri

Matthew A. Ciorba, MD
Associate Professor
Division of Gastroenterology
Washington University School of Medicine
St. Louis, Missouri

Jeffrey S. Crippin, MD
Professor
Division of Gastroenterology
Washington University School of Medicine
St. Louis, Missouri

Kelly C. Cushing, MD
Fellow
Division of Gastroenterology
Washington University School of Medicine
St. Louis, Missouri

Koushik K. Das, MD
Assistant Professor
Division of Gastroenterology
Washington University School of Medicine
St. Louis, Missouri

Dayna S. Early, MD
Professor
Division of Gastroenterology
Washington University School of Medicine
St. Louis, Missouri

Avegail Flores, MD
Assistant Professor
Division of Gastroenterology
Washington University School of Medicine
St. Louis, Missouri

Martin H. Gregory, MD
Fellow
Division of Gastroenterology
Washington University School of Medicine
St. Louis, Missouri

C. Prakash Gyawali, MD, MRCP
Professor
Division of Gastroenterology
Washington University School of Medicine
St. Louis, Missouri

Stephen Hasak, MD
Fellow
Division of Gastroenterology
Washington University School of Medicine
St. Louis, Missouri

Kevin M. Korenblat, MD
Professor
Division of Gastroenterology
Washington University School of Medicine
St. Louis, Missouri

Vladimir M. Kushnir, MD
Associate Professor
Division of Gastroenterology
Washington University School of Medicine
St. Louis, Missouri

Gabriel D. Lang, MD
Assistant Professor
Division of Gastroenterology
Washington University School of Medicine
St. Louis, Missouri

Mauricio Lisker-Melman, MD
Professor
Division of Gastroenterology
Washington University School of Medicine
St. Louis, Missouri

Scott A. McHenry, MD
Fellow
Division of Gastroenterology
Washington University School of Medicine
St. Louis, Missouri

Claire Meyer, MD
Fellow
Division of Gastroenterology
Washington University School of Medicine
St. Louis, Missouri

Daniel K. Mullady, MD
Professor
Division of Gastroenterology
Washington University School of Medicine
St. Louis, Missouri

Farhan Quader, MD
Fellow
Division of Gastroenterology
Washington University School of Medicine
St. Louis, Missouri

Rajeev Ramgopal, MD
Fellow
Division of Gastroenterology
Washington University School of Medicine
St. Louis, Missouri

Dominic N. Reeds, MD
Associate Professor
Division of Nutritional Science
Division of Gastroenterology
Washington University School of Medicine
St. Louis, Missouri

Benjamin D. Rogers, MD
Fellow
Division of Gastroenterology
Washington University School of Medicine
St. Louis, Missouri

Deborah C. Rubin, MD
Professor
Division of Gastroenterology
Washington University School of Medicine
St. Louis, Missouri

Jose B. Saenz, MD, PhD
Instructor
Division of Gastroenterology
Washington University School of Medicine
St. Louis, Missouri

Gregory S. Sayuk, MD, MPH
Associate Professor
Division of Gastroenterology
Washington University School of Medicine
St. Louis, Missouri

Yeshika Sharma, MD
Resident
Department of Medicine
Washington University School of Medicine
St. Louis, Missouri

Zachary L. Smith, MD
Assistant Professor
Department of Surgery
Washington University School of Medicine
St. Louis, Missouri

Rama Suresh, MD
Associate Professor
Medical Oncology
Washington University School of Medicine
St. Louis, Missouri

Ted Walker, MD
Fellow
Division of Gastroenterology
Washington University School of Medicine
St. Louis, Missouri

Michael J. Weaver, MD
Fellow
Division of Gastroenterology
Washington University School of Medicine
St. Louis, Missouri

Chairman's Note

I t is a pleasure to present the new edition of *The Washington Manual*® Subspecialty Consult Series: *Gastroenterology Subspecialty Consult*. This pocket-size book continues to be a primary reference for medical students, interns, residents, and other practitioners who need ready access to practical clinical information to diagnose and treat patients with a wide variety of disorders. Medical knowledge continues to increase at an astounding rate, which creates a challenge for physicians to keep up with the biomedical discoveries, genetic and genomic information, and novel therapeutics that can positively affect patient outcomes. *The Washington Manual* Subspecialty Consult Series addresses this challenge by concisely and practically providing current scientific information for clinicians to aid them in the diagnosis, investigation, and treatment of common medical conditions.

I want to personally thank the authors, which include house officers, fellows, and attendings at the Washington University School of Medicine and Barnes Jewish Hospital. Their commitment to patient care and education is unsurpassed, and their efforts and skill in compiling this manual are evident in the quality of the final product. In particular, I would like to acknowledge our editor Dr. C. Prakash Gyawali and executive editor Dr. Thomas Ciesielski, who have worked tirelessly to produce another outstanding edition of this manual. I believe this manual will meet its desired goal of providing practical knowledge that can be directly applied at the bedside and in outpatient settings to improve patient care.

Victoria J. Fraser, MD
Adolphus Busch Professor of Medicine
Chair of Medicine
Washington University School of Medicine

Preface

Advances in the field of gastroenterology since the last edition of this manual have been incorporated into the chapters in this edition. The manual continues to provide succinct, precise recommendations on the evaluation and management of common gastrointestinal symptoms and disorders. Each chapter has been thoroughly revised, and some chapters have been rewritten, to update content to modern concepts and guidelines. The chapters were written predominantly by Washington University subspecialty fellows, with support and guidance from their faculty mentors. Similar to previous editions, the fourth edition of the manual is targeted to medical students, novice and advanced trainees, physician extenders, nurse practitioners, other health care providers, and physicians, and will provide easy access to clinically relevant recommendations for diagnosis and management of gastrointestinal disorders.

I would like dedicate this edition of the manual to all the trainees who aspire to become gastroenterologists, and I sincerely hope reading the manual will further inspire them to pursue training within the field of gastroenterology.

—C.P.G.

Contents

PART II. APPROACH TO SPECIFIC DISEASES

Dysphagia

Farhan Quader and C. Prakash Gyawali

GENERAL PRINCIPLES

Dysphagia is the sensation of impairment in transit of food or liquid to the stomach. This can lead to significant morbidity, and complications like weight loss and pulmonary aspiration.

Definition

- Dysphagia is defined as **difficulty in swallowing or the sensation of an obstruction in the passage of food** (semisolid, solid, and/or liquid) anywhere from the mouth to the stomach.[1]
- Dysphagia should be distinguished from the following:
    - **Odynophagia:** painful swallowing that can be present with or without dysphagia.
    - **Globus:** also known as globus pharyngeus or idiopathic globus, a persistent or intermittent nonpainful sensation of fullness or tightness in the throat, without pain and without impairment of swallowing.
    - **Aphagia:** inability to swallow, which can result when a food bolus gets impacted in the esophagus, thus blocking passage of any further boluses. Aphagia can also result from pharyngeal muscle paralysis from lower cranial nerve involvement.
    - **Xerostomia:** dryness of the mouth from decreased salivation (from Sjögren syndrome, radiation to head and neck, medication side effects, etc.), which can cause trouble initiating a swallow because of poor lubrication of the food bolus.

Classification

- Dysphagia can be classified as oropharyngeal or esophageal.[1]
- **Oropharyngeal dysphagia**
    - This arises from disorders that affect the function of the oropharynx, larynx, and upper esophageal sphincter (UES), and is typically caused by lesions of the swallowing center, cranial nerves, or oropharyngeal muscles, mucosa, or teeth.[2]
    - There is dysfunction in oral and pharyngeal phases of swallowing.[3]
    - These disorders cause difficulties with preparing the food for swallowing or with transferring a bolus of food from oral cavity to esophagus.
    - Patients with oropharyngeal dysphagia may report difficulty initiating a swallow, coughing, choking, drooling, or nasal regurgitation. This sensation is typically reported within 1 second of initiating a swallow.[3]
- **Esophageal dysphagia**
    - This arises commonly from structural or motor defects within the body of the esophagus, the lower esophageal sphincter (LES), or gastric cardia.[2]
    - Mechanical processes in the distal esophagus with lumen narrowing, often related to GERD, are the most common conditions causing esophageal dysphagia. Dysphagia is typically reported with solid foods initially.
    - Motor abnormalities in LES relaxation or the esophageal phase of swallowing can also cause esophageal dysphagia, which is reported with both solids and liquids.
    - Patients may describe the sensation of food sticking in the throat or the chest, retrosternal chest pain, or regurgitation soon after swallowing. The regurgitate may

taste similar to food just eaten and not sour or bitter (which implicates retrograde transit from the stomach, as in reflux disease or emesis).

Determining location of obstruction based on symptoms is not always reliable due to lack of site-specific sensory receptors.[4]

Epidemiology

As many as 16–22% of individuals older than 50 years describe symptoms of dysphagia.[3]

Etiology

- Oropharyngeal dysphagia is most commonly caused by neurogenic and myogenic disorders and rarely occurs as a result of oropharyngeal or base-of-skull tumors.
- Esophageal dysphagia is either the result of a structural esophageal (luminal, intramural, or extraluminal) lesion or a neuromuscular disorder of esophageal peristalsis. Eosinophilic esophagitis, an idiopathic eosinophilic inflammatory disease with remodeling of the esophagus, is becoming increasingly recognized as a cause for esophageal dysphagia, particularly in young adults.

Pathophysiology

- **The normal swallowing process can be divided into three phases[5]:**
  - **Oral:** The food bolus is first mechanically prepared by the muscles of the jaw, face, and tongue, and propelled posteriorly and superiorly by the tongue and the palate. This process lasts 1–2 seconds.
  - **Pharyngeal:** This phase begins when the bolus passes the anterior tonsillar pillars. The soft palate closes the nasopharynx, and the lips and the jaws remain closed. The larynx elevates and closes the laryngeal valves (epiglottis and vocal cords). This also opens the UES, allowing passage of the bolus into the esophagus. The entire process lasts <1 second.
  - **Esophageal:** This phase begins with the entry of the bolus into the esophagus. The UES closes, and bolus is propelled efficiently through the esophagus to the stomach. In the upright position, this is facilitated by gravity, with the esophageal muscle contraction stripping the remnants of the bolus through an open LES. Secondary esophageal peristalsis may initiate in response to esophageal distension if the primary peristaltic effort is insufficient in propelling the bolus.
- **Dysphagia is caused by a disruption in this process.**
  - **Oropharyngeal dysphagia:** occurs when there is a disruption in the oral or pharyngeal phases of swallowing.
  - **Esophageal dysphagia:** occurs when there is a disruption in the esophageal phase of swallowing.

DIAGNOSIS

Clinical Presentation

- **Oropharyngeal**
  - Oropharyngeal dysphagia is commonly a manifestation of a **neurologic or systemic disorder** (Table 1-1). A careful and directed history specifically intended to include or rule out neurologic, muscular, collagen vascular, and local structural disorders is essential.
  - Patients complain of difficulty initiating a swallow, coughing, choking, drooling, or nasal regurgitation within 1 second of initiating a swallow.
  - Patients have difficulty with swallowing solids and/or liquids.
  - Evidence of neurologic dysfunction in the lower cranial nerves, or of generalized muscle weakness or dystrophy may be evident on physical examination.

TABLE 1-1 CAUSES OF OROPHARYNGEAL DYSPHAGIA

Neuromuscular Disorders
Cerebrovascular accident
Parkinson disease
Amyotrophic lateral sclerosis
Poliomyelitis
Polymyositis
Myasthenia gravis
Brain tumors
Hypothyroidism
Abnormal upper esophageal sphincter relaxation

Structural Lesions
Neoplasm
Inflammation (pharyngitis, radiation)
Plummer–Vinson syndrome
Cervical hyperostosis
Thyromegaly
Lymphadenopathy
Prior oropharyngeal surgery
Zenker diverticulum

- **Esophageal**
  - Esophageal dysphagia is typically related to an esophageal process, either structural or neuromuscular.
  - Patients complain of food sticking in the throat or the chest.
  - Symptoms start a few seconds to minutes after swallowing.
  - Esophageal dysphagia can start as difficulty in swallowing solid foods, but can progress to both solids and liquids.
  - Regurgitation and chest pain may be associated symptoms.

History
- A carefully taken symptom history can provide clues to the underlying cause of dysphagia.[3]
- It is important to determine whether the patient has esophageal or oropharyngeal dysphagia.[3] The following are factors important in making this determination:
  - Onset and duration of symptoms, including chronicity
  - Quality of symptoms, including chest pain, heartburn, regurgitation
  - Nocturnal symptoms, including water brash, waking up at night with heartburn or regurgitation
  - Prescribed and over-the-counter medications, including herbal supplements
  - Past medical history, including asthma and abdominal surgeries
  - Coughing while swallowing
  - Regurgitation of food through the nose, drooling, or food spilling from the corners of the mouth
  - Food items that typically cause difficulty (specifically, solids, liquids, or both)
  - History of radiation therapy to head and neck
  - The presence of weight loss[1]

Physical Examination
- General examination: evaluate nutritional status (including body weight).

- Complete neurologic examination (attention to resting tremor, cranial nerves, and muscle strength).
- Examine oral cavity, head, and neck, including assessment for pharyngeal erythema and Mallampati classification of the oropharynx.
- Observe the patient's gait and balance to assess for neurologic disorders. If concern for premature muscle fatigue, have patient perform repetitive tasks.[3]
- Examine the nails for pitting and the skin for thickening or texture changes, especially palms of hands and the soles of feet (tylosis, associated with squamous esophageal cancer).[1]
- Evaluate the neck for thyromegaly or other mass.
- Inspect the muscles for wasting and fasciculations and palpate for tenderness to detect an underlying motor neuron disease.[3]

Differential Diagnosis

- **Oropharyngeal dysphagia**
  - Neuromuscular causes are more frequent than structural causes for this type of dysphagia. This is mainly because the nerves that control the muscles in this region have a direct connection to the brain through cranial nerves and can be damaged in accidents or diseases that affect the brain or the cranial nerves.[3]
  - Table 1-1 refers to some of the more frequent causes of oropharyngeal dysphagia.
- **Esophageal dysphagia**
  - Structural causes are a more frequent cause of esophageal dysphagia than disorders involving nerves and muscles.
  - Eosinophilic esophagitis can present with intermittent food bolus impactions.
  - Patients with a neuromuscular disorder commonly report dysphagia to both solids and liquids from the onset of symptoms.[1]
  - Table 1-2 refers to some of the more frequent causes of esophageal dysphagia.

Diagnostic Testing

- **If oropharyngeal dysphagia is suspected:**
  - **A careful neurologic examination is the first step in evaluation.**
  - **Modified barium swallow/videofluoroscopy**[5]: This consists of a radiographic study in which the oral and pharyngeal phases are observed in real time while the patient

TABLE 1-2 CAUSES OF ESOPHAGEAL DYSPHAGIA

Structural Causes

Benign stricture
Esophageal cancer
Schatzki ring
Esophageal webs
Foreign bodies
Extrinsic (vascular, cervical osteoarthritis, adenopathy)

Motility Disorders

Achalasia
Scleroderma
Abnormal lower esophageal sphincter relaxation
Diffuse esophageal spasm
Chagas disease
Jackhammer esophagus

swallows barium of varying consistencies, such as thin liquids, thick liquids, and barium cookies, or a cracker. This study helps identify abnormalities of the oropharyngeal phases and may direct therapy. Patients may tolerate certain consistencies better than others, and the diet can be modified accordingly.

Laryngoscopy: If structural lesions are identified, direct laryngoscopy should be performed for further evaluation.

High-resolution manometry (HRM): Esophageal manometry may have value in evaluation of pharyngeal muscle and UES function. HRM can also be utilized if a spastic process of the UES is suspected.

- **If esophageal dysphagia is suspected:**

  Upper endoscopy: This is the most useful initial test and should be the first test ordered for patients presenting with dysphagia. Upper endoscopy allows for evaluation of mucosa as well as structural restrictions, including stricture, ring, web, and hiatus hernia. It also allows for therapeutic intervention, such as dilation, and mucosal biopsies, such as in the case of eosinophilic esophagitis or Barrett esophagus, if needed.[6] One study reported a diagnostic yield of 54% with EGD in the initial evaluation of dysphagia in patients aged >40 years.[7]

  Esophagram (barium swallow): Alternate test that is useful when subtle strictures or narrowings are suspected or when road mapping of a tight or complicated stricture is desired before endoscopic evaluation. This test can also provide information on the length and degree of narrowing of a structural lesion.[6] An esophagogram commonly reveals structural esophageal abnormalities such as tumors, webs, and rings, or aids in the detection of subtle abnormalities. Motility disorders, such as achalasia, diffuse esophageal spasm, and scleroderma esophagus, have typical esophagram findings, but esophageal manometry is typically required for a definitive diagnosis. Esophagram should not be performed if there's concern for significant obstruction or food impaction.

  Esophageal manometry: This test is performed when no structural or obstructive process is identified on upper endoscopy or barium esophagram in patients presenting with dysphagia, or the diagnosis of achalasia is suspected.[1] High-resolution esophageal manometry involves using a solid state catheter with 36 circumferential sensors 1 cm apart and provides high-fidelity topograms (Clouse plots) of esophageal peristalsis and sphincter function. The catheter is passed through an anesthetized nasal canal, down the esophagus, and past the LES into the stomach. Pressure measurements are then obtained over the full length of the esophagus, including the UES and the LES, both at rest and during test water swallows.[8] Esophageal manometry has been demonstrated to substantially improve the sensitivity of diagnosis of LES relaxation abnormalities. The addition of stationary impedance to HRM, the administration of solid boluses, and the provocative tests with multiple rapid swallows and rapid drink challenge to the manometry protocol may improve the yield for a motor diagnosis in the evaluation of dysphagia.

  Endoluminal functional lumen imaging probe (EndoFLIP): This is a newer technique that measures the distensibility of the esophagus to evaluate for abnormal biomechanics not otherwise evident on alternate testing. The EndoFLIP system uses impedance planimetry for real-time measurement of the cross-sectional area and distensibility of the esophagus and esophagogastric junction. Hydraulic dilation (similar to pneumatic dilation) can also be performed using the EndoFLIP system using special catheters when indicated.[9]

TREATMENT

Medications

Medications are useful only if they can treat the underlying condition causing dysphagia.

Nonpharmacologic Therapies

- **Oropharyngeal dysphagia**
  - When possible, treatment should be directed at the underlying disorder.
  - However, many patients have irreversible or progressive neurologic diseases, which can lead to worsening oropharyngeal dysphagia.
  - **Consultation with a speech therapist** is often helpful in modifying eating behaviors and food consistency.[5]
  - Despite these interventions, some patients will still experience oropharyngeal dysphagia placing them at a high risk for aspiration or inadequate caloric intake.
  - If significant improvement of oropharyngeal dysphagia is not expected, alternative sources of **nutritional support** should be pursued. Options may include nasogastric feeding tube, or long-term options such as enteral feeding through percutaneous gastrostomy or jejunostomy tubes.
  - Excessive drooling or troublesome oropharyngeal secretions can sometimes be suppressed using anticholinergic agents or tricyclic antidepressants.
- **Esophageal dysphagia**
  - Management of esophageal dysphagia should be tailored to the underlying disorder (see Chapter 13 for more detail).
  - **Endoscopic therapies**, including dilation of strictures and disruption of esophageal rings, can be helpful in the management of structural causes of esophageal dysphagia.
  - Eosinophilic esophagitis can be treated with PPI, topical steroids, and exclusion diets; intermittent dilation of dominant strictures may be sometimes necessary.
  - **Empiric endoscopic dilation** with a large caliber dilator is often performed in patients wherein a definitive etiology for esophageal-type dysphagia is not apparent on routine investigation. This approach may result in symptomatic improvement of varying durations.
  - Obstructing tumors can be treated with dilation or by placement of an endoscopic stent.
  - Some motility disorders are amenable to endoscopic therapy, including botulinum toxin injection into the LES and pneumatic or hydraulic dilation in disorders of LES relaxation.
  - Surgical myotomy and pneumatic dilation are durable options in achalasia.
  - **Gastrostomy tube placement** may be indicated in patients with large, obstructing esophageal tumors that are not amenable to dilation or stent placement.

Lifestyle/Risk Modification

Diet

Treatment of dysphagia can include a change in the patient's diet or the consistency of the diet to aid swallowing. A **modified barium swallow** may help identify food consistencies that can be swallowed better than others. This is particularly relevant in oropharyngeal dysphagia from neuromuscular disease and in esophageal dysphagia where there is residual dysphagia after treatment.

Activity

A speech–language pathologist can help a patient learn different exercises and head and neck positions that may help facilitate swallowing.[3]

SPECIAL CONSIDERATIONS

Functional dysphagia: A disorder that is characterized by a sensation of abnormal bolus transits through the esophagus in the absence of structural lesions, GERD, and histopathology-based esophageal motility disorders. Functional dysphagia includes the sense of solid and/or liquid foods sticking, lodging, or passing through esophagus.[10] This is related to increased perception of esophageal sensation, sometimes triggered by noxious triggers like gastroesophageal reflux disease. In addition to treating associated reflux disease, neuromodulators (e.g., low-dose tricyclic antidepressants) may be of value.

COMPLICATIONS

The most common complications with dysphagia include **aspiration, pneumonia, and dehydration.**[11] Prolonged dysphagia can lead to weight loss and malnutrition. Aggressive dilation of esophageal strictures can rarely result in esophageal perforation.

REFERRAL

Treating a patient with dysphagia is often a joint effort of a team of specialists including a gastroenterologist, radiologist, speech–language therapist, neurologist, otolaryngologist, and nutritionist.[3]

OUTCOME/PROGNOSIS

- The improvement of symptoms often depends on the type of dysphagia.
- In the case of strictures, tumors, and cervical webs, surgery, dilation, antineoplastic therapy, or a combination of these treatments may be used.[3] An alternative option, especially with untreatable tumors, is stent placement.
- Certain types of dysphagia such as those caused by acid reflux disease, esophageal infections, and eosinophilic esophagitis may be treated with medical therapy.
- Dysphagia caused by achalasia can be treated with pneumatic balloon dilation, botulinum toxin injection, or myotomy.[6]

REFERENCES

1. Trate DM, Parkman HP, Fisher RS. Dysphagia. Evaluation, diagnosis and treatment. *Prim Care.* 1996;23:417–432.
2. Schechter GL. Systemic causes of dysphagia in adults. *Otolaryngol Clin North Am.* 1998;31:525–535.
3. Cook IJ, Kahrilas PJ. AGA technical review on management of oropharyngeal dysphagia. *Gastroenterology.* 1999;116:455–478.
4. Abdel Jalil AA, Katzka DA, Castell DO. Approach to the patient with dysphagia. *Am J Med.* 2015;128:1138.e17–1138.e23.
5. Logemann JA. Swallowing disorders. *Best Pract Res Clin Gastroenterol.* 2007;21:563–573.
6. Spechler SJ. AGA technical review on treatment of patients with dysphagia caused by benign disorders of distal esophagus. *Gastroenterology.* 1999;117:233–254.
7. ASGE Standards of Practice Committee; Pasha SF, Acosta RD, Chandrasekhara V, et al. The role of endoscopy in the evaluation and management of dysphagia. *Gastrointest Endosc.* 2014;79:191–201.
8. Roman S, Pandolfino J, Mion F. High-resolution manometry: a new gold standard to diagnose esophageal dysmotility? *Gastroenterol Clin Biol.* 2009;33:1061–1067.
9. Carlson DA, Kahrilas PJ, Lin Z, et al. Evaluation of esophageal motility utilizing the functional lumen imaging Probe. *Am J Gastroenterol.* 2016;111:1726–1735.
10. Galmiche JP, Clouse RE, Balint A, et al. Functional esophageal disorders. *Gastroenterology.* 2006;130:1459–1465.
11. Schindler A, Ginocchio D, Ruoppolo G. What we don't know about dysphagia complications? *Rev Laryngol Otol Rhinol (Bord).* 2008;129:75–78.

Nausea and Vomiting

Benjamin D. Rogers and C. Prakash Gyawali

GENERAL PRINCIPLES

- Nausea is one of the most common gastrointestinal (GI) symptoms and can be related to a wide variety of GI, systemic, and neurologic disorders.
- Nausea encompasses a heterogeneous group of symptoms ranging from upper abdominal discomfort to urge to vomit.
- Nausea can precede the act of emesis, occur concurrently with emesis, or occur on its own.
- Altered autonomic activity and decreased function of the upper GI tract can accompany severe nausea.

Definitions

- Nausea refers to an unpleasant subjective sensation of an imminent urge to vomit and is usually sensed in the throat or epigastrium. It can be accompanied by autonomic changes such as hypersalivation, light-headedness, dizziness, sweating, tachycardia, or increased blood pressure.[1]
- **Vomiting** (or emesis) denotes the forceful ejection of GI contents through the mouth. The act of emesis is a highly coordinated event requiring the integration of both central and peripheral nervous systems.[1]

Epidemiology

Nausea and vomiting are commonly reported symptoms, and are more common in women than in men. Prevalence in the community is estimated at 10%.[2] Nausea and vomiting are frequent reasons for consultation with a gastroenterologist and contribute significantly to hospital costs and physician visits, with an annual economic burden of 4–16 billion dollars in the United States.

Etiology

- Clinically important etiologies of nausea and vomiting are listed in Table 2-1.
- **Medications**
  - **Antiparkinsonian agents** (e.g., L-DOPA, bromocriptine), nicotine, and digoxin produce nausea and vomiting through direct action on receptors in the chemoreceptor trigger zone.
  - **Nonsteroidal anti-inflammatory drugs (NSAIDs)** and **antibiotics**, such as erythromycin, stimulate peripheral afferent pathways to activate the vomiting center directly.[3]
  - **Opioid analgesics** cause nausea in >25% of patients. Multiple mechanisms have been implicated, including direct stimulation of the chemoreceptor trigger zone, reduced GI motility, or enhanced vestibular sensitivity.
  - **Chemotherapeutic agents** frequently cause nausea and vomiting. Acute vomiting, usually caused by agents such as cisplatin, nitrogen mustard, and dacarbazine, is generally mediated through serotonergic pathways, both centrally and peripherally. Delayed and anticipatory vomiting is serotonin independent.

TABLE 2-1 DIFFERENTIAL DIAGNOSIS OF NAUSEA AND VOMITING

Medications

Chemotherapy: cisplatin, dacarbazine, nitrogen mustard

Analgesics

Oral contraceptives

Cardiovascular: digoxin, antiarrhythmics, β-blockers, antihypertensives, calcium channel blockers

Antibiotics: erythromycin, tetracycline, sulfonamides

Sulfasalazine

Azathioprine

Antiparkinsonian agents

Theophylline

Narcotic agents

Infections

Gastroenteritis

Viral: rotavirus, Norwalk virus, adenovirus, Reovirus

Bacterial: *Staphylococcus aureus, Salmonella, Bacillus cereus,* and *Clostridium perfringens* (toxins)

Systemic nongastrointestinal infections

Other

Pregnancy

Uremia

Diabetic ketoacidosis

Addison's disease

Postoperative nausea and vomiting

Cardiac ischemia or infarction

Gastrointestinal and Peritoneal Disorders

Peptic ulcer disease

Appendicitis

Hepatitis

Mesenteric ischemia

Pancreatitis

Cholecystitis

Gastric outlet obstruction

Small bowel obstruction

Inflammatory bowel disease

Gastroparesis

Nonulcer dyspepsia

Central Nervous System Disorders

Increased intracranial pressure: tumor, hemorrhage, pseudotumor cerebri

Migraine

Psychogenic vomiting

Cyclic vomiting syndrome

Anorexia Nervosa

Bulimia nervosa

Labyrinthine disorders

- **Cannabis**, when used on a long-term basis, can result in an illness that resembles cyclic vomiting syndrome, termed cannabinoid hyperemesis. Cannabis-induced autonomic dysregulation and abnormal gastric emptying are thought to be contributing to this process.[4]
- **Infections**
  - **Viral gastroenteritis** is a common cause of acute nausea and vomiting, particularly in the pediatric population. Causative agents include *rotavirus, Norwalk virus, Reovirus,* and *adenovirus.*
  - **Bacterial infections** with *Staphylococcus aureus, Salmonella, Bacillus cereus,* and *Clostridium perfringens* are commonly associated with "food poisoning." Enterotoxins act both centrally and peripherally.
  - **Miscellaneous infectious processes**, such as *otitis media, meningitis, urinary tract infections,* and *acute hepatitis* also commonly produce nausea and vomiting.[3]
- **Endocrine and metabolic disorders**
  - **Pregnancy** is an important cause of nausea and vomiting in women of reproductive age. Nausea and vomiting occurs in 70–80% of women during the first trimester.[5]

Symptoms typically peak around the ninth week and subside by the end of the first trimester. Nausea in pregnancy is related to fluctuations in hormone levels, as the symptoms parallel the rise and fall of β-human chorionic gonadotropin (β-hCG) levels. Hyperemesis gravidarum complicates 1–5% of pregnancies, causing intractable vomiting. This condition is serious and can result in significant weight loss and fetal loss.[6]

Uremia, diabetic ketoacidosis, and **hypercalcemia** are postulated to cause nausea and vomiting through direct action on the area postrema. **Parathyroid, thyroid**, and **adrenal disease** act by disruption of GI motility.

Practically any **electrolyte imbalance** can result in nausea and vomiting.

- **Gastrointestinal and peritoneal disorders**

  Nausea can be caused by **gastroesophageal reflux disease (GERD)** or **peptic ulcer disease**.

  Functional disorders, such as *chronic nausea/vomiting syndrome* and *cyclic vomiting syndrome,* account for a large proportion of chronic nausea and vomiting.[7] Alterations in motility (e.g., abnormal gastric emptying) may be present but correlate poorly with symptoms.

  Gastroparesis, where altered gastric motility leads to a failure or near failure of gastric emptying, is associated with a multitude of systemic disorders, notably diabetes mellitus, systemic lupus erythematosus, scleroderma, and amyloidosis. Upper abdominal fullness, nausea, vomiting (particularly delayed vomiting of food ingested hours or days earlier), and weight loss can be seen.[8]

  Inflammation of any viscus can cause nausea and vomiting through activation of afferent pathways. *Pancreatitis, diverticulitis, colitis, appendicitis, cholecystitis*, and *biliary pain* (colic) are common causes. Peritoneal inflammation is usually associated with severe abdominal pain in addition to nausea and vomiting.

  Mechanical obstruction at any level in the GI tract can be the cause of nausea and vomiting. Distention of the bowel lumen causes activation of afferent pathways and emesis ensues in an attempt to decrease pressure.

  Intestinal pseudo-obstruction usually results from disorders of neuromuscular function in the colon and small bowel. Clinical presentation is similar to that of mechanical bowel obstruction, but no anatomic obstruction is evident on investigation.

- **Central nervous system (CNS) disorders**

  Increased intracranial pressure from any cause (malignancy, infection, cerebrovascular accident, hemorrhage) can induce emesis with or without nausea.

  Vestibular disorders, including labyrinthitis, cerebellopontine angle tumors, Ménière disease, and motion sickness, are common causes of nausea and vomiting.[3]

Pathophysiology

- **Initiation of emesis**

  The *vomiting center,* in the dorsal portion of the lateral reticular formation of the medulla oblongata, serves as the point of integration and initiation of emesis.

  Afferent stimuli are received by the vomiting center principally from four sources: the vestibular system, peripheral GI tract neural pathways, the chemoreceptor trigger zone, and the cortex.

  The vestibular system, particularly the labyrinthine apparatus located in the inner ear, sends afferent signals through the vestibular nucleus and the cerebellum to the vomiting center.[9]

  Peripheral neural pathways from the GI tract play a significant role in the initiation of emesis. Afferent vagal fibers project to the nucleus tractus solitarius and from there to the vomiting center. Serotonergic pathways are also believed to play a large role in peripheral stimulation via 5-hydroxytryptamine (5-HT_3) receptors located on the afferent vagal nerves.

The chemoreceptor trigger zone, located in the area postrema on the floor of the fourth ventricle, is a major mediator of the initiation of emesis. A number of drugs and toxins activate the zone via dopamine D_2, muscarinic M_1, histaminergic H_1, serotonergic 5-HT_3, neurokinin NK-1, and vasopressinergic receptors. Several metabolic abnormalities also affect the trigger zone. Once activated, efferent signals are sent on to the vomiting center, where the physical act of emesis is initiated.

Several areas of the cerebral cortex interact to modulate a parasympathetic to sympathetic shift, potentiating emesis during states of anxiety, stress, or elevation of intracranial pressure, primarily via GABA and histaminergic H_1 receptors.

- **Mechanisms of emesis**
  - Efferent pathways from the vomiting center serve to initiate vomiting. Important pathways include the phrenic nerves to the diaphragm, the spinal nerves to the abdominal musculature, and visceral efferent vagal fibers to the larynx, pharynx, esophagus, and stomach.[9]
  - The act of emesis involves a coordinated sequence of events that includes the abdominal wall musculature and smooth muscle of the GI tract. While the lower esophageal sphincter and the gastric body relax, a combination of forceful contractions of the abdominal wall muscles, diaphragm, and gastric smooth muscle causes the expulsion of gastric contents into the esophagus. Reverse peristalsis propels these contents into the mouth, whereas reflex closure of the glottis prevents aspiration and elevation of the soft palate prevents reflux into the nasopharynx.

DIAGNOSIS

In general, a three-step approach is recommended for the evaluation of nausea and vomiting[1]:

1. Assess the degree to which symptoms impair the patient's quality of life and ability to function. Patients with refractory symptoms, significant metabolic abnormalities, or evidence of an acute emergency require hospitalization for expedited evaluation and treatment.
2. Investigate and treat the cause of nausea and vomiting.
3. If no cause can be determined, therapy to improve symptoms is initiated.

Clinical Presentation

History

- **Acute vomiting** suggests bowel obstruction or infarction, infection, medication-induced cause, or an accumulation of toxins as in uremia or diabetic ketoacidosis.[1] Pregnancy needs to be considered in the appropriate setting.
- **Chronic vomiting**, defined as emesis for ≥1 month, suggests a chronic medical or functional basis for the symptom; rarely, the etiology is psychogenic.
- **Abdominal pain** is commonly associated with nausea and vomiting. This may indicate an inflammatory condition, such as appendicitis or pancreatitis; pain can also occur from violent retching and bruising of abdominal wall musculature.
- **Acute diarrhea** or **fever** suggests an infectious process.
- **Weight loss** occurs when nutrition is affected in chronic and severe situations; it can also be seen with gastroparesis.
- **Mental status changes** and **headache** indicate meningitis or other CNS abnormalities.
- **Vertigo** and **tinnitus** suggest a labyrinthine process.
- **Timing of vomiting** can offer clues to the etiology of nausea and vomiting:
  - Vomiting that occurs within minutes of a meal can be caused by an obstructive process in the proximal GI tract.

- Inflammatory conditions generally produce vomiting within approximately 1 hour after meals.
- Vomiting from gastroparesis can occur several hours after a meal and can be associated with weight loss.
- Early morning vomiting often occurs with first-trimester pregnancy and uremia.
- Neurogenic vomiting is typically projectile and brought on by positions that increase intracranial pressure.
- **The nature of the vomited material** can point to a diagnosis:
  - Vomiting of undigested or partially digested foods suggests gastric retention caused by obstruction or gastroparesis.
  - Blood or the appearance of "coffee grounds" in the emesis indicates an upper GI bleed.
  - Bile rules out the possibility of obstruction proximal to the duodenal papilla.
  - Foul odor can indicate a distal obstruction, coloenteric fistula, or bacterial overgrowth.
  - If the patient reports emesis of food that looks and tastes just like the food they just ate, consider regurgitation of esophageal content instead of emesis, and an obstructive distal esophageal process (e.g., achalasia) needs to be excluded.

Physical Examination

- **Assessment of volume status** should be the initial focus of the physical examination. Orthostatic hypotension and tachycardia indicate hypovolemia and should be corrected immediately with volume resuscitation.[1,3]
- **Examination of the oropharynx** may reveal loss of dental enamel in situations associated with chronic emesis such as bulimia or functional nausea and vomiting. Patients with bulimia may also have callus formation over their knuckles from repetitively inducing vomiting.
- **Abdominal tenderness** suggests an inflammatory condition, and rebound tenderness suggests peritonitis.
- Absence of **bowel sounds** is consistent with ileus, whereas obstruction classically presents with high-pitched, hyperactive bowel sounds.
- **Hepatomegaly** or a tender liver edge may indicate hepatitis.
- **Neurologic examination** can reveal signs of meningitis and other nervous system disorders.

Differential Diagnosis

- Table 2-1 lists the common etiologies of nausea and vomiting.
- Vomiting needs to be distinguished from regurgitation and rumination.
  - **Regurgitation** is the passive retrograde flow of esophageal contents into the mouth, commonly seen in gastroesophageal reflux.
  - **Rumination** is the effortless regurgitation of recently ingested food into the mouth, followed by rechewing and swallowing. In adults, rumination can be seen in association with psychiatric disorders and in individuals with developmental disability.
  - **Retching** and **dry heaving** are terms applied to spasmodic respiratory and abdominal muscle contraction with a closed glottis. This typically occurs in the setting of intense nausea, and may eventually progress to vomiting.

Diagnostic Testing

Laboratory Testing

- **Basic metabolic panel** evaluates for electrolyte imbalances, especially hyponatremia, elevated blood urea nitrogen, and creatinine. This can be seen with uremia and dehydration. Hypokalemia and alkalosis can also occur with prolonged vomiting.
- **Liver chemistries** may reveal acute hepatitis or cholestasis.
- Elevated **lipase** and **amylase** levels indicate pancreatitis.

- **Complete blood cell count** may reveal an elevated white blood cell count, suggesting an infectious or inflammatory process. Blood counts show decreased hemoglobin and hematocrit in situations associated with blood loss.
- **Urinalysis** may reveal evidence of urinary tract infection; additionally, ketonuria can be seen in the setting of prolonged fasting or diabetic ketoacidosis.
- Urine or serum β-**hCG** levels are mandatory in women of reproductive age with acute vomiting to evaluate for pregnancy.

Imaging
- **Plan abdominal radiograph.** Flat and upright plain x-ray films of the abdomen can be obtained, typically termed "obstructive x-ray series." The presence of air–fluid levels and small bowel dilatation indicates ileus or obstruction. Free air under the diaphragm indicates bowel perforation.
- **Computed tomography** of the abdomen may be useful for evaluating hollow viscus for evidence of dilatation and obstruction, evaluating for inflammatory conditions, as well as in looking for structural abnormalities of the liver, the pancreas, and the biliary system.
- An **upper GI x-ray series**, sometimes performed with small bowel follow-through with barium contrast, can further evaluate subtle obstruction and mucosal lesions.
- **Nuclear medicine gastric emptying study** may be useful in cases when gastroparesis or functionally delayed gastric emptying is suspected.
- **SmartPill®** is an ingestible, wireless capsule that measures pressure, pH, and temperature as it transits the GI tract. The SmartPill may be useful in the evaluation of nausea and vomiting when gastroparesis, small bowel, or colonic dysmotility are suspected as the etiology.[10]

Diagnostic Procedures
- **Esophagogastroduodenoscopy (EGD)** allows for direct visualization of the foregut mucosa. An EGD is typically considered if the history points toward a GI etiology for chronic nausea and vomiting; it can also be a key test to exclude mucosal disease when an etiology is not apparent. A number of disorders including reflux esophagitis, peptic ulcer disease, gastric outlet obstruction, and foregut malignancy can be diagnosed during EGD.[3]

TREATMENT

- **General principles**
  - Orthostatic hypotension and sinus tachycardia are signs of hypovolemia (with loss of approximately 10% of circulating blood volume) and should be corrected immediately with administration of intravenous (IV) fluids.[3]
  - Emesis caused by peptic ulcer disease can be treated with acid suppression and eradication of *Helicobacter pylori*.
  - Many inflammatory conditions, including appendicitis and cholecystitis, as well as mechanical small bowel or gastric outlet obstruction, require surgical intervention. Antiemetic and promotility agents are useful for symptomatic relief.
  - Patients with acute, self-limited nausea and vomiting may only require observation, antiemetics, and hydration.
- **Antiemetic medications**
  - **Antihistamines:** *Meclizine* (25 mg PO QID) is used for labyrinthitis, whereas *promethazine* (12.5–25 mg PO/IM q6h) is very useful for treating the nausea caused by uremia.
  - **Anticholinergics:** *Scopolamine* (1.5-mg transdermal patch every 3 days) is used for the nausea of motion sickness.
  - **Dopamine receptor antagonists:** *Prochlorperazine* (5–10 mg PO/IM/IV q6h) and *chlorpromazine* (10–50 mg PO/IM q8h) are commonly used in both chronic and

acute vomiting. Side effects, which are caused by the action on dopamine receptors throughout the CNS, include drowsiness, insomnia, anxiety, mood changes, confusion, dystonic reactions, tardive dyskinesia, and parkinsonian symptoms.

5-HT$_3$ receptor antagonists: Included in the class of 5-HT$_3$ receptor antagonists are *ondansetron* (4 to 8 mg PO/IV q8h) and *granisetron* (1 mg PO q12h), *palonosetron* (0.25 mg PO/IV once a week), which are very useful in nausea caused by chemotherapeutic agents, particularly cisplatin.[11]

Neurokinin-1 receptor antagonists: *Aprepitant* (40–125 mg PO) and *fosaprepitant* (150 mg IV) are used in the prevention of chemotherapy-related nausea and vomiting.

Miscellaneous agents: *Corticosteroids* and *cannabinoids* exert potent antiemetic effects in patients undergoing chemotherapy.

- **Prokinetic medications**

  Metoclopramide (5–20 mg PO QID), which acts on both 5-HT$_4$ and peripheral dopamine receptors, is used for treating nausea. Although it is also used to accelerate gastric emptying in gastroparesis and functional dyspepsia, its promotility action is subject to tachyphylaxis with continued use. Its antiemetic properties, through its central action, may allow suppression of nausea and vomiting despite continued use. Jitteriness, tremors, parkinsonism, and the risk of tardive dyskinesia limit its long-term use. It also carries a black box warning related to the risk of irreversible neurologic complications associated with prolonged use.[12]

  Erythromycin, a macrolide antibiotic, is a motilin receptor agonist that improves gastric emptying but without significant suppression of nausea. It can be administered intravenously for acute gastric distension to stimulate gastric emptying. Its promotility action is subject to tachyphylaxis and therefore it is not useful for long-term management.

  Cisapride is no longer available in the United States because of its proarrhythmic effects.

  Domperidone, also a peripheral dopamine receptor antagonist, is a potent prokinetic agent but is not currently available in the United States.

  Tegaserod, a 5-HT$_4$ receptor agonist, primarily used in the treatment of irritable bowel syndrome, has modest promotility action in the stomach and can be used to improve gastric emptying. This medication is now reemerging as an option for clinical use, after being withdrawn for several years due to cardiovascular side effects.[13]

- **Complementary and alternative therapy**

  Ginger (*Zingiber officinale*) root extract has been evaluated in the treatment of nausea and vomiting in multiple settings. It appears to act via inhibition of serotonin receptors in the GI tract and in the CNS. It has been most extensively studied and effective in pregnancy-related nausea and vomiting. The typical dose of ginger root extract is 250 mg QID.[14]

  Acupuncture has been shown to be an efficacious therapy for acute as well as chronic nausea and vomiting related to a wide variety of etiologies. Acupoint PC6 (Nei Guan) has been the most commonly evaluated acupuncture point.[15] Acupressure bands that apply pressure on the ventral aspect of the wrist have also been used in this setting.

  Hypnosis has been used for the treatment of functional nausea and vomiting as well as nausea and vomiting related to pregnancy and chemotherapy.[6,16]

SPECIAL CONSIDERATIONS

- **Refractory nausea and vomiting**
  Nausea and vomiting are considered refractory if investigation fails to reveal a treatable etiology and if routine measures do not result in symptomatic improvement.

Three patterns of symptoms are recognized according to Rome IV.[17]

Chronic nausea and vomiting syndrome is associated with nausea and/or vomiting occurring at least 1 day per week for at least 3 months. This syndrome is part of the spectrum of functional nausea and vomiting, and it can be effectively treated with neuromodulators, including tricyclic antidepressants, selective serotonin reuptake inhibitors (SSRIs), and to a lesser extent, bupropion and buspirone.[18]

Cyclic vomiting syndrome (CVS) is a unique disorder characterized by short periods of abdominal pain and violent nausea and vomiting that are separated by symptom-free intervals during which patients are relatively asymptomatic.[17]

- Current understanding of this condition links it to migraine headaches. The treatment approach is similar to that used for migraine headaches, with both abortive and prophylactic medications.[19]
- Associated complaints during symptom "attacks" include upper abdominal pain, diarrhea, flushing, and sweating. Some patients report a prodrome lasting several minutes to hours.
- Abortive therapy could include triptans during the prodromal period and combinations of antiemetic medications, anxiolytics, and narcotic analgesics, in addition to IV hydration, during symptomatic periods.
- Prophylactic approaches include not only tricyclic antidepressants as first-line medications but also antiepileptic medications such as zonisamide, levetiracetam, or even topiramate.[19,20]

Cannabis hyperemesis syndrome presents in the setting of either acute or chronic use of cannabinoid agents. Abdominal pain may be present. Symptoms may be relieved by hot showers. Definitive treatment consists of cessation of use of cannabinoids.[21] Benzodiazepines have been used for acute treatment, and haloperidol may be beneficial in refractory cases. Tricyclic antidepressants have been used effectively for prophylaxis.[22]

Treatment of refractory nausea and vomiting

- **Low-dose tricyclic antidepressants**, such as amitriptyline or nortriptyline (10–50 mg PO at bedtime), are useful in functional vomiting syndrome and as prophylaxis in CVS.[23]
- **SSRIs**, which are generally used for depression and anxiety disorders, may also block presynaptic serotonin receptors on sensory vagal fibers, helping to control nausea. Use of SSRIs for functional nausea and vomiting is largely based on anecdotal evidence; however, these agents are sometimes better tolerated than tricyclic antidepressants. Their role in CVS has not been established.[24]
- **Bupropion**, an inhibitor of neuronal uptake of norepinephrine and dopamine, is an antidepressant and may additionally help relieve nausea and vomiting. It can be considered if side effects from tricyclic antidepressants (especially anticholinergic effects, sexual side effects, and weight gain) are poorly tolerated.
- **Buspirone** is an anxiolytic drug that binds to serotonin and dopamine receptors. This drug may increase the compliance of the gastric antrum and is useful in functional dyspepsia associated with nausea and vomiting.
- **Sumatriptan** activates 5-HT_1 receptors and is used as an abortive therapy for migraines. It can be used as part of abortive therapy early during a cyclic vomiting attack, especially during the prodrome.[18]
- **Zonisamide**, an antiepileptic agent, has multiple mechanisms of action, including blockade of voltage-dependent sodium and T-type calcium channels, binding to the γ-aminobutyric acid receptor, and facilitating dopaminergic and serotoninergic neurotransmission. It has been used with some success as a prophylactic agent in the treatment of CVS.[20]

- **Levetiracetam**, another antiepileptic drug with a less well-understood mechanism of action, appears to inhibit bursts of neuronal firing without affecting normal neuronal excitability. It may also be of benefit as prophylactic therapy in CVS.[20]
- **Surgical therapy is considered a last resort** in refractory nausea and vomiting, specifically when significant weight loss results from the symptomatic state or from impaired gastric emptying.
- **Enteral feeding** can be maintained through a *jejunostomy tube*, which can be placed endoscopically, surgically, or with radiologic guidance (depending on local expertise).
- **Gastric stimulator**, a device that delivers electrical stimulation through electrodes implanted into the gastric wall, can be an option for patients with refractory persistent nausea and vomiting. It does not appear to improve gastric emptying and therefore may not benefit advanced gastroparesis wherein impaired gastric emptying leads to weight loss and nutritional issues.[25]

COMPLICATIONS

- Vomiting, particularly when protracted, can lead to a number of life-threatening complications.
- **Metabolic and electrolyte alterations** can develop rapidly; dehydration with resultant hypotension may lead to syncope and prerenal azotemia. Hypochloremic alkalosis is typically the first electrolyte abnormality to appear due to loss of hydrogen and chloride ions; this is followed by development of hypokalemia due to renal potassium wasting in response to alkalosis. The resulting metabolic derangement can lead to rhabdomyolysis and cardiac arrhythmias.
- **Nutritional deficiencies and weight loss** may result in decreased oral intake. Enteral (via jejunostomy or nasojejunal tube) or parenteral nutrition may be needed in both the acute and chronic settings. A more detailed discussion of nutritional issues can be found in Chapter 11.
- **Dental erosions** may develop in patients with chronic vomiting syndromes as a result of acid- and bile-induced erosion of the dental enamel.
- **Erosive esophagitis** can develop as a result of protracted vomiting and may range from mild to severe. It is important to distinguish esophagitis that is due to vomiting from that associated with GERD. On endoscopy, esophagitis related to protracted vomiting extends uniformly up to the proximal esophageal body whereas GERD-related esophagitis is most pronounced in the distal esophagus.
- **Mallory–Weiss syndrome** can result from forceful and prolonged vomiting episodes and is characterized by longitudinal lacerations of the mucosa near the gastroesophageal junction. These tears can lead to GI bleeding, which is typically self-limited.
- **Boerhaave syndrome** refers to free perforation of the esophagus into the mediastinum due to vomiting. It is most often seen in alcoholics and patients with binge-eating disorders. It should be suspected in any patient presenting with severe chest pain and subcutaneous emphysema after an episode of vomiting (Mackler triad). The diagnosis can be made on the basis of chest computed tomography or esophagram (with water-soluble contrast). Even with prompt surgical repair, *Boerhaave syndrome* carries a 25–50% mortality rate.[26]

REFERENCES

1. Quigley EM, Hasler WL, Parkman HP. AGA technical review on nausea and vomiting. *Gastroenterology*. 2001;120:263–286.
2. Almario CV, Ballal ML, Chey WD, et al. Burden of gastrointestinal symptoms in the United States: results of a nationally representative survey of over 71,000 Americans. *Am J Gastroenterol*. 2018;113:1701–1710.

3. Hasler WL, Chey WD. Nausea and vomiting. *Gastroenterology*. 2003;125:1860–1867.
4. Sullivan S. Cannabinoid hyperemesis. *Can J Gastroenterol*. 2010;24:284–285.
5. Flaxman SM, Sherman PW. Morning sickness: a mechanism for protecting mother and embryo. *Q Rev Biol*. 2000;75:113–148.
6. Niebyl JR. Clinical practice. Nausea and vomiting in pregnancy. *N Engl J Med*. 2010;363: 1544–1550.
7. Prakash C, Clouse RE. Cyclic vomiting syndrome in adults: clinical features and response to tricyclic antidepressants. *Am J Gastroenterol*. 1999;94:2855–2860.
8. Parkman HP, Yates K, Hasler WL, et al. Clinical features of idiopathic gastroparesis vary with sex, body mass, symptom onset, delay in gastric emptying, and gastroparesis severity. *Gastroenterology*. 2011;140:101–115.
9. Horn CC. Why is the neurobiology of nausea and vomiting so important? *Appetite*. 2008;50: 430–434.
10. Sarosiek I, Selover KH, Katz LA, et al. The assessment of regional gut transit times in healthy controls and patients with gastroparesis using wireless motility technology. *Aliment Pharmacol Ther*. 2010;31:313–322.
11. Aapro M. 5-HT(3)-receptor antagonists in the management of nausea and vomiting in cancer and cancer treatment. *Oncology*. 2005;69:97–109.
12. Camilleri M, Parkman HP, Shafi MA, et al.; American College of Gastroenterology. Clinical guideline: management of gastroparesis. *Am J Gastroenterol*. 2013;108:18–37; quiz 38.
13. Degen L, Petrig C, Studer D, et al. Effect of tegaserod on gut transit in male and female subjects. *Neurogastroenterol Motil*. 2005;17:821–826.
14. White B. Ginger: an overview. *Am Fam Physician*. 2007;75:1689–1691.
15. Ouyang H, Chen JD. Review article: therapeutic roles of acupuncture in functional gastrointestinal disorders. *Aliment Pharmacol Ther*. 2004;20:831–841.
16. Chiarioni G, Palsson OS, Whitehead WE. Hypnosis and upper digestive function and disease. *World J Gastroenterol*. 2008;14:6276–6284.
17. Stanghellini V, Chan FK, Hasler WL, et al. Gastroduodenal disorders. *Gastroenterology*. 2016;150:1380–1392.
18. Talley NJ. Functional nausea and vomiting. *Aust Fam Physician*. 2007;36:694–697.
19. Hayes WJ, VanGilder D, Berendse J, et al. Cyclic vomiting syndrome: diagnostic approach and current management strategies. *Clin Exp Gastroenterol*. 2018;11:77–84.
20. Clouse RE, Sayuk GS, Lustman PJ, et al. Zonisamide or levetiracetam for adults with cyclic vomiting syndrome: a case series. *Clin Gastroenterol Hepatol*. 2007;5:44–48.
21. Ruffle JK, Bajgoric S, Samra K, et al. Cannabinoid hyperemesis syndrome: an important differential diagnosis of persistent unexplained vomiting. *Eur J Gastroenterol Hepatol*. 2015;27:1403–1408.
22. Richards JR, Gordon BK, Danielson AR, et al. Pharmacologic treatment of cannabinoid hyperemesis syndrome: a systematic review. *Pharmacotherapy*. 2017;37:725–734.
23. Prakash C, Lustman PJ, Freedland KE, et al. Tricyclic antidepressants for functional nausea and vomiting: clinical outcome in 37 patients. *Dig Dis Sci*. 1998;43:1951–1956.
24. Talley NJ, Ford AC. Functional dyspepsia. *N Engl J Med*. 2015;373:1853–1863.
25. McCallum RW, Lin Z, Forster J, et al. Gastric electrical stimulation improves outcomes of patients with gastroparesis for up to 10 years. *Clin Gastroenterol Hepatol*. 2011;9:314–319.e1.
26. Atallah FN, Riu BM, Nguyen LB, et al. Boerhaave's syndrome after postoperative vomiting. *Anesth Analg*. 2004;98:1164–1166, table of contents.

Diarrhea

Adeeti J. Chiplunker

3

GENERAL PRINCIPLES

Definition

- Diarrhea is defined as increased liquidity/decreased consistency of stools, which may be associated with increased frequency of bowel movements, specifically more than three stools per day.
- The small intestine and colon are highly efficient in reabsorption of water.[1,2]
  - 10 L of intestinal fluid enters the jejunum on a daily basis
  - 1–1.5 L of intestinal fluid is passed into the colon
  - 100 mL/day passes out of the colon as stool
- Diarrhea results from the inability or inefficiency of the digestive tract to perform this reabsorptive function.

Classification

- Diarrhea can be classified into acute and chronic, based on the duration of symptoms. **Acute diarrhea** is typically <2 weeks in duration, although some acute diarrheal illnesses may continue to improve over 3–4 weeks. Diarrhea lasting longer than 4 weeks can be designated **chronic**.
- Diarrhea can be categorized into several types, based on pathophysiology of the causative process.[1,2]
- **Osmotic**
  - Large amounts of poorly absorbed solute within the intestinal lumen cause osmotic retention of water in the stool.
  - Osmotic diarrhea is characterized by cessation of diarrhea with fasting and an abnormally elevated stool osmotic gap (>125 mOsm/kg).
  - The body maintains equal fecal and serum osmolality, which is approximately 290 mOsm/kg.
    - Stool osmotic gap is calculated using the formula: $290 - 2 \, (Na^+ + K^+)$.
    - Poorly absorbed substances within the intestinal lumen require that additional water be retained in the stool to maintain this value, resulting in an osmotic gap.
    - An osmotic gap <50 mOsm/kg is considered normal.
    - An osmotic gap >125 mOsm/kg is consistent with a pure osmotic diarrhea.
- **Secretory**
  - Intestinal secretion overcomes the absorptive capability of the small intestine and colon.
  - Secretion of incompletely absorbed electrolytes leads to retention of intraluminal water.
  - Intestinal secretion is a constant process. The diarrhea is incessant regardless of fasting state or time of the day.
  - Characterized by large amounts of watery diarrhea (1–10 L/24 hrs).
  - The stool osmotic gap is normal.
- **Inflammatory**
  - Inflammation and ulceration impair the absorptive and digestive functions of normal mucosa.

- Inflammation itself often adds to stool volume through addition of mucus, proteins, fluid, and blood into the bowel lumen. Secretory mechanisms may be coexistent.
- Clinical presentation includes nocturnal diarrhea and systemic signs such as fatigue or fever.

- **Steatorrhea**
  - Any process that affects digestion and absorption of fats can lead to steatorrhea. Etiologies range from celiac disease to pancreatic insufficiency.
  - Inadequate contact time of bowel contents with the digestive juices and absorptive intestinal mucosa, as with altered intestinal motility, can also contribute to steatorrhea.
- **Dysmotility/Functional**
  - Gut dysmotility may cause increased intestinal and colonic transit time as well as decreased contact time with intestinal absorptive mucosa.
  - Functional syndromes such as irritable bowel syndrome (IBS) include a pain component as well as a change in bowel habits.

Epidemiology

- **Acute diarrhea**
  - Worldwide, >2 billion people experience at least one episode of acute diarrhea each year.
  - Acute infectious diarrhea remains one of the most common causes of death in developing countries, accounting for >5 million childhood deaths per year and is attributable to poor sanitation and limited access to health care.
  - In the United States, nearly 179 million people are affected by acute diarrhea annually. Approximately 330,000 require hospitalization and over 4000 people die with most deaths occurring in the debilitated and elderly.[3,4]
- **Chronic diarrhea**
  - Chronic diarrhea has an estimated prevalence of 5% in the United States, which may be an underestimation since many patients do not seek medical attention.[1]
  - According to the AGA Burden of Illness study, direct costs of chronic diarrhea associated with GI conditions is $2.8 billion per year, with $385 million per year for indirect costs.[4,5]
  - Although it is a major cause of disability, there are limited studies on the economic impact or effect on quality of life that results from chronic diarrhea, diagnostic testing, and treatment.

Etiology

Etiologies of acute infectious diarrhea[3,6,7] and chronic diarrhea[1,8–11] are listed in Tables 3-1 and 3-2.

DIAGNOSIS

Clinical Presentation

- **Acute**
  - Most cases of acute diarrhea are mild and are caused by self-limited processes/infections, typically lasting <5 days. In some circumstances, symptoms may continue to improve for 2–3 weeks after onset.
  - Nearly 90% of cases require no diagnostic evaluation and respond to simple rehydration.
- **Chronic**
  - Patients may present with symptoms that have been present anywhere from 4 weeks to many years.

TABLE 3-1 CAUSES OF ACUTE INFECTIOUS DIARRHEA

Viruses	Preformed Toxins
Rotavirus	*Staphylococcus aureus*
Norwalk virus	*Clostridium perfringens*
Adenovirus	*Bacillus cereus*
Astrovirus	**Parasites**
Hepatitis A	*Giardia lamblia*
Bacteria	*Entamoeba histolytica*
Campylobacter	*Cyclospora*
Salmonella	*Isospora*
Shigella	*Cryptosporidium*
Clostridium difficile	*Strongyloides*
Enterohemorrhagic *Escherichia coli* (EHEC, 0157:H7)	**Opportunistic**
Enterotoxigenic *E. coli* (ETEC)	Microsporidia
Enteroinvasive *E. coli* (EIEC)	*Mycobacterium avium intracellulare*
Vibrio cholerae	Cytomegalovirus
Vibrio parahaemolyticus	Herpes simplex virus
Yersinia	
Listeria	
Aeromonas	
Plesiomonas	

There are a wide variety of causes (Table 3-2). A careful and detailed history and physical examination, along with judicious use of laboratory tests and investigative procedures, often yield an accurate diagnosis.

In contrast to acute diarrhea, chronic diarrhea often has a noninfectious etiology.

- **Noninflammatory versus inflammatory**
  - **Noninflammatory**
    - Noninflammatory diarrhea typically presents with watery, nonbloody loose bowel movements associated with periumbilical cramps, bloating, nausea, or vomiting.
    - This is usually caused by disruption of normal absorption or secretory processes in the small intestine, as can be seen with certain bacterial toxins.
    - In most cases, the diarrhea is mild but it may become voluminous, ranging from 10–200 mL/kg/24 hrs, which can result in dehydration and electrolyte abnormalities.
  - **Inflammatory**
    - Inflammatory diarrhea may present with fever, bloody diarrhea, abdominal pain, and tenesmus.
    - Infectious agents preferentially involve the colon, leading to a small-volume diarrhea defined as <1 L/day. Fecal leukocytes can be present as these infectious agents are often invasive.

History

- Special attention should be paid to the following details when obtaining **history of diarrhea**[11,12]:
  - Onset, duration, pattern/frequency
  - Stool characteristics: watery, fatty, or inflammatory (blood or mucus)
  - Systemic symptoms: fever, fatigue
  - Abdominal pain: postprandial?

TABLE 3-2 CAUSES OF CHRONIC DIARRHEA

Osmotic

Medications: antibiotics, lactulose, antacids, sorbitol, laxative abuse, Mg ingestion

Carbohydrate malabsorption/disaccharidase deficiencies (i.e., lactose intolerance)

High ingestion of sugar substitutes or fructose

Secretory

Medications: nonosmotic laxatives, stimulants, selective serotonin reuptake inhibitors

Bile salt–induced diarrhea (bacterial breakdown of bile acids stimulates secretion from colonic mucosa): postcholecystectomy or ileal malabsorption

Colitis: inflammatory bowel disease, microscopic colitis, diverticulitis

Bacterial toxins

Neuroendocrine tumors: carcinoid syndrome, insulinoma, Zollinger–Ellison/gastrinoma, VIPoma, medullary carcinoma of the thyroid, somatostatinoma, pheochromocytoma, glucagonoma, mastocytosis

Endocrinopathies: hyperthyroidism, diabetes mellitus, Addison's, hyperparathyroidism

Miscellaneous: villous adenoma (chloride secreting), colon cancer, lymphoma, multiple myeloma, HIV/AIDS, amyloidosis, vasculitis, cholera, congenital chloridorrhea

Inflammatory

Infection: *C. difficile*, tuberculosis, *Yersinia*, cytomegalovirus, herpes simplex virus, amebiasis

Inflammatory bowel disease

Ischemic colitis

Radiation enterocolitis

Eosinophilic enterocolitis

Colon cancer, lymphoma

Steatorrhea

Maldigestion: pancreatic exocrine insufficiency, bile acid deficiency, abetalipoproteinemia

Malabsorption: celiac sprue, tropical sprue, Whipple disease, short bowel syndrome, small intestinal bacterial overgrowth—bacterial deconjugation of bile acids, mesenteric ischemia, protein-losing enteropathy

Altered intestinal motility: hyperthyroidism, diabetes mellitus, scleroderma, medications (i.e., metoclopramide, erythromycin)

Dysmotility/Functional

Irritable bowel syndrome

Fecal impaction (overflow diarrhea)

Enteric fistula

Systemic disease: diabetes mellitus, hyperthyroidism, Addison's, amyloidosis, scleroderma

---

- Fecal incontinence
- Weight loss, if present, suggests decreased intake (potentially volitional to decrease diarrhea), malabsorption, neoplasm, or ischemia. Significant weight loss (>10 lb) is more worrisome and often points to nutrient malabsorption.
- Nocturnal/fasting symptoms
- Aggravating/mitigating factors such as diet, stress, medications
- Recent exposure to hospitals or antibiotic use
- Sick contacts/regional outbreak: food related
- **Past medical and surgical conditions** may be relevant to the history as follows:
  - Systemic disease: diabetes mellitus, thyroid disease, inflammatory/autoimmune disorder, HIV, immunocompromised state, cancer
  - History of an eating disorder, malingering, or secondary gain

○ Previous surgery: gastrectomy, vagotomy, bowel resection, cholecystectomy
○ Previous radiation therapy
- A **family history** of inflammatory bowel disease (IBD), celiac sprue, or multiple endocrine neoplasia (MEN) syndromes may be helpful.
- A detailed medication history is especially important regarding the use of laxatives, antibiotics, over-the-counter medications, and any new medications prior to the onset of symptoms.
- A **diet history** may be relevant, especially the following:
  ○ Recent changes or associated foods.
  ○ Intake of sugar-free substitutes, lactose, or fructose.
  ○ Exposure to contaminated food or water. Time from ingestion: <6 hours suggests a preformed toxin, 8–16 hours suggests *Clostridium perfringens* infection, and >16 hours suggests an enteroinvasive viral or bacterial infection.
- **Social history**
  ○ Alcohol, tobacco, illicit drug use
  ○ Travel/immigration history
    ■ Recent travel to endemic areas may suggest traveler's diarrhea, *Giardia* infection, tropical sprue.
    ■ Recent immigration from a developing country raises the possibility of a parasitic infection.
  ○ Sexual history, including any history of anal intercourse

Physical Examination
- Vital signs are obtained to assess for patient has fever, tachycardia, or hypotension. Orthostatic blood pressure changes may be evident with severe volume depletion from fluid loss.
- General examination takes into account whether the patient is toxic appearing and acutely ill. Cachexia and muscle wasting may indicate a chronic process.
- Volume status is assessed by examining orthostatic hemodynamics, mucus membranes, and skin turgor. A history of oliguria supports volume loss.
- Head and neck examination evaluates for findings of hyperthyroidism (thyroid mass, exophthalmos) and extraintestinal manifestations of IBD (eye pain or conjunctival injection, mouth ulcers).
- Flushing, wheezing, and cardiac murmurs can rarely be seen in secretory diarrhea, especially carcinoid syndrome.
- A detailed abdominal examination assesses for tenderness, peritoneal signs, hepatomegaly, masses, and ascites. Surgical scars indicate past surgery. Bowel sounds are evaluated for hyper- and hypoactivity.
- Anorectal examination focuses on sphincter tone/contractility, fistulas, fissures, perianal abscess, and blood on the examining finger.
- Other areas examined include the peripheries for edema, arthritis, lymphadenopathy; a skin examination for rashes and flushing, and a neurologic examination for neurologic deficits and peripheral neuropathy.

Differential Diagnosis

Clinical patterns can help determine pathophysiologic mechanisms of diarrhea as follows:
- **Watery diarrhea**
  ○ Osmotic diarrhea decreases with fasting.
  ○ Secretory diarrhea is voluminous, with no change with fasting. Patients may have nocturnal symptoms.
- **Bloody diarrhea with or without mucus:** This suggests inflammatory or infectious etiologies. Patients may also manifest systemic symptoms, fevers, fatigue, abdominal pain, tenesmus, and nocturnal symptoms.

- **Fatty stool** suggests steatorrhea. Diarrhea typically decreases with fasting and can be foul smelling. Stool may adhere to the toilet bowl, and the patient may report oil droplets in the toilet water.
- **Functional etiologies:** In IBS and other functional disorders, there is a predominance of abdominal pain, lack of nocturnal symptoms, and lack of significant weight loss.

Diagnostic Testing

- **In acute diarrhea**, testing is indicated in the presence of severe symptoms (hypovolemia, fever, severe abdominal pain, bloody diarrhea), in the elderly, in immunocompromised individuals, or in IBD.[3,13,14]
- **In osmotic diarrhea**[1,8–11]:
  - Osmotic gap can be checked and is typically >125 mOsm/kg.
  - Stool pH indicates carbohydrate malabsorption if it is acidic (pH <5.6).
  - Stool magnesium level can assess for excessive intake of magnesium, such as in laxative abuse.
- **Secretory diarrhea**
  - Osmotic gap is usually normal (<50 mOsm/kg).
  - Infectious etiologies need to be excluded, as some acute infections can induce a transient secretory pattern.
  - Imaging studies and endoscopy can evaluate for structural and inflammatory diseases of the small intestine and colon.
  - Specialized tests can be performed to investigate for endocrinopathies and neuroendocrine tumors.
- **Inflammatory diarrhea**
  - Fecal occult blood test (FOBT) and/or fecal leukocytes can be assessed in chronic diarrhea wherein both inflammatory and secretory etiologies are being considered. These tests are consistently positive in bloody diarrhea or where other features suggest an inflammatory etiology. If the history, physical examination, and other testing are convincing for an inflammatory etiology, these tests are redundant and should not be performed.
  - Infectious etiologies need to be excluded, even when IBD is suspected, as infectious superinfection can be seen.
  - Imaging studies and endoscopy are useful to evaluate for structural and/or inflammatory diseases of the small intestine and colon.
- **Steatorrhea**
  - Fecal fat assays are typically abnormal and the osmotic gap is >50 mOsm/kg.
  - Imaging studies and endoscopy are useful for evaluating structural and/or inflammatory diseases of the small intestine and pancreas.
  - Investigation can be performed for evaluating pancreatic exocrine insufficiency.

Laboratory Testing
*Indicates initial testing.
- ***Complete blood cell count with differential.** This may show anemia, leukocytosis (infection), or eosinophilia (neoplasm, allergies, parasites, eosinophilic gastroenterocolitis).
- ***Comprehensive metabolic panel.** This evaluates for electrolyte abnormalities, coexistent liver disease, hypoalbuminemia/dysproteinemia (malnutrition, protein-losing enteropathy), or diabetes.
- ***TSH, FT4.** This evaluates for hyperthyroidism, which can rarely cause diarrhea on its own but can potentiate diarrhea from other causes.
- **Stool studies.** The following studies can be performed:
  - *Osmolarity, electrolytes (Na, K) to calculate osmotic gap
  - *Infectious, bacterial culture, *Clostridium difficile* toxin ×3, O&P ± microscopy ×3, stool wet mount for amebiasis in sexually active male homosexuals or travel to endemic areas

○ Leukocytes, lactoferrin, calprotectin if there is suspicion of inflammatory diarrhea
○ FOBT
○ Fat: qualitative/Sudan stain versus 24-, 48-, or 72-hour quantitative collection on a 100-g fat/day diet (<6 g/24 hrs is normal, >14 g/24 hrs suggests malabsorption/maldigestion, >8% suggests pancreatic insufficiency)
○ pH <5.6 suggests carbohydrate malabsorption (colonic fermentation by bacteria)
○ Mg level
○ Laxative screen
○ α_1-Antitrypsin. This is typically elevated in protein-losing enteropathy
○ Chymotrypsin or elastase concentration: These are elevated in in pancreatic insufficiency
- **Urine studies**
  ○ Urinalysis: for protein loss in the urine
  ○ Laxative screen
- **Secretory diarrhea.** Hormonal work-up for secretory diarrhea can include serum levels of VIP, gastrin, calcitonin, pancreatic polypeptide, somatostatin, tryptase, serum protein electrophoresis, immunoglobulins; urinary excretion of 5-hydroxyindoleacetic acid, metanephrines, and histamine; and an adrenocorticotropin stimulation test.
- **Celiac disease.** Testing for celiac disease should be performed early in the evaluation of chronic diarrhea: antitissue transglutaminase antibody (IgA, preferred test for patients >2 years of age), deamidated gliadin peptide (IgA and IgG, alternative test in high probability patients or supplementary in children <2 years of age), and serum IgA levels (up to 10% of patients will be IgA deficient and have a false-negative result).[15] HLA-DQ2/DQ8 testing should only be used to rule out the disease in patients with equivocal small bowel histology, those on a gluten free diet at the time of testing, those with serology/history discrepancies, refractory cases, or in patients with Down syndrome.
- **IBD and immunocompromised patients.** Cytomegalovirus (CMV) DNA polymerase chain reaction (PCR) and *C. difficile* toxins. PCR testing for *C. difficile* is preferred over EIA/ELISA testing due to increased sensitivity and sensitivity for both tests increases with ≥3 performed tests (100% for PCR, 86% for EIA).[14,16]
- **Rectal swab** in those active in anal intercourse (gonorrhea, *Chlamydia,* herpes simplex virus [HSV])

Imaging

The following can be performed to assess for structural/inflammatory disease of the small intestine and pancreas:
- Small bowel follow-through
- CT enterography
- MR enterography
- Dual-phase CT scan of the pancreas
- Abdominal ultrasonography
- Endoscopic ultrasonography

Diagnostic Procedures
- **Endoscopy with biopsies**[12,17]
  ○ Upper endoscopy with small bowel biopsies for the evaluation of celiac disease (minimum of four duodenal biopsies), Whipple disease, protein-losing enteropathy, eosinophilic gastroenteritis, giardiasis, amyloidosis. Small bowel aspirate may be useful to evaluate for small intestinal bacterial overgrowth (SIBO)
  ○ Flexible sigmoidoscopy or colonoscopy with random biopsies
    ▪ Flexible sigmoidoscopy is acceptable in cases of acute diarrhea with suspicion for diffuse colitis, such as graft-versus-host disease, or chronic diarrhea in patients with significant comorbidities or pregnancy.

- Colonoscopy is preferred for evaluation of IBD, microscopic colitis, eosinophilic colitis, amyloidosis, colorectal neoplasia or screening, HIV patients, or in cases with significant blood loss.
- **Endoscopic ultrasonography** to evaluate for chronic pancreatitis
- **Breath tests** for specific carbohydrate malabsorption (lactose, sucrose) and SIBO (glucose, lactulose, ^{14}C-xylose, ^{14}C-glycocholate)
- **Secretin test** to assess for pancreatic exocrine insufficiency[18]

TREATMENT

Medications

- Acute diarrhea
  - **Volume status and electrolyte disturbances need to be assessed first.**
    - Uncomplicated, mild acute diarrhea is treated with oral fluids containing carbohydrates and electrolytes.
      - World Health Organization oral rehydration solution (2.6 g NaCl, 2.9 g trisodium citrate, 1.5 g KCl, and 13.5 g glucose per L) is recommended.
      - Pedialyte, Gatorade, and similar sports drinks may also be taken, but the carbohydrate load is greater and the sodium content is lower.
    - In severe diarrhea, intravenous fluids (Lactated Ringer or 0.9% normal saline) may be necessary to restore volume and to keep up with ongoing losses.
  - **Antidiarrheal agents** are safe in mild to moderate diarrhea and may improve patient comfort.
    - Loperamide 4 mg followed by 2 mg after each loose stool up to a maximum daily dose of 16 mg.
    - Diphenoxylate plus atropine (Lomotil) 4 mg QID has combined opioid and anticholinergic effects.
    - Antidiarrheal agents are not recommended in bloody or febrile cases.
  - **Traveler's diarrhea:** Bismuth subsalicylate 30 mL QID may reduce symptoms through anti-inflammatory and antibacterial properties.
    - The addition of a fluoroquinolone or rifaximin ×3 days may lessen the duration and severity of the illness. Azithromycin is also effective, especially against *Campylobacter, Shigella,* and noninvasive *E. coli* infections.
    - **Antibiotics.** Empiric treatment with antibiotics is only recommended when invasive bacterial infection is suspected suggested by high fever, tenesmus, bloody diarrhea, or fecal leukocytes or severe illness is present. Use must be weighed against possible risks including antibiotic resistance or other possible complications (Table 3-3).[3,13]
      - **First line.** Fluoroquinolones ×3 days (i.e., ciprofloxacin 500 mg BID, norfloxacin 400 mg BID, levofloxacin 400 mg daily)
      - **Alternatives.** Trimethoprim-sulfamethoxazole, azithromycin, or erythromycin
      - **Giardia/Amebiasis.** Metronidazole 250 to 750 mg TID ×7–10 days
      - **Cyclospora/Isospora.** Trimethoprim-sulfamethoxazole DS BID ×7–10 days
      - Antibiotic treatment is also recommended in **infectious diarrhea caused by sexually transmitted diseases**, such as *Chlamydia* infection, gonorrhea, HSV infection, and syphilis.
      - **Enterohemorrhagic *E. coli* (EHEC) or *E. coli* O157:H7.** Antibiotics are NOT recommended as they have not been shown to hasten recovery or decrease the contagious period. In addition, their use may precipitate the hemolytic–uremic syndrome. Clinical clues to EHEC infection include recent ingestion of raw/undercooked ground meat, bloody diarrhea, abdominal pain, and minimal or lack of fever.

TABLE 3-3 TREATMENT OF BACTERIAL DIARRHEA

Campylobacter	Azithromycin 500 mg daily ×3 days or 1000 mg ×1 dose
Salmonella	Ciprofloxacin 500 mg BID ×3–7 days Azithromycin 1000 mg ×1 followed by 500 mg daily ×5–7 days
Shigella	Ciprofloxacin 500 mg BID or 750 mg daily ×3 days Azithromycin 500 mg daily ×3 days Cefixime 200 mg BID or 400 mg qday OR Ceftriaxone 1000 mg IV daily for patients at high risk for resistance
Clostridium difficile	Metronidazole 500 mg TID ×14 days Vancomycin 125 mg PO QID ×14 days in severe/recurrent cases
Enterohemorrhagic *E. coli*	NOT RECOMMENDED
Enterotoxigenic *E. coli*	Ciprofloxacin 500 mg BID or 750 mg daily ×3 days Azithromycin 1000 mg ×1 or 500 mg qday ×3 days
Enteroinvasive *E. coli*	As for *Shigella* with the exception of azithromycin, which is not recommended
Vibrio cholerae	Doxycycline 300 mg ×1 Azithromycin 1000 mg ×1 dose Ciprofloxacin 1000 mg ×1 dose
Vibrio parahaemolyticus	As for *Vibrio cholerae*
Aeromonas	Trimethoprim-sulfamethoxazole DS ×5 days or a fluoroquinolone or third-generation cephalosporin as for *Shigella*
Plesiomonas	Ciprofloxacin 500 mg BID ×3 days

- Chronic diarrhea
  - **Volume status, electrolyte disturbances, and vitamin deficiencies** need to be addressed.
    - Uncomplicated, mild diarrhea is treated with oral fluids similar to that in acute diarrhea.
    - In cases of severe diarrhea, intravenous fluids (lactated Ringer or 0.9% normal saline) may be necessary to restore volume depletion and to keep up with ongoing losses. Rarely, patients may require intravenous fluids long term, administered through a permanent indwelling catheter with the assistance of home healthcare nursing.
    - Total parenteral nutrition may be required in the hospital or long term at home, requiring an indwelling catheter and home healthcare nursing.
    - Vitamin deficiencies may occur due to decreased oral intake or malabsorption. Vitamin levels should be monitored and supplemented if deficient, especially the fat-soluble vitamins in those with chronic steatorrhea.
  - The **underlying cause needs to be treated** whenever possible.[1,8–11]

If there is a reversible cause such as infection, dietary precipitant, medication, or tumors, then chronic diarrhea may potentially be resolved with treatment or by removal of the offending agent.

Microscopic (collagenous/lymphocytic) colitis. Budesonide 9 mg daily with slow taper can be used when clinically appropriate. Bismuth subsalicylate, cholestyramine, and mesalamine may also be used. In severe or refractory cases, immunomodulators such as azathioprine or systemic steroids may be required.

Bile acid–induced diarrhea. An empiric trial of cholestyramine (a binding resin) is both diagnostic and therapeutic. Recommended dose is 4 g TID. Alternatively, colestipol may be used.[19]

Lactose intolerance. Empiric trial of avoiding dairy products is both diagnostic and therapeutic. Lactase enzyme supplements may also be efficacious.

SIBO. Clinical response to antibiotics is often rapid; cyclical antibiotics are often necessary unless the predisposing cause for bacterial overgrowth has been addressed.

Pancreatic enzyme replacement. A therapeutic trial may be beneficial in steatorrhea.

Opiate antidiarrheal agents are safe in mild to moderate diarrhea.

- **Loperamide** (Imodium) 2–4 mg QID or 4 mg followed by 2 mg after each loose stool up to a maximum daily dose of 16 mg.
- **Diphenoxylate plus atropine** (Lomotil) 4 mg QID has combined opioid and anticholinergic effects.
- Other more potent options include combinations of opiates with antispasmodics, such as tincture of opium (2–20 drops QID) with belladonna or hyoscyamine.

Empiric treatment with antidiarrheals without extensive investigation is appropriate for patients without alarm findings such as those with IBS.

Psyllium can be used to increase stool bulk in those with fecal incontinence.

Octreotide (a somatostatin analog) may be used in secretory diarrhea to decrease the volume of stool.

- Octreotide can be used parenterally at 50–250 µg subcutaneous BID to TID.
- Octreotide may also be used in acute postoperative diarrhea, such as with high ostomy output. In this scenario, a fluid-filled bowel is often mistaken for postoperative ileus. Clues to this diagnosis are abdominal distention on examination in the presence of significant diarrhea. Cross-sectional imaging reveals a distended, fluid-filled bowel. Symptoms resolve rapidly with decompression by a nasogastric tube and initiation of subcutaneous octreotide.

Antibiotics

- Empiric treatment can be considered if the patient is at high risk for dehydration or systemic complications, in the setting of a high suspicion of infectious cause, or if there is high prevalence of infectious diarrhea in the community.
- Metronidazole or fluoroquinolone may be used.

Surgical Management

Surgery may be indicated to treat the underlying cause, such as with neuroendocrine tumor, severe colitis, or malignancy.

Lifestyle/Risk Modification

- Malnutrition and vitamin deficiencies may occur due to decreased oral intake or malabsorption.
- Enteral feeds are always recommended when the gut is healthy and functioning, but additional intravenous fluids and total parenteral nutrition may be necessary either temporarily or long term.
- In acute diarrhea, bowel rest or a change to a clear liquid or bland diet that avoids high-fiber foods, fats, milk products, caffeine, and alcohol may improve the patient's symptoms in the short term.

- If there is an underlying mucosal cause for malabsorption, such as celiac disease or disaccharidase deficiency, diet should exclude the offending agent (i.e., gluten- or lactose-free diets).
- Vitamin levels should be evaluated and supplemented if deficient. Prophylactic supplementation may be recommended with daily multivitamin, calcium, vitamin D, and B complex.
- Probiotics are not routinely recommended at this time, given the lack of regulations and consensus on their benefits. However, these agents may be beneficial in chronic diarrhea in the setting of IBS. Anecdotal evidence exists for benefit in other types of chronic diarrhea.

SPECIAL CONSIDERATIONS

- **HIV/AIDS**
  - Patients who are HIV positive with low CD4 counts have high risk of chronic infectious diarrhea. Etiologies include common infectious agents as well as opportunistic infections such as CMV and *Mycobacterium avium intracellulare*. Other causes include intestinal malignancies such as lymphoma and Kaposi sarcoma, AIDS enteropathy, and medication-induced symptoms from HAART treatment such as with nelfinavir and ritonavir. The lack of simple diagnostic tools and directed treatment, however, often relegates these patients to symptomatic therapy.
- **IBD**
  - Antimotility agents should be used with caution in patients with severe IBD because of the potential complication of toxic megacolon; patients with bloody diarrhea, high fever, or systemic toxicity should not be given antidiarrheals. Anticholinergic agents are absolutely contraindicated in acute diarrhea because of the rare complication of toxic megacolon.
  - The initial clinical presentation of IBD may be unmasked by acute infectious diarrhea.
  - CMV and *C. difficile* infection should always be ruled out first in IBD patients.
- **Pediatrics**
  - Patients with symptoms suggestive of EHEC/*E. coli* O157:H7 should not be treated with antibiotics, given the risk of precipitating hemolytic–uremic syndrome.
  - Clinical clues to EHEC infection include recent ingestion of raw/undercooked ground meat, bloody diarrhea, and abdominal pain but no or minimal fever.
- **Pregnancy**
  - *Listeria* with or without systemic symptoms should be considered in pregnant women.

COMPLICATIONS

- Dehydration
- Acute renal failure
- Electrolyte abnormalities such as metabolic acidosis, hypokalemia
- Weight loss and wasting
- Malnutrition such as fat-soluble vitamin A, D, E, and K deficiencies with steatorrhea
- Transient acquired mucosal digestive insufficiency such as a secondary lactose malabsorption, following an acute gastroenteritis. This phenomenon often manifests as persistent diarrhea, abdominal cramps, and bloating until normal mucosal enzymatic activity is restored. These symptoms may persist for weeks to months.
- A subset of patients with an acute gastroenteritis develop a chronic postinfectious IBS.

REFERRAL

Referral to a gastroenterologist/specialist is indicated depending on the following:
- Severity of disease
- Diagnosis
- Need for endoscopy
- Long-term management (IBD, chronic pancreatitis)

REFERENCES

1. Fine KD, Schiller LR. AGA technical review on the evaluation and management of chronic diarrhea. *Gastroenterology.* 1999;116:1464–1486.
2. Camilleri M. Chronic diarrhea: a review on pathophysiology and management for the clinical gastroenterologist. *Clin Gastroenterol Hepatol.* 2004;2:198–206.
3. DuPont HL. Acute infectious diarrhea in immunocompetent adults. *N Engl J Med.* 2014;370:1532–1540.
4. Peery AF, Dellon ES, Lund J, et al. Burden of gastrointestinal disease in the United States: 2012 update. *Gastroenterology.* 2012;143:1179–1187.
5. Everhart JE, Ruhl CE. Burden of digestive diseases in the United States part I: overall and upper gastrointestinal diseases. *Gastroenterology.* 2009;136:376 386.
6. Pawlowski SW, Warren CA, Guerrant R. Diagnosis and treatment of acute or persistent diarrhea. *Gastroenterology.* 2009;136:1874–1886.
7. Thielman NM, Guerrant RL. Clinical practice. Acute infectious diarrhea. *N Engl J Med.* 2004;350:38–47.
8. Schiller LR. Chronic diarrhea. *Gastroenterology.* 2004;127:287–293.
9. Schiller LR. Diarrhea. *Med Clin North Am.* 2000;84:1259–1274.
10. Donowitz M, Kokke FT, Saidi R. Evaluation of patients with chronic diarrhea. *N Engl J Med.* 1995;332:725–729.
11. Headstrom PD, Surawicz CM. Chronic diarrhea. *Clin Gastroenterol Hepatol.* 2005;3:734–737.
12. American Gastroenterological Association medical position statement: guidelines for the evaluation and management of chronic diarrhea. *Gastroenterology.* 1999;116:1461–1463.
13. Riddle MS, DuPont HL, Connor BA. ACG clinical guideline: diagnosis, treatment, and prevention of acute diarrhea infections in adults. *Am J Gastroenterol.* 2016;111:602–622.
14. Surawicz CM, Brandt LJ, Binion DG, et al. Guidelines for diagnosis, treatment, and prevention of *Clostridium difficile* infections. *Am J Gastroenterol.* 2013;108:478–498.
15. Rubio-Tapia A, Hill ID, Kelly CP, et al. ACG clinical guidelines: diagnosis and management of celiac disease. *Am J Gastroenterol.* 2013;108:656–676.
16. Peterson LR, Manson RU, Paule SM, et al. Detection of toxigenic Clostridium difficile in stool samples by real-time polymerase chain reaction for the diagnosis of C. difficile-associated diarrhea. *Clin Infect Dis.* 2007;45:1152–1160.
17. ASGE Standards of Practice Committee; Shen B, Khan K, Ikenberry SO, et al. The role of endoscopy in the management of patients with diarrhea. *Gastrointest Endosc.* 2010;71:887–892.
18. ASGE Standards of Practice Committee; Chandrasekhara V, Chathadi KV, Ruben D. The role of endoscopy benign pancreatic disease. *Gastrointest Endosc.* 2015;82:203–214.
19. Wilcox C, Turner J, Green J. Systematic review: the management of chronic diarrhea due to bile acid malabsorption. *Aliment Pharmacol Ther.* 2014;39:923–939.

Constipation

Jeffrey W. Brown and Ghadah Al Ismail

4

GENERAL PRINCIPLES

- Constipation is one of the most common gastrointestinal complaints in the general population and is associated with decreased work productivity,[1] decreased quality of life,[1,2] and increased anxiety and depression.[3]
- Constipation encompasses a multitude of disorders and symptoms that affect colonic and anorectal function, and a careful understanding of this heterogeneity is essential for proper patient management.

Definition

Constipation is a symptomatically defined disorder, characterized by infrequent stools, difficult stool passage, or both.[4-6] Thus, normal bowel movement frequency (which can range from a bowel movement every 3 days to 3 bowel movements a day) does not preclude this diagnosis. Associated symptoms often include passage of hard stools, straining, unproductive urges, and tenesmus.

Classification

- **Primary versus secondary.** Secondary constipation occurs as a side effect of various conditions and medications and is important to rule out before embarking on a complex evaluation (Table 4-1).
- **Acute versus chronic.** A consensus definition has been established to address the varied components of chronic constipation (Table 4-2).[7]

Epidemiology

- The median adult prevalence of constipation is 16% (range 2–27%); however, this increases to 33% in adults older than 60.[5,6] It is the primary diagnosis or reason for visit in approximately 2.8 million outpatient and emergency department visits annually.[8]
- Greater than $800 million is spent annually in the United States on over-the-counter laxatives.[9]

Etiology

The potential etiologies of primary constipation can be generally categorized into normal transit constipation, slow transit constipation, pelvic floor dyssynergia, and constipation-predominant irritable bowel syndrome. It is important to note that there is considerable overlap between these categories.[4-6]

- Patients with **normal transit constipation** have symptoms without evidence of delayed colonic transit.
- **Slow transit constipation** is an idiopathic entity with delayed transit from the proximal to distal colon.
- **Pelvic floor dyssynergia** occurs when the puborectalis and anal sphincter muscles fail to relax or paradoxically contract with attempted defecation, leading to an inability to defecate at the level of the anorectum; colonic transit to the rectum can be normal in this disorder.

TABLE 4-1 DIFFERENTIAL DIAGNOSIS OF CONSTIPATION

Endocrine	Diabetes mellitus, hypothyroidism, hyperparathyroidism, pregnancy, pheochromocytoma
Metabolic	Chronic kidney disease, hypercalcemia, hypokalemia, hypomagnesemia, porphyria, heavy metal poisoning
Neurogenic	Hirschsprung disease, Chagas disease, Parkinson disease, spinal cord injuries or tumors, autonomic neuropathy, intestinal pseudo-obstruction, stroke, multiple sclerosis, dementia
Myopathies	Scleroderma, amyloidosis, myotonic dystrophy
Structural	Colon cancer, stricture, external compression, rectocele, fissure, hemorrhoids
Medications	Opiates, analgesics, tricyclic antidepressants, antiemetics anticholinergics, antihistamines, antipsychotics, antiparkinsonian agents, antidiarrheals, antacids, calcium channel blockers, diuretics, anticonvulsants, cation-containing agents (e.g., iron, bismuth), bile acid resins
Other	Irritable bowel syndrome, anal spasm, rectal prolapse, depression, low-fiber diet, sedentary lifestyle, slow-transit constipation, pelvic floor dysfunction

- **Irritable bowel syndrome** is considered **constipation predominant** if the patient has ≥25% hard or lumpy stools with Bristol Stool Scale Types 1–2 and <25% loose or watery stools with Types 6–7. This diagnosis should be entertained when abdominal pain or discomfort is a predominant complaint in a patient without concerning warning signs (see below), especially in those with comorbid affective disorders such as anxiety and depression.

Pathophysiology

Colonic and anorectal function are incompletely understood but are thought to be influenced by various factors, including intrinsic reflexes and autonomic processes, neurotransmitters, diurnal variation, and learned behaviors.[6,10]

TABLE 4-2 ROME IV DIAGNOSTIC CRITERIA FOR FUNCTIONAL CONSTIPATION

At least 3 mo (with symptom onset at least 6 mo prior to diagnosis) of two or more of the following:
- Straining with ≥25% of defecations
- Lumpy or hard stools with ≥25% of defecations
- Sensation of incomplete evacuation with ≥25% of defecations
- Sensation of anorectal obstruction or blockage with ≥25% of defecations
- Manual maneuvers to facilitate ≥25% of defecations
- Fewer than three spontaneous defecations per week

Loose stools are absent without use of laxatives
Insufficient criteria for the diagnosis of constipation-predominant IBS (IBS-C)

Adapted from Lacy BE, Mearin F, Chang L, et al. Functional bowel disorders. *Gastroenterology.* 2016;150:1393–1407.

Risk Factors

- Women tend to have more self-reported constipation than men, and the prevalence of constipation increases with age.[11] Over 50% of the elderly living in the community are estimated to suffer from constipation.[12,13]
- Other risk factors include physical inactivity, malnutrition, restricted diets, polypharmacy, recent abdominal or pelvic surgery, travel, and known comorbid conditions.

DIAGNOSIS

The workup of the constipated patient requires a thorough history and physical examination. Though not always necessary, diagnostic tests are available to evaluate colonic transit, to document colonic and anorectal motor function, and to exclude obstructive processes.

Clinical Presentation

Patients with constipation present with a wide range of complaints, many of which may create substantial embarrassment for them. A trusting relationship will aid in obtaining a clear and well-defined history.

History

- A well-performed defecation history elicits whether the patient has infrequent stools, hard stools, a sense of incomplete evacuation, straining, need for digital disimpaction, and associated abdominal pain. Onset and duration of symptoms are also important. For instance, lifelong abdominal discomfort may suggest overlap with irritable bowel syndrome.
- The **Bristol Stool Scale** is a frequently used descriptor of stool form and consistency, and can be a very useful tool; please see Figure 4-1.[14]
- A complete review of symptoms will help narrow the differential diagnosis. For example, if the patient reports cold intolerance and weight gain, hypothyroidism should be considered. The triad of kidney stones, confusion, and constipation suggests hypercalcemia. Current diuretic use or vomiting may predispose to constipation through hypokalemia and ileus. Esophageal dysmotility associated with constipation can be seen in systemic sclerosis.
- Colon cancer can present with obstructive symptoms, but this is typically a late manifestation; important questions include a history of weight loss, bloody stools, family history of colon cancer, and prior screening colonoscopy.
- A careful medication history should be obtained before embarking on an involved workup of constipation. Numerous medications can be associated with constipation, and simple discontinuation can lead to resolution of symptoms.

Physical Examination

- The physical examination can help identify both gastrointestinal and extraintestinal causes of constipation. For instance, the presence of a thyroid goiter or peripheral neuropathy may suggest an endocrine or neurologic etiology.
- **Abdominal examination** includes inspection for signs of previous surgery; auscultation for the presence and frequency of bowel sounds; and palpation to assess for distention, masses, or retained stool.
- The **perineal and rectal examination** can provide invaluable information. Close inspection helps detect internal hemorrhoids, fissures, or masses. Perineal sensation and the anal wink reflex should also be assessed. Anorectal neuromuscular function can be evaluated on digital examination by checking the sphincter tone both at rest and with squeeze. Gaping of the anal canal on immediate withdrawal of the finger may suggest external anal sphincter denervation. Asking the patient to bear down may reveal rectal prolapse, rectocele, or paradoxical contraction. Significant pain on digital examination can imply a fissure or ulceration.

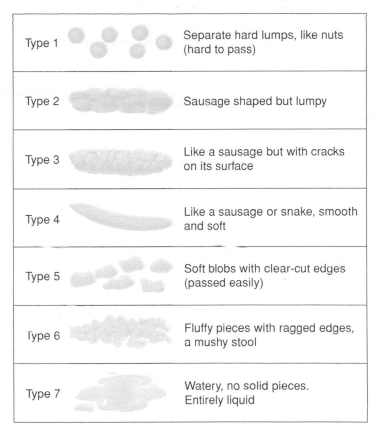

Type 1	Separate hard lumps, like nuts (hard to pass)
Type 2	Sausage shaped but lumpy
Type 3	Like a sausage but with cracks on its surface
Type 4	Like a sausage or snake, smooth and soft
Type 5	Soft blobs with clear-cut edges (passed easily)
Type 6	Fluffy pieces with ragged edges, a mushy stool
Type 7	Watery, no solid pieces. Entirely liquid

Figure 4-1. Bristol Stool Chart. (Adapted from Lewis SJ, Heaton KW. Stool form scale as a useful guide to intestinal transit time. *Scand J Gastroenterol.* 1997;32: 920–924.)

Differential Diagnosis

Differential diagnosis is broad and includes myriad conditions and medications as listed in Table 4-1.

Diagnostic Testing

No single test makes a clear diagnosis, so patients must be assessed thoroughly on an individual basis.

Laboratory Testing

- Initial laboratory tests include **basic chemistry panel with glucose, calcium, thyroid-stimulating hormone**, and **complete blood cell count**. Stool should be checked for occult blood.
- More specific testing for rare endocrinopathies, metabolic disorders, or collagen vascular disorders should be performed when a high suspicion exists.

Imaging

- **Plain radiographs** can be helpful to investigate possible ileus or obstruction as well as to look for stool retention or megacolon. **Barium radiography** can be performed if plain radiographs are suggestive of megacolon, megarectum, or structural disease with luminal narrowing.
- **Defecography** typically involves placing a small amount of barium into the patient's rectum and then having him or her perform a series of maneuvers. **Dynamic MRI** may be used instead of fluoroscopic techniques to view the pelvis in greater detail. This can prove helpful when previous studies are inconclusive or inconsistent with the clinical scenario.[15]

Diagnostic Procedures

- **Flexible sigmoidoscopy** and **colonoscopy** are typically reserved for new-onset constipation of unclear etiology, especially in the presence of warning signs, such as weight loss, anemia, bloody stools, family history of colon cancer, or hemoccult-positive stools. When seen in patients older than 50 years, these signs should prompt a full workup to rule out colorectal cancer. Other processes that can be detected on colonoscopy, such as hemorrhoids, fissures, and stercoral ulcers, may be the result of long-standing constipation. Melanosis coli, a brownish-black discoloration of the bowel mucosa, is sometimes seen in the presence of chronic anthraquinone laxative use.
- **Colonic transit studies** can be performed to distinguish causes of primary constipation. Ingestion of radio-opaque markers is a simple method to evaluate colonic transit, with plain radiography performed 5 days later. If six or more markers are left scattered throughout the colon, slow transit is suggested. If those markers are confined to the rectosigmoid colon, there may be an element of obstructive defecation. A wireless capsule technique, called the SmartPill, can provide similar information while also assessing transit and pH in the stomach and small bowel.
- **Anorectal manometry** provides an assessment of both pressure activity and sensation of the anorectum and its sphincters. These measures are carefully evaluated during rest, squeeze, and bear down maneuvers. A balloon inflation test measures the patient's symptoms at various pressures. Finally, a balloon expulsion test can be performed to assess the patient's ability to expel a simulated bowel movement within an allotted amount of time, typically within 2 minutes in normal subjects.

TREATMENT

- Initial therapy for chronic constipation involves use of dietary fiber supplementation and laxatives.
- In the event that first-line therapy fails, assessment of colonic and/or anorectal function may be appropriate before trialing further medications.

Medications

First Line

- **Fiber supplementation** can begin at 10 g/day and increased by approximately 5 g/day each week to a total intake of approximately 25 g/day. It is important to instruct patients to maintain adequate hydration during trials of increased fiber, as constipation can potentially worsen. Bloating, abdominal distention, and flatulence are side effects seen with fiber supplementation.
- **Osmotic laxatives**, such as polyethylene glycol, lactulose, sorbitol, and magnesium-containing products work by delivering poorly absorbed polymers or ions to the colon, which osmotically draws water into the bowel lumen. Adverse effects include cramping and incontinence due to fluid being delivered to the rectum. Magnesium toxicity can occur in children and in those with renal dysfunction.

- **Stimulant laxatives** are the most frequently prescribed laxatives. They work by increasing colonic motility. Anthraquinones additionally increase fluid and electrolyte content in the distal ileum and colon. Examples are senna and bisacodyl. Adverse effects include abdominal cramping and cathartic colon.
- **Emollients** consist of mineral oils and docusate salts. Mineral oil penetrates the stool and softens it, whereas docusate salts lower surface tension of stool, allowing more water through. Adverse effects include malabsorption of fat-soluble vitamins and lipid pneumonia if aspirated.
- **Enemas** (tap water, saline, mineral oil, or sodium phosphate) cause distal colonic and rectal distension and reflex evacuation of luminal contents. Adverse effects include mechanical trauma, damage to rectal mucosa with chronic use, and rarely acute phosphate nephropathy which primarily occurs in older individuals with compromised renal function who use phosphate-containing products.
- **Glycerin suppositories** can act as a lubricant; glycerin expands at body temperature, and can provide additional volume in the rectum to initiate defecation. Stimulant suppositories are also available.

Second Line

- **5-hydroxytryptamine-4 (5-HT$_4$)** receptor agonists have been studied extensively for their prokinetic value. The older drugs in this class, cisapride and tegaserod, have been taken off the market due to potential cardiovascular adverse events. Instead, attention has shifted to newer drugs in this class, such as prucalopride and potentially velusetrag.[16]
- **Lubiprostone**, a chloride channel activator that increases intestinal water secretion, has been approved for use in constipation-predominant IBS (IBS-C), chronic constipation,[17] as well as opioid-induced constipation.[18] Nausea is the most commonly seen adverse effect.
- **Linaclotide and plecanatide** are guanylate cyclase C activators that lead to intestinal chloride and bicarbonate secretion.[19] In addition to treating constipation, linaclotide also appears to decrease pain in patients with IBS.[20,21] Loose stool is the most common side effect for this class of medications.
- **μ-Receptor antagonists** work in the periphery by blocking the constipating effects of opiates without altering the pain relief. **Naloxegol** and **naldemedine** are oral formulations approved for opioid-induced constipation.[22] **Methylnaltrexone** works similarly but is only available as a subcutaneous injection and thus is primarily used for inpatients. **Alvimopan** has been used successfully in postoperative ileus.
- **Probiotics** can be trialed. The mechanism of action is unknown.

Nonpharmacologic Therapies

- **Biofeedback** is a type of behavioral training that has shown benefit in the setting of defecatory disorders, both in improving symptoms and anorectal function.[23] Patients are retrained to relax their pelvic floor muscles and restore normal anorectal synergy during defecation. This method appears to be beneficial primarily in those with outlet dysfunction.[24]
- Other behavioral training includes **ritualization of bowel movement timing**.[10]

Surgical Management

Surgical intervention can be used in patients with a structural reason for obstructed defecation (e.g., rectocele). It is rarely used in chronic constipation, except in the patient with colonic inertia who has failed prolonged medical therapy.

Lifestyle/Risk Modification

Proper fluid intake[25] and **exercise** could be beneficial in patients with constipation.

SPECIAL CONSIDERATIONS

- In the elderly, the etiology of constipation is often multifactorial and can include comorbid illnesses, medications, and decreased mobility.[26] Care should be taken to monitor hydration and electrolytes closely, especially in those with renal disease.
- Constipation is a commonly encountered problem in pregnancy. Oftentimes, patients can be treated with simple reassurance and proper education.[27]

COMPLICATIONS

- Early recognition and management of constipation is important because chronic constipation can lead to **fecal impaction, pudendal nerve damage, fecal incontinence, rectal prolapse, stercoral ulcers** with perforation or bleeding, **volvulus, hemorrhoids,** or **anal fissures**.
  - These complications tend to occur more frequently in the elderly and nursing home residents. Early recognition of these complications is an effective strategy to reduce morbidity in these patients.
  - Some complications can require surgical management, such as stercoral ulcers with perforation, or anatomic abnormalities that obstruct defecation (e.g., enterocele, rectocele, cystocele). Refractory slow transit constipation or colonic inertia is sometimes managed with total colectomy and ileorectal anastomosis, but pelvic floor dyssynergia is first excluded in these instances.
  - Endoscopic therapy of stercoral ulcers may be necessary to achieve hemostasis in the setting of rectal bleeding.
  - Fecal impaction should always be considered in patients with chronic constipation regardless of whether presentation involves constipation or incontinence. Fecal impaction can lead to incontinence by invoking the rectoanal inhibitory reflex, that is, the tendency for the internal anal sphincter to relax in the presence of stool in the rectum. A quick digital rectal examination can often help detect stool in the rectum. However, fecal impaction sometimes occurs higher than the rectum, and absence of stool in the rectum does not exclude the diagnosis. A plain x-ray film of the abdomen may reveal obstructive features and lack of rectal air. Management involves disimpaction, sometimes manually. Oil-based enemas (cottonseed enema, mineral oil enema) may help soften the stool and ease evacuation. Hypaque enemas may provide both diagnosis and therapy of fecal impaction. After disimpaction, an effective oral laxative regimen with or without rectal suppositories or enemas needs to be established.
- Abdominal pain associated with constipation can sometimes lead to unnecessary surgeries, such as appendectomy, hysterectomy, or ovarian cystectomy.

REFERRAL

Referral to a gastroenterologist may be warranted, especially if specialized studies, such as anorectal manometry, are needed.

REFERENCES

1. Sun SX, Dibonaventura M, Purayidathil FW, et al. Impact of chronic constipation on health-related quality of life, work productivity, and healthcare resource use: an analysis of the National Health and Wellness Survey. *Dig Dis Sci.* 2011;56:2688–2695.
2. Irvine EJ, Ferazzi S, Pare P, et al. Health-related quality of life in functional GI disorders: focus on constipation and resource utilization. *Am J Gastroenterol.* 2002;97:1986–1993.
3. Cheng C, Chan AOO, Hui WM, et al. Coping strategies, illness perception, anxiety and depression of patients with idiopathic constipation: a population-based study. *Aliment Pharmacol Ther.* 2003;18:319–326.

4. Ford AC, Moayyedi P, Lacy BE, et al. American College of Gastroenterology Monograph on the management of irritable bowel syndrome and chronic idiopathic constipation. *Am J Gastroenterol.* 2014;109:S2–S26.

5. Bharucha AE, Dorn SD, Lembo AJ, et al. American Gastroenterological Association medical position statement on constipation. *Gastroenterology.* 2013;144:211–217.

6. Rao SSC, Rattanakovit K, Patcharatrakul T. Diagnosis and management of chronic constipation in adults. *Nat Rev Gastroenterol Hepatol.* 2016;13:295–305.

7. Lacy BE, Mearin F, Chang L, et al. Functional bowel disorders. *Gastroenterology.* 2016;150:1393–1407.

8. Perry AF, Crockett SD, Barritt AS, et al. Burden of gastrointestinal, liver, and pancreatic diseases in the United States. *Gastroenterology.* 2015;149:1731–1741.

9. Rao SS. Constipation: evaluation and treatment of colonic and anorectal motility disorders. *Gastroenterol Clin N Am.* 2007;36:687–711.

10. Rao SS. Constipation: evaluation and treatment of colonic and anorectal motility disorders. *Gastrointest Endosc Clin N Am.* 2009;19:117–139.

11. Cook IJ, Talley NJ, Benninga MA, et al. Chronic constipation: overview and challenges. *Neurogastroenterol Motil.* 2009;21(Suppl 2):1–8.

12. Bouras EP, Tangalos EG. Chronic constipation in the elderly. *Gastroenterol Clin North Am.* 2009;38:463–480.

13. Gallegos-Orozco JF, Foxx-Orenstein AE, Sterler SM, et al. Chronic constipation in the elderly. *Am J Gastroenterol.* 2012;107:18–25.

14. Lewis SJ, Heaton KW. Stool form scale as a useful guide to intestinal transit time. *Scand J Gastroenterol.* 1997;32:920–924.

15. Camilleri M, Bharucha AE. Behavioural and new pharmacological treatments for constipation: getting the balance right. *Gut.* 2010;59:1288–1296.

16. Nelson AD, Camilleri M, Chirapongsathorn S. Comparison of efficacy of pharmacological treatments for chronic idiopathic constipation: a systemic review and network meta-analysis. *Gut.* 2017;66:611-622.

17. Barish CF, Drossman D, Johanson JF, et al. Efficacy and safety of lubiprostone in patients with chronic constipation. *Dig Dis Sci.* 2010;55:1090–1097.

18. Jamal MM, Adams AB, Jensen JP, et al. A randomized, placebo controlled trial of lubiprostone for opioid induced constipation in chronic noncancer pain. *Am J Gastroenterol.* 2015;110:725–732.

19. Lembo AJ, Kurtz CB, Macdougall JE, et al. Efficacy of linaclotide for patients with chronic constipation. *Gastroenterology.* 2010;138:886–895.

20. Chey WD, Lembo AJ, Lavins BJ, et al. Linaclotide for irritable bowel syndrome with constipation: a 26-week, randomized, double-blind, placebo-controlled trial to evaluate efficacy and safety. *Am J Gastroenterol.* 2012;107:1702–1712.

21. Weinberg DS, Smalley W, Heidelbaugh JJ, et al. American Gastroenterological Association Institute guideline on the pharmacological management of irritable bowel syndrome. *Gastroenterology.* 2014;147:1146–1148.

22. Chey WD, Webster L, Sostek M, et al. Naloxegol for opioid-induced constipation in patients with noncancer pain. *N Engl J Med.* 2014;370:2387–2396.

23. Enck P, Van der Voort IR, Klosterhalfen S. Biofeedback therapy in fecal incontinence and constipation. *Neurogastroenterol Motil.* 2009;21:1133–1141.

24. Chiaroni G, Salandini L, Whitehead WE. Biofeedback benefits only patients with outlet dysfunction, not patients with isolated slow transit constipation. *Gastroenterology.* 2005;129:86–97.

25. Markland AD, Palson O, Goode PS. Association of low dietary intake of fiber and liquids with constipation: evidence from the national health and nutrition examination survey. *Am J Gastroenterol.* 2013;108:796–803.

26. Rao SS, Go JT. Update on the management of constipation in the elderly: new treatment options. *Clin Interv Aging.* 2010;5:163–171.

27. Cullen G, O'Donoghue D. Constipation and pregnancy. *Best Pract Res Clin Gastroenterol.* 2007;21:807–818.

GENERAL PRINCIPLES

- Abdominal pain is one of the most common complaints for which patients visit primary care providers, and one of the most common reasons for a gastroenterology consult.[1,2]
- The ability to diagnose and treat abdominal pain accurately and efficiently is of great importance.
- A general understanding of anatomy and physiology is important in formulating a differential diagnosis.
- An orderly approach is essential in the evaluation of abdominal pain, particularly in avoiding unnecessary repetitive testing and potential harmful delays in making the diagnosis.

Classification

- **Parietal pain**
  - The parietal peritoneum lining the abdominal cavity is innervated by somatic nerve fibers.
  - The pain is **usually sharp, well localized, and lateralizes to the site of irritation**.
  - The **most frequent stimulus is inflammation**, often from an inflamed adjacent organ or viscus.
  - Other stimuli that can irritate the parietal peritoneum are blood, gastric acid, or stool.
  - The pain is **constant and worse with motion** of the peritoneum.
  - Pain severity depends on the specific irritating agent and the rate of development.
  - There is open associated reflex muscle spasm of the abdominal muscles referred to as "**involuntary guarding.**"
  - When bowel perforates or when blood collects in the peritoneal cavity, extensive stimulation of the parietal peritoneum results in a boardlike **rigid abdomen**, with **diffuse and excruciating pain made worse by even minimal movement**.
- **Visceral pain**
  - Noxious stimuli affecting the abdominal viscera result in the perception of visceral pain.
  - This can result from traction on the peritoneum, distension of a hollow viscus, or muscular contraction.
  - The pain fibers innervating the visceral structures are bilateral, so pain is typically perceived in the midline.
  - Visceral pain is **dull and poorly localized, often remote from the location of the abnormality**.
  - The pain is **often intermittent or colicky**.
  - Pain is often associated with autonomic symptoms such as nausea, vomiting, or diaphoresis.
- **Referred pain**
  - Pain is **felt in areas distant to the diseased organ**.
  - The pain can be well localized and felt in the skin or deeper tissues.

Examples include diaphragmatic irritation from a subphrenic hematoma or abscess resulting in shoulder pain, pain in the thigh from a psoas abscess, and radiation of renal colic from loin to groin. Gallbladder and bile duct pain can also be referred to the shoulder or scapular area, particularly on the right side.

Pathophysiology

- Noxious stimuli can result in pain within the abdomen by various mechanisms, and the characteristics of these mechanisms can help in identifying the underlying disease process.[1,2]
- The two principal mechanisms of pain, parietal pain and visceral pain, are discussed below.
- Other mechanisms of pain that may be relevant include ischemia, musculoskeletal pain, referred pain, metabolic derangements, neurogenic pain, and functional pain. A single-diseased organ can produce pain through multiple mechanisms.[1,3]

DIAGNOSIS

Clinical Presentation

- A thorough, detailed history and physical examination are keys to efficient evaluation of patients with abdominal pain.
- An accurate diagnosis often depends on a meticulous history and physical examination; however, diagnosis can remain elusive regardless of the extensive history and physical examination, in which case admission, serial examinations, follow-up calls, or surgical exploration should be considered.

History

- This is the **most important part of the evaluation**, thus an organized approach is essential.
- Attempts should be made to identify the pain onset, duration, character, location, severity, exacerbating or alleviating factors, and associated symptoms.[4]
- Other key aspects of the history should include underlying medical conditions, prior surgeries, medications, allergies, family history, travel, contact with animals or sick individuals, and social history including occupation and substance abuse. Some general features regarding these aspects of the history are described here.[3,4]
- **Onset of pain**
  - It is important to **differentiate acute versus chronic pain**.
  - Severe pain that begins abruptly may indicate an intra-abdominal catastrophe, including ruptured abdominal vasculature, occluded mesenteric vasculature, or perforated viscus. Urgent or immediate surgery may be essential in certain situations for a good patient outcome.
  - Pain that develops rapidly over minutes suggests inflammation or luminal obstruction.
  - Gradual onset over hours may also suggest inflammation.
- **Duration**
  - Pain caused by irritation of the parietal peritoneum is constant.
  - Obstruction of a hollow viscus typically results in crampy or colicky pain that waxes and wanes and is associated with abdominal distension, nausea, and vomiting.
  - Pain lasting more than 6 months is generally considered as chronic abdominal pain and can remain undiagnosed despite extensive workup.
- **Character**
  - Parietal pain is usually severe and well localized.
  - Pain associated with visceral noxious stimuli is dull or gnawing and poorly localized.

- **Location**
  - This is often the most important characteristic in parietal pain. The parietal peritoneum is supplied by somatic nerves; thus pain is perceived in the area where the peritoneum is irritated.
  - Visceral pain is usually midline and poorly localized, but the location may provide useful information regarding the involved organ.
  - Radiation of pain may also help identify the affected organ.
  - Table 5-1 lists the commonly affected organs and perceived areas of pain.
- **Severity/Intensity**
  - This is very subjective and difficult to measure because it is dependent on the individual patients' point of reference, based on past experience of pain, personality traits, or cultural differences.
  - Severe pain suggests ruptured abdominal viscus or vascular structure.
  - Pain that is severe in the setting of a benign examination may suggest mesenteric ischemia.
- **Exacerbating and alleviating factors**
  - Pain caused by inflammation of the peritoneum is worse with coughing or movement.
  - Patients with renal or intestinal colic may move around in an attempt to get into a comfortable position.
  - Eating exacerbates pain caused by gastric ulcer, chronic mesenteric ischemia, or biliary pain but may alleviate pain caused by duodenal ulcer.
  - The pain associated with pancreatitis is classically relieved by bending forward or curling up in the fetal position.
- **Associated symptoms**
  - Nausea, vomiting, diaphoresis, hematemesis, hematochezia, melena, diarrhea, obstipation, hematuria, and fever may further focus the diagnostic evaluation.

Physical Examination

- As with the history, an organized approach to the physical examination, particularly of the abdomen, increases the likelihood of an accurate diagnosis.
- In addition, focusing on key extra-abdominal physical examination findings is crucial because they may provide valuable clues as to the diagnosis.
- An exhaustive review of all the signs is beyond the scope of this chapter; however, several points deserve emphasis.

TABLE 5-1 ORGAN INVOLVEMENT AND PERCEIVED LOCATION OF PAIN

Esophagus	Chest, epigastrium
Stomach	Epigastrium, Left upper quadrant
Small intestine	Periumbilical region
Colon	Lower abdomen
Gallbladder	Right upper quadrant, radiation to scapula, shoulder, back
Liver	Right upper quadrant
Spleen	Left upper quadrant
Kidney or ureter	Costovertebral angle, flank, radiation to groin
Bladder	Suprapubic region
Aorta	Mid-back region

- **Vital signs**
  - Particular attention must be given to frequent hemodynamic monitoring.
  - The presence of ***tachycardia or orthostatic hypotension*** suggests significant volume depletion and should prompt an immediate search for the underlying cause (hemorrhage, vomiting, diarrhea, or third spacing).
  - ***Tachycardia*** may be the only sign of impending hemodynamic collapse in a patient with vascular catastrophe.
  - ***Fever*** suggests an inflammatory process, such us infection or inflammatory bowel disease.
  - ***Tachypnea*** is often the earlier sign of sepsis.
- **General appearance**
  - Much information can be determined by observing the patients' general appearance.
  - This includes an assessment of their overall appearance, respiratory pattern, and ability to converse, position in bed, posture, and facial expression. Facial expression should be noted also while palpating the abdomen.
  - Patients with peritonitis often lie still, whereas those with renal or intestinal colic writhe in bed.
  - Generalized pallor suggests severe anemia, potentially from acute blood loss.
- **Abdominal examination**
  - Patients with acute abdominal pain are very apprehensive; hence, it is important to take a gentle, reassuring approach to the abdominal examination.
  - The abdomen should be examined with the patients' knees and hips flexed to relax the abdominal muscles.
  - First, the abdomen should be visually inspected for surgical scars, distension, bulging flanks, or other obvious abnormalities.
  - Next, auscultate for the presence or absence of bowel sounds or bruits.
  - Gentle pressure with the stethoscope allows assessment of tenderness without alarming the patient.
  - Palpation should begin at the site furthest away from the area of pain and additionally noting any visceral enlargement or masses.
  - The presence or absence of guarding, rigidity, or rebound tenderness should be noted, because these may signify peritoneal irritation.
  - Peritoneal inflammation is best determined by light percussion on the abdomen, gently shaking the bed or asking the patient to cough.
  - Hernial orifices should be inspected and palpated in all instances, and the patient is asked to cough to determine whether an impulse is felt on coughing.
  - Digital rectal examinations may have value, not just in anal/rectal palpation and inspecting rectal content on the examining finger but in localizing pain.
  - External genitalia should be inspected, particularly the scrotum in males.
  - Female patients should have pelvic examinations performed when appropriate.

Differential Diagnosis

- The list of diagnoses that can cause abdominal pain is extensive and includes inflammatory, mechanical, ischemic, metabolic, and neurologic conditions.[1–3,5]
- This emphasizes the need for a careful and systematic history and physical examination to narrow the possible diagnoses. Table 5-2 lists some of the common causes of abdominal pain.

Diagnostic Testing

- The differential diagnosis in patients presenting with acute abdominal pain can be determined with a careful history and physical examination; further diagnostic evaluation should be targeted to ruling in or excluding these conditions.[3]

TABLE 5-2 CAUSES OF ABDOMINAL PAIN

Inflammation	Mechanical	Ischemic	Metabolic	Other
Cholecystitis	Small or large bowel obstruction	Mesenteric ischemia	Diabetic ketoacidosis	Thoracic disorders
Pancreatitis	Volvulus	Ischemic colitis	Uremia	Herpes zoster
Appendicitis	Biliary obstruction	Splenic infarction	Porphyria	SLE
Diverticulitis	Ureteral stones	Testicular torsion	Lead poisoning	Musculoskeletal disorders
Hepatitis	Adhesions	Ovarian cyst torsion	Angioedema	Functional abdominal pain
PID	Ruptured aortic aneurysm	Incarcerated hernia	Familial Mediterranean fever	Constipation
Peptic ulcer	Ruptured ectopic pregnancy	Arcuate ligament syndrome		Ovarian cyst
Gastroenteritis	Intussusception			Endometriosis
Acute colitis	Retroperitoneal fibrosis			Abdominal migraine
Pyelonephritis				
Acute cholangitis				

PID, pelvic inflammatory disease; SLE, systemic lupus erythematosus.

- Excessive, undirected testing increases the costs and may cause unnecessary delays in diagnosis and treatment.
- While elaborating all potential tests in the workup of abdominal pain is beyond the scope of this handbook, a few specific tests deserve special mention.

Laboratory Testing
- A **complete blood cell count with differential count** should be ordered in all patients to evaluate for leukocytosis or anemia.
- **Serum electrolytes** (including blood urea nitrogen, creatinine, and glucose) are important to assess fluid status, acid–base status, and renal function.
- **Lipase** is useful in patients with suspected pancreatic disease.
- **Lactate** levels may be elevated in bowel infarction.
- **Liver chemistries** help evaluate causes of right upper quadrant pain such us hepatic injury or biliary obstruction.
- **Coagulation profile** should be checked in those with suspected liver disease.

- **Acute phase reactants** such as C-reactive protein (CRP) or erythrocyte sedimentation rate (ESR) can point to underlined inflammatory conditions such as Crohn disease.
- All female patients of childbearing age should have β-human chorionic gonadotropin (**β-hCG**) to exclude pregnancy.

Imaging
- **Standard radiography**
  - Not all patients with acute abdominal pain require plain or upright films of the abdomen. However, if ordered they should include two views of the abdomen: one in supine and one in the upright position or lateral decubitus with left side down.
  - Abdominal x-ray films are **useful for diagnosing perforated viscus** (identified as free air under the diaphragm), **ileus, or bowel obstruction**.
  - Abdominal films may also demonstrate the calcific changes associated with chronic pancreatitis as well as calcium-containing renal stones.
  - The sensitivity of abdominal radiography in the diagnosis of abdominal pathology in the setting of acute abdominal pain is about 10%. Therefore, abdominal plain films are often used for monitoring ileus, small bowel obstruction, and colonic dilation in hospitalized patients with established diagnosis.[6]
- **Ultrasonography**
  - This is the **preferred initial imaging test in biliary tract disease and gallstones**. It is frequently obtained in patients with suspected acute cholecystitis, biliary colic, choledocholithiasis, and cholangitis. It has a sensitivity and specificity of (85% and 81%, respectively).[6]
  - Transabdominal ultrasound is also useful for patients with abdominal aortic aneurysms, ectopic pregnancy, tubo-ovarian abscess, and ovarian or testicular torsion.
  - Ultrasonography is safe and can be performed at the bedside in most cases.
- **Computed tomography (CT)**
  - Abdominal CT, especially with rapid spiral scanning techniques, provides a powerful imaging tool.[6,7]
  - CT allows "three-dimensional" imaging of the entire abdomen and pelvis.
  - CT is less operator dependent than the ultrasound; it provides more consistent results and it has a reported sensitivity and specificity (91% and 90%, respectively).[8]
  - CT is a sensitive test for identifying bowel obstruction, inflammatory processes (appendicitis, necrotizing pancreatitis, diverticulitis, intra-abdominal abscess), vascular lesion (ruptured aortic aneurysm, portal vein thrombosis), and abdominal or retroperitoneal hemorrhage.
  - Organ-specific protocols require focused helical CT, which requires coordination of oral/IV contrast and image attainment. This is useful to assess perforated viscus or differentiate ischemic, traumatic, or neoplastic lesions of the pancreas or the liver.
  - CT arteriography is another useful tool in assessing the aorta and visceral vasculature.
  - Patient selection for CT imaging is of great importance, as this can be costly and unnecessarily delay diagnosis and treatment especially in patients who require urgent surgery. There is also the risk of nephrotoxicity and anaphylactic reaction that can occur with iodinated contrast dye.
- **Magnetic resonance imaging (MRI)**
  - This is a multiplanar imaging modality using the different intrinsic soft tissue contrast properties to distinguish areas with different degrees of enhancement.[6]
  - MRI can detect subtle lesions that do not conform to organ contours with high sensitivity.
  - MRI is an excellent modality in the evaluation and differentiation of liver and pancreatic lesions.
  - MRI is highly sensitive in evaluating the mesenteric vessels in suspected ischemia.
  - MR cholangiopancreatography (MRCP) has become the noninvasive imaging modality of choice for evaluating abnormalities of the biliary and pancreatic ducts.

MRI enterography has been used to image the small bowel and colon to detect inflammation, strictures, and fistulae and is a very useful study in patient suspected of having Crohn disease.

Advantages over CT:

- MRI is safer in children and pregnant women because of lack of ionizing radiation.
- The intravenous contrast medium typically used (gadolinium) is not nephrotoxic. In patients with severe kidney disease, gadolinium is associated with rare nephrogenic systemic fibrosis manifested by localized skin thickening and contractures.

Disadvantages:

- MRI cannot be used in patients with permanent pacemakers, defibrillators, aneurysm clips, or metallic implants/devices.
- MRI is not suited for patients with severe claustrophobia because it is performed in a "closed tube"; open MRIs can be considered in such situations.
- MRI is more costly, time consuming, and requires greater patient cooperation thus making it less desirable in an urgent setting.

Diagnostic Procedures

- **Endoscopy** is useful in evaluation of the esophagus, stomach, small bowel, and colon for ulceration, neoplasia, ischemia, or inflammation. However, bowel integrity has to be intact before performing endoscopy, as air and intestinal content can be pushed into the peritoneal cavity if endoscopy is performed where bowel integrity is compromised by perforation or extensive inflammation. Procedure risk needs to be balanced with potential benefits before performing endoscopy in acute abdominal pain presentations; it remains a very useful test in patients with chronic pain.[9]
- **Peritoneal aspiration or lavage**
  - A peritoneal tap is a useful adjunct for detecting hemoperitoneum from trauma or feculent material from hollow viscus injury/perforation.
  - Peritoneal taps are also performed for evaluation of peritoneal fluid accumulation, particularly in determining portal hypertension as an etiology, and in evaluating for infectious or spontaneous bacterial peritonitis (see also Chapters 10 and 20).
- **Urgent surgical intervention via laparoscopy or exploratory laparotomy** is warranted in patients with intra-abdominal catastrophes such as ruptured abdominal aortic aneurysm or ruptured intra-abdominal organ. Surgical exploration is sometimes performed in severe abdominal pain presentations wherein significant pathology is suspected, especially mesenteric ischemia.

REFERENCES

1. Kasper DL, ed. *Harrison's Principles of Internal Medicine*. 19th ed. New York: McGraw-Hill; 2015:1610–1627; Chapter 13.
2. Podolsky DK, ed. *Yamada's Textbook of Gastroenterology*. 6th ed. Philadelphia, PA: Lippincott Williams & Wilkins; 2003:695–722.
3. Spiller RC, Thompson WG. Bowel disorders. *Am J Gastroenterol*. 2010;105(4):775–785.
4. Cartwright AL, Knudson MP. Evaluation of acute abdominal pain in adults. *Am Fam Physician*. 2008;77(7):971–978.
5. Sleisenger MH, Fordtran JS. *Gastrointestinal Disease: Pathophysiology, Diagnosis, Management*. 10th ed. Philadelphia, PA: WB Saunders; 2015:161–175.
6. Cartwright SL, Knudson MP. Diagnostic imaging of acute abdominal pain in adults. *Am Fam Physician*. 2015;91(7):452–459.
7. Stoker J, van Randen A, Lameris W, et al. Imaging patients with acute abdominal pain. *Radiology*. 2009;253(1):31–46.
8. Srinivasan R, Greenbaum DS. Chronic abdominal wall pain: a frequently overlooked problem. *Am J Gastroenterol*. 2002;97(4):824–830.
9. ASGE Standards of Practice Committee; Early DS, Ben-Menachem T, Decker GA, et al. Appropriate use of GI endoscopy. *Gastrointest Endosc*. 2012;75(6):1127–1131.

Acute Gastrointestinal Bleeding

Jason G. Bill

6

- Acute gastrointestinal bleeding (GIB) is a common medical emergency resulting in significant morbidity, mortality, and >300,000 hospitalizations in the United States per year.[1]
- GIB involves a spectrum of clinical presentations based on the cause and site of bleeding. It can occur anywhere in the gastrointestinal (GI) tract from the mouth to the anus.
- This chapter discusses the etiologies, diagnostic strategies, and management of acute GIB.

Classification

GIB can be subdivided into **upper gastrointestinal bleeding** (UGIB) and **lower gastrointestinal bleeding** (LGIB). Historically this was based on location of the source in relationship to the ligament of Treitz. However, with the advent of newer investigative modalities targeting the small bowel, LGIB can be further characterized to **small bowel bleeding (middle GIB)** and **colonic bleeding**.

Epidemiology

- Most GIB episodes are self-limited and require only supportive therapy. Despite this, GIB accounts for 16,000–20,000 deaths annually.[1]
- The annual incidence of hospitalization for UGIB has declined over the past decade; incidence is 47 per 100,000 population. In contrast, given the increase in clinical indications for use of antiplatelet and anticoagulation therapies, the incidence of LGIB has increased; and currently is 33 per 100,000 population.[2]
- It is well established that hospitalization and mortality rates for both UGIB and LGIB increase with age, and with number of comorbid conditions but data also suggest gender differences, with males having higher incidence of UGIB than females, and females being older than males at the time of LGIB occurrence.[2]

Etiology

- **Upper gastrointestinal bleeding**
  - **Erosive/Ulcerative disease**
    - **Peptic ulcer disease.** This includes gastric and duodenal ulcers. Peptic ulcer disease (PUD) is the most common cause of acute UGIB accounting for up to 50% of cases.
      - Risk factors include *Helicobacter pylori* infection, nonsteroidal anti-inflammatory drug (NSAID) use, acetylsalicylic acid (ASA) use, and acid hypersecretion as in Zollinger–Ellison syndrome. *H. pylori* infection and NSAID use are the two most common causes of PUD.
      - In patients taking NSAIDs, cofactors such as age (>75 years), concurrent coronary artery disease, previous GIB, and a history of PUD may be independent risk factors for ulcer bleeding.
      - Predictors for mortality include age >70 years, multiple comorbidities, systolic blood pressure <100 mm Hg, hematemesis on presentation, ulcer rebleeding, and requirement for surgery.

TABLE 6-1 ENDOSCOPIC CLASSIFICATION AND OUTCOME OF BLEEDING PEPTIC ULCERS

	Description	Forrest Classification	Prevalence (%)	Rebleeding Rate (%)	Need for Surgery (%)	Mortality (%)
Acute bleeding	Spurting	Ia	18	55	35	11
	Oozing	Ib				
Stigmata of recent bleeding	NBVV*	IIa	17	43	34	11
	Adherent clot	IIb	17	22	10	7
	Flat pigmented spot	IIc	20	10	6	3
No stigmata of bleeding	Clean ulcer base	III	42	5	0.5	2

*NBVV, nonbleeding visible vessel.
Modified from Forrest JA, Finlayson ND, Shearman DJ. Endoscopy in gastrointestinal bleeding. *Lancet.* 1974;2(7877):394–397; Laine L, Peterson WL. Bleeding peptic ulcer. *N Engl J Med.* 1994;331:717–727.

Studies have shown that the endoscopic appearance of ulcers is strongly associated with rebleeding, need for surgery, and mortality (Table 6-1). Despite therapeutic advances, bleeding ulcer–related mortality rate has remained at approximately 10%.[3,4]

- **Erosive and hemorrhagic gastropathy.** Gastric erosions can be defined as a 3–5-mm breaks in the mucosa that do not penetrate to the muscularis mucosa. This is most commonly the result of medications such as NSAIDs or ASA, which can cause a hemorrhagic gastropathy within 24 hours of administration.

- **Stress ulcers** are distinct from peptic ulcers and occur in the setting of severe medical illness/physiologic stress. The pathophysiology is thought to be related to gastric hypoperfusion as a result of splanchnic vasoconstriction during physiologic stress.[3]

- **Esophagitis.** Causes include gastric reflux, infections (i.e., Cytomegalovirus, herpes simplex virus, *Candida albicans* infection), medications/pill induced (quinidine, tetracycline, alendronate), radiation therapy, and eosinophilic infiltration. This rarely leads to severe bleeding. Common presenting symptoms include heartburn, nausea, epigastric discomfort, dysphagia, odynophagia, and chest pain.[3]

Portal hypertension

- **Variceal bleeding.** Variceal hemorrhage can originate from esophageal, gastric, and duodenal varices.

- Varices are the result of portosystemic collateral circulation in patients with cirrhosis, portal or hepatic vein thrombosis, congenital hepatic fibrosis, and schistosomiasis resulting in subsequent portal hypertension.

- In the United States, alcoholic cirrhosis is the most common cause of portal hypertension.

- Esophageal varices account for 5–30% of UGIB cases. The 1-year incidence rate of a first variceal hemorrhage is 5% for large varices and 15% for small varices.

- Primary risk factors for bleeding from varices include size and wall thickness, presence of endoscopic stigmata such as red signs, severity of liver disease, and portal pressure.

- The estimated 6-week mortality from an episode of variceal bleeding has decreased over the past 2 decades from 30–50% to 15–25%.[5,6]
- **Portal hypertensive gastropathy.** This is characterized by congestion of the gastric mucosa from dilated arterioles and venules mainly in the gastric fundus and cardia. Erythema, petechiae, multiple bleeding areas, vascular ectasias, and congestion are hallmarks. The endoscopic appearance is often described as a mosaic pattern.[7]
- **Vascular malformations**
  - **Vascular ectasias** account for 5–10% of UGIB.
    - Vascular ectasias include isolated arteriovenous malformations and diffuse linear vascular ectasia known as gastric antral vascular ectasia or "watermelon stomach."
    - Vascular ectasia are formed by a complex tangle of arteries and veins connected by one or more fistulae. The vascular complex is known as the nidus, which is lacking a capillary bed and, therefore, arteries directly drain into veins. The draining veins are known to dilate secondary to high-velocity blood flow and can eventually rupture, resulting in a bleed.
    - Vascular ectasias have been associated with various medical conditions including chronic renal failure, valvular heart disease, congestive heart failure, hereditary hemorrhagic telangiectasia, and von Willebrand disease.[8]
  - **Dieulafoy lesion.** This is an aberrant vessel protruding through the mucosa without an underlying ulcer. This represents <5% of UGIB cases.[8]
- **Traumatic. Mallory–Weiss tear** is classically associated with vomiting or retching and is characterized by mucosal disruption at the gastroesophageal junction. This is responsible for 5–15% of all cases of UGIB and is self-limited in the majority of cases with a recurrence rate estimated to be 6%.[3] The tear usually heals within a few days; however, continued vomiting and retching can lead to esophageal rupture (Boerhaave syndrome).
- **Other etiologies**
  - **Foreign body ingestion**
  - **Hemobilia.** This is characterized by bleeding into the duodenum from the biliary tract. It is usually caused by trauma but can be seen in malignant tumors, cholelithiasis, acalculous inflammatory disease, or vascular disorders.
  - **Tumors.** Benign tumors such as GI stromal tumors can bleed when the tumor outgrows its blood supply and ulcerates. Malignant tumors such as esophageal, gastric, and duodenal cancers can also bleed. Bleeding from malignant tumors may not be amenable to endoscopic therapeutic measures or vascular embolization, and surgical resection or radiation therapy may be required.
  - **Aortoenteric fistulas.** These can occur as a late complication after aortic graft surgery and usually involve the third and fourth parts of the duodenum. The fistulas can be difficult to diagnose because visualization of the graft eroding through the intestinal wall is uncommon. The classic "herald bleed" is a small bleed that can occur days to weeks before massive fatal hemorrhage.
  - **Hemosuccus pancreaticus.** This is characterized by hemorrhage into the pancreatic duct and occurs primarily in patients with chronic pancreatitis, pseudocyst, pancreatic cancer, aneurysms of the splenic artery, or trauma.[8]
- **Lower gastrointestinal bleeding (Table 6-2)**[9]
  - **Diverticular bleeding.** It is the most common cause of major LGIB in the United States, related to the high prevalence of diverticulosis. Diverticula form at sites of weakness in the muscle wall of the colon where arteries can penetrate the muscularis layer to reach the mucosa or submucosa.
  - **Anorectal disease. Hemorrhoids** and **anal fissures** are common causes of minor intermittent LGIB. The characteristic clinical history of hemorrhoidal bleeding is bright red blood on the toilet tissue or around the stool but not mixed in the stool. Bleeding often occurs with straining or passage of hard stool. A similar history is

TABLE 6-2 SOURCES OF LOWER GASTROINTESTINAL BLEEDING

Source	Frequency (%)	Painless Hematochezia	Comments
Diverticulosis	30–65	Yes	Large volume; ~80% stop spontaneously
Angiodysplasia	4–15	Yes	Frequently multifocal; mostly right colon
Hemorrhoids	4–12	Yes	Typically intermittent and small volume
Ischemic colitis	4–11	No	Primarily affects watershed areas of colon
Colitis, other	3–15	No	Includes infection, radiation, and IBD
Neoplasia	2–11	Yes	Rarely causes brisk bleeding
Postpolypectomy	2–7	Yes	Typically occurs within 2 wks
Rectal ulcer	0–8	Yes	Can result in massive hemorrhage
Dieulafoy lesion, rare		Yes	Usually located in the rectum
Rectal varices, rare		Yes	Commonly linked to chronic liver disease

IBD, inflammatory bowel disease.
Adapted from Strate LL, Naumann CR. The role of colonoscopy and radiological procedures in the management of acute lower intestinal bleeding. *Clin Gastroenterol Hepatol.* 2010;8:333–343.

common in patients with bleeding from anal fissures, with the exception that anal fissures are often painful.

Ischemic colitis. It is typically caused by "low flow states" and small vessel disease rather than large vessel occlusion and most commonly involves the splenic flexure, descending colon, and sigmoid colon. Most cases resolve spontaneously with observation and medical support. Surgery is reserved for the rare circumstance of clinical deterioration with fever and rising leukocyte count or persistent hemorrhage.

Infectious colitis. Pathogens such as *Campylobacter jejuni*, *Shigella* species, invasive *Escherichia coli* or *E. coli* O157:H7, and, rarely, *Clostridium difficile* may cause bloody diarrhea. Cytomegalovirus can cause invasive disease characterized by ulcers that can bleed but limited to immunocompromised states (immunosuppressive of biologic therapy for inflammatory bowel disease, after organ transplant, AIDS, etc.). The degree of blood loss is variable and rarely significant except with anticoagulation or coagulopathy.

Radiation-induced proctopathy and colopathy. Radiation injury is a chronic or recurrent problem that may follow irradiation immediately or present several years later. Radiation impairs the normal course of repopulation of surface epithelium within the GI tract. The loss of absorptive surface can often lead to malabsorption and diarrhea, but microulcerations can also form. These **microulcerations** can coalesce and form bigger lesions and eventually result in a GI bleed. Alternatively, **telangiectasia** can form in the mucosa, which can also bleed—this mechanism is typically seen as radiation proctopathy after radiation for prostate cancer. Blood loss is rarely massive but can cause iron deficiency or the need for intermittent blood transfusion.

Inflammatory bowel disease. It usually causes a small to moderate degree of bleeding, although rarely it can be massive. The blood is usually mixed with the stool and is associated with other symptoms of the disease, such as diarrhea, tenesmus, and pain.

Other less common causes

- **Meckel diverticulum.** Meckel diverticulum is the most frequent congenital anomaly of the intestinal tract, with an incidence of 0.3–3.0% in autopsy reports. It develops from incomplete obliteration of the vitelline duct, leaving an ileal diverticulum. Patients present with painless bleeding that may be melenic or bright red. The diagnosis can be made by radiolabeled technetium scanning. Barium filling of the diverticulum may occur, especially with enteroclysis. Surgical excision is the treatment of choice.

- **Intussusception.** Uncommon in adults, it usually has a leading point, such as a polyp or malignancy. Patients often present with bloody stools mixed with mucus, often described as "currant jelly." The diagnosis may be made by plain abdominal x-ray films and a sausage-shaped mass found during physical examination. Barium enema may be useful for diagnosis; in children, it may be used for therapeutic reduction. Treatment of intussusception in adults is usually surgical.[10,11]

DIAGNOSIS

Clinical Presentation

The localization of acute GIB should begin with an assessment of the patient's hemodynamic status, and a focused history and physical examination (Table 6-3). However, these

TABLE 6-3 ASSESSMENT OF ACUTE GASTROINTESTINAL BLEEDING

Hemodynamics	Intravascular Volume Loss (%)	Pertinent History	Physical Examination
Normal	<10	Description of bleeding	Vital signs
Orthostatic hypotension	10–20	Duration and frequency	Orthostatic blood pressure
Shock	20–25	Prior bleeding	Stigmata of liver disease
		Comorbidities	Abdominal tenderness
		Medications	Stool color
		Previous surgery	Rectal examination
		Recent polypectomy	
		Prior radiation	
		Associated symptoms	

measures will not be diagnostic of the source of blood loss and further investigation, typically including endoscopy and/or radiologic imaging may be required.[12]

- **Digital rectal examination.** This has been recommended as a part of the initial evaluation in patients with acute LGIB and, in fact, may prove helpful in providing information regarding anorectal pathology prior to any endoscopic intervention. However, a digital examination does not preclude the need for endoscopic evaluation. One study found that 40% of rectal carcinomas diagnosed by proctoscopy were palpable on digital rectal examination.[13]

- **Nasogastric aspiration.** This should be performed if an upper GI source is suspected or if patients have hematochezia with hemodynamic compromise (as UGIB is detected in 10–15% of patients presenting with severe hematochezia). A positive gastric aspirate (frank blood) that does not clear may identify patients with high-risk lesions that may benefit from urgent endoscopy. A negative aspirate does not rule out an UGIB. In fact, up to 18% of patients with UGIB have a nonbloody aspirate.[14] Hemoccult testing of a clear or nonbloody gastric aspirate does not add to the evaluation, and visual inspection has better value.

Diagnostic Testing

- **Upper endoscopy.** Esophagogastroduodenoscopy (EGD) is the **preferred method for evaluating patients with UGIB**. Endoscopy allows direct visualization of the mucosa and identification of the bleeding site.
  - Endoscopy within the first 24 hours of presentation is the goal in UGIB, and endoscopy is recommended as soon as the patient is clinically stable when active ongoing bleeding is suspected. Since 10% of severe hematochezia presentations with hemodynamic compromise can be the result of UGIB, upper endoscopy is indicated as the first step in the evaluation of such presentations.
  - Total cost of hospitalization, length of hospitalization, rate of rebleeding, and need for emergent surgery have all been greatly reduced with early endoscopy, largely because of the therapeutic options available to the endoscopist (i.e., heater probe, argon plasma coagulation, epinephrine injection, band ligation). Definitive diagnosis is made when active bleeding, stigmata of bleeding, or significant lesions are seen.[8]
  - Early endoscopy (i.e., within 24 hours of admission) has not been demonstrated to decrease mortality.
  - It is important that the hemodynamically unstable patient be adequately volume resuscitated and any coagulopathy be corrected before performing upper endoscopy.
  - Morbidity and mortality rates from upper endoscopy have been reported at 1% and 0.1%, respectively.
  - Contraindications for endoscopy include an agitated patient, perforated viscous, and severe cardiopulmonary disease.

- **Colonoscopy.** Colonoscopy is the **most frequently used diagnostic tool for evaluating LGIB**.
  - A diagnosis is made in 48–90% of patients depending on the definition of the bleeding source, patient selection criteria, and timing of colonoscopy.[9,15]
  - For an optimal procedure, patients should be adequately resuscitated, hemodynamically stable, and free of stool and debris with bowel preparation.
  - With regard to timing of colonoscopy, patients with high-risk clinical features and signs or symptoms of ongoing bleeding should have colonoscopy performed within 24 hours of patient presentation after adequate bowel preparation in order to potentially improve diagnostic and therapeutic yield.[15] It still remains unclear whether urgent colonoscopy truly improves clinical outcomes or lowers hospital costs.

- As many as 10% of hematochezia presentations associated with hemodynamic compromise may be due to an upper GI bleeding source. Therefore, under these circumstances, an **upper endoscopy** may be indicated as the first step in the evaluation of severe hematochezia. It is widely accepted that once an upper GI source has been excluded, the next step in evaluation of a patient with severe hematochezia is generally colonoscopy. Although upper endoscopy and colonoscopy are the standard tools utilized to evaluate acute GIB, visualization of the entire small bowel is not possible with standard endoscopy.

- **Capsule endoscopy serves a crucial role in the initial evaluation of the small bowel.** In cases when small bowel bleeding is suspected, or when findings on upper endoscopy and colonoscopy are negative, capsule endoscopy can be used for further visualization of the small bowel. The diagnostic yield in patients with overt obscure GI bleeding ranges from 50–72%.[16]
- **Tagged red blood cell (RBC) scan.** The technetium 99m–labeled RBC scan can be used as a bedside evaluation of active lower GIB. Bleeding must exceed a rate of 0.1 mL/min to be detected. The procedure is of very low risk; however, the test is positive <50% of the time. One use of this procedure is as a **screening test before angiography**. A patient with a negative tagged RBC scan is unlikely to have a positive angiogram. If the test is negative, a colonoscopy is usually performed, followed by capsule endoscopy to evaluate the small bowel if colonoscopy is unrevealing.
- **Angiography.** Angiography offers accurate diagnosis and therapy in the rapidly bleeding patient. Bleeding rates of 0.5 to 1 mL/min are required to detect extravasation into the bowel from a bleeding site. The overall diagnostic yield from arteriography ranges from 40–78%. If a bleeding source is identified, therapeutic modalities, such as infusion of vasopressin or selective embolization, can be used to stop bleeding. Complications of this procedure include contrast allergy, bleeding from arterial puncture, and embolism from dislodged thrombus. Arteriography should be reserved for those patients with massive, ongoing LGIB for which colonoscopy is not feasible, for suspected massive small bowel bleeding, and for UGIB where endoscopy either fails or is unable to localize the source because of rapid bleeding.[9]
- **Computerized tomography angiography** is an emerging tool in the evaluation of the actively bleeding patient with suspected small bowel or colonic bleeding. The sensitivity to detect ongoing bleeding appears slightly lower when compared to a tagged RBC scan, however, has the advantage of being more expedient and accurate. Therefore, this modality has utility as the initial test in clinically unstable patients who cannot be sedated for endoscopy. Please see Table 6-4.[6]

TABLE 6-4	MANAGEMENT OF ACUTE VARICEAL HEMORRHAGE
Resuscitation	Cautious transfusion of fluid and blood products with goal hemoglobin of ~7–9 g/dL
	Ensure airway is protected
Pharmacologic therapy	Octreotide 50 mcg IV bolus followed by continuous infusion 50 μg/hr (3–5 days)
	Ciprofloxacin 400 mg BID IV or 500 mg BID PO or ceftriaxone 1 g/day IV (3–7 days)
Diagnosis and treatment	Endoscopy (within 12 hrs of admission) with endoscopic therapy, preferably ligation
Rescue management	TIPS or shunt therapy in patients with esophageal varices who have failed pharmacologic and endoscopic therapy or in patients with bleeding gastric fundic varices

Adapted from Garcia-Tsao G, Abraldes JG, Berzigotti A, et al. Portal hypertensive bleeding in cirrhosis: risk stratification, diagnosis, and management: 2016 practice guidance by the American Association for the study of liver diseases. *Hepatology*. 2017;65:310–335.

TREATMENT

- **Resuscitation is key.**
- **Intravascular volume should be restored initially with either isotonic saline or lactated Ringer solution.** Two large-bore (≥18-gauge) intravenous (IV) lines should be in place at all times. Centrally inserted, triple lumen catheters are typically placed. Although these may not confer an advantage over peripheral IV lines in terms of rate of fluid administration, they may be easier to place in the setting of vascular collapse or hypotension where peripheral veins are collapsed.
- **Blood transfusion with packed RBCs** is the method of choice for volume resuscitation in patients with severe GI hemorrhage.
  - All patients who are admitted for GIB should be typed and crossed, and cross-matched blood should be transfused when possible. In the case of catastrophic bleeding, however, O-negative units should be used without delay.
  - In the setting of acute upper GI bleeding, recent data clearly demonstrate the benefit of a restrictive approach when administering blood transfusions. The target hemoglobin is 7–9 g/dL with a threshold of <7 g/dL for administering PRBCs unless a patient continues to have ongoing clinical evidence of intravascular volume depletion or comorbidities such as coronary artery disease.[17,22] (Please also see Table 6-4.)
- Coagulopathy should be corrected with fresh frozen plasma in the unstable patient, but subcutaneous vitamin K (5–10 mg) can be used if the patient is hemodynamically stable. Heparin drips and other anticoagulants should be discontinued and protamine used for reversal, if necessary.
- If the patient is at risk for aspiration, consider endotracheal intubation to protect the airway prior to endoscopic intervention.

Medications

- **Nonvariceal UGIB**
  - **IV histamine-2 receptor antagonists.** These have not been shown to reduce surgery requirements or mortality rates. These agents are, therefore, **not recommended in the actively bleeding patient**.
  - **Proton pump inhibitors (PPIs).** PPIs have been found to **reduce rates of further bleeding, surgery, and deaths** caused by ulcer complications. The current standard of care is to administer IV PPIs either as intermittent bolus doses or as an infusion for the first 48–72 hours. High-dose (double-dose bid) oral PPI therapy is also of value and can be used when IV PPI is unavailable, or if clinical active bleeding has ceased. It is unclear whether PPI therapy affects mortality despite obvious benefits to morbidity from UGIB.[18]
    - **PPIs in prophylaxis of GIB in NSAID and ASA users.** Therapy should be tailored according to risk. American College of Gastroenterology practice guidelines recommend treatment according to risk stratification: low-, moderate-, and high-risk groups.
      - Included in this risk stratification are factors such as age >65, concurrent medications (ASA, high-dose NSAIDs, corticosteroids, or anticoagulants), history of ulcer(s), and *H. pylori* infection.
      - Low-risk patients, those without risk factors, should not receive prophylactic PPI therapy.
      - Conversely, PPIs are indicated in those patients at moderate (one to two risk factors) and high risk (more than two risk factors or history of ulcer complications) for peptic ulcer(s) and associated complications.[19]
    - **PPIs in prophylaxis of GIB in clopidogrel and ASA users:** A randomized, double-blinded, placebo-controlled trial found a significant reduction in UGIB in patients on dual therapy with clopidogrel and ASA who were randomized to

receive prophylactic omeprazole. Importantly, there was no significant increase in cardiovascular events or mortality with the use of combination clopidogrel and PPI in this study.[20]

- **Variceal UGIB**

  Vasoconstrictors. Several vasoconstricting agents are available and are uniformly effective in reducing variceal bleeding rates in the short term (Table 6-4). These agents produce splanchnic vasoconstriction and thus decrease portal blood inflow. Randomized controlled trials comparing different vasoconstrictor agents (vasopressin, somatostatin, terlipressin, octreotide, vapreotide), show no difference in control of hemorrhage and early rebleeding. Octreotide has the most favorable side effect profile and is therefore the agent of choice in the United States. The recommended dose is 50 µg IV bolus, followed by continuous infusion of 50 µg/hr for 3–5 days (Table 6-4).

  Antibiotic prophylaxis. It is recommended that all patients with cirrhosis and GIB receive antibiotic prophylaxis for 3–7 days to prevent development of spontaneous bacterial peritonitis. Regimens typically include ciprofloxacin or ceftriaxone.

Nonpharmacologic Therapies

- **Variceal UGIB**

  Endoscopic variceal ligation, which involves banding of the base of the varix, is the treatment of choice in acute variceal bleeding. Rubber bands are placed using a device attached through the instrument channel of the upper endoscope, which interrupt blood flow in the variceal column. This mode of therapy is used both for hemostasis in actively bleeding esophageal varices and for prophylaxis of variceal bleeding in patients with large varices. In the latter instance, repeat band ligation is performed every 4–8 weeks till all visible varices are obliterated, following which the patient is screened for recurrence every 6–12 months. Band ligation is easy to perform and is associated with lower complication rates than sclerotherapy, although rebleeding rates and mortality may not be different.[21]

  Sclerotherapy. This involves injection of a variety of sclerosing agents (ethanolamine oleate, sodium tetradecyl sulfate, polidocanol, morrhuate sodium, or ethanol) directly into the varix, achieves hemostasis in >90% of cases. Recurrent bleeding within 10 days occurs in up to 50% of patients, however, and side effects of therapy include fever, ulceration, strictures, perforation, acute respiratory distress syndrome, and sepsis. This form of therapy is currently limited to refractory bleeding, unavailability of endoscopic band ligation, or gastric varices where band ligation cannot be performed.

  Rescue management of variceal hemorrhage

  - **Balloon tamponade.** Balloon tamponade should be restricted to patients with uncontrollable bleeding for whom definitive therapy is planned within 24 hours. Either the Sengstaken–Blakemore tube or the Minnesota tube, both of which have gastric and esophageal balloons, can be used. In contrast, the Linton–Nachlas tube has only a large gastric balloon and can be considered for isolated gastric variceal bleeding. Hemostasis is achieved 70–90% of the time. Complications can be severe and include esophageal perforation, aspiration, chest pain, erosion, agitation, and death from asphyxiation from balloon migration with airway occlusion.

  - **Transjugular intrahepatic portosystemic shunt (TIPS).** This is reserved for patients with intractable variceal bleeding or if bleeding recurs after two or more unsuccessful endoscopic attempts at treatment of esophageal varices. TIPS creates a direct portosystemic shunt, thereby decreasing pressure within the portal system. Technical success is achieved >90% of the time, but complications include hepatic encephalopathy (in as many as 25% of patients), shunt stenosis, shunt thrombosis, and rebleeding. When TIPS is used in emergency situations, inhospital mortality is around 10%, and 30-day mortality rate as high as 40%. Contraindications for

TIPS include portal vein thrombosis, inferior vena cava obstruction, and polycystic liver disease.

- **Balloon-occluded retrograde transvenous obliteration (BRTO).** BRTO is a procedure for treatment of gastric varices associated with large gastro-/splenorenal collaterals. The technique involves retrograde cannulation of the left renal vein followed by balloon occlusion and slow infusion of sclerosant to obliterate the gastro-/splenorenal shunt supplying the gastric varix. This procedure should not be used in the presence of coinciding esophageal varices as it does not divert portal blood inflow and therefore may increase portal pressure leading to an increased bleeding risk.[6]

- **Surgical shunts.** These are rarely used because of the availability of TIPS procedures. Portacaval and distal splenorenal shunts achieve hemostasis 95% of the time but are associated with a high rate of postprocedural encephalopathy; mortality rates of 50–80% are reported, largely because of severe underlying liver disease. Surgical shunts are sometimes considered in noncirrhotic portal hypertension and patients with Child's A cirrhosis.[21]

- **Therapeutic upper endoscopy**
  - There are myriad techniques employed to achieve hemostasis and prevent recurrence of UGIB, namely, injection, ablative, and/or mechanical therapy (Table 6-5).[22] Use of a combination of any two of these methods, most commonly injection therapy followed by either ablative or mechanical therapy, has been associated with a dramatic reduction in the risk of ongoing and recurrent bleeding. Studies suggest a risk reduction from 80% to approximately 15% for an actively bleeding ulcer and from 50–10% for an ulcer with nonbleeding visible vessel.[23,24]

- **Therapeutic colonoscopy**
  - Endoscopic therapy is applied in 10–40% of patients undergoing colonoscopy, and immediate hemostasis is achieved in 50–100% of these cases.[9]
  - Endoscopic therapy options are similar to those used in upper endoscopy and include thermal coagulation (heater probe, bipolar or multipolar coagulation, argon plasma

TABLE 6-5 COMMON THERAPIES FOR UPPER GASTROINTESTINAL BLEEDING

Injection Therapy Action

Dilute epinephrine tamponade, vasospasm, thrombosis

Sclerosants tamponade and thrombosis

Ablative Therapy

Thermocoagulation—heater probe tissue ablation via direct compressive contact

Electrocoagulation—BICAP, Gold Probe™ tissue ablation via direct compressive contact

Argon plasma coagulation—noncontact tissue coagulation via argon gas

Mechanical Therapy

Hemoclips	Joins two sides of a vessel to occlude and arrest bleeding
Band ligation	Entrapment of a varix with a rubber band or elastic ring

Adapted from Cappell MS. Therapeutic endoscopy for acute upper gastrointestinal bleeding. *Nat Rev Gastroenterol Hepatol.* 2010;7:214–229.

coagulation), and injection of vasoconstrictors and sclerosants. Placement of metallic hemoclips has also been successful in the treatment of diverticular bleeding.

- **Angiotherapy**
  - When angiographic localization of bleeding is achieved, two modalities of therapy can be instituted directly into the bleeding vessel: vasopressin infusion and embolization. Vasopressin infusion is typically used in bleeding sources in the colon or small bowel, with the intent to induce vasospasm and, consequently, clotting and hemostasis. With superselective cannulation of the bleeding vessel, embolization with coils or Gelfoam can be highly successful in both UGIB and LGIB, with low risk of ischemic changes in the affected bowel segment.

Surgical Management

- The role of surgery is as a salvage therapy in the small group of patients in whom bleeding cannot be controlled with endoscopic therapy and/or angiotherapy. In both UGIB and LGIB, surgery should not be postponed excessively in the patient with persistent bleeding and hemodynamic instability because morbidity and mortality increase with delay.
- **Surgery for UGIB.** Surgery is indicated in patients in whom arterial bleeding cannot be controlled during initial endoscopy. However, in patients in whom bleeding recurs after initial endoscopic hemostasis, the management decision is more challenging and the data are conflicting. Some studies support a second endoscopic attempt at hemostasis, whereas others support immediate surgery or angiographic embolization. Surgical series have suggested that high-risk patients (ulcers ≥ 2 cm located at the lesser curvature or posterior duodenum, shock at presentation, and/or elderly with comorbidities) require aggressive postendoscopic management. Operative mortality following failed endoscopic therapy in some series has been as high as 25%. However, this varies with operator and institution experience in management of bleeding peptic ulcers.[25]
- **Surgery for LGIB.** Accurate preoperative localization of LGIB reduces postoperative rebleeding rates. Surgical mortality rates from recent series are 5–10%. For the difficult situation of recurrent massive bleeding without demonstration of a bleeding site, a subtotal colectomy may be indicated in patients with a good overall prognosis. When the patient is a high-risk surgical candidate, angiotherapy or a percutaneously or surgically placed portal-hepatic shunt for variceal bleeding can be considered as alternatives.[11,26]

SPECIAL CONSIDERATIONS

- **Prokinetics in UGIB.**
  - Pre-endoscopic administration of **IV erythromycin or metoclopramide** 20–120 minutes before EGD significantly reduces the need for a repeat EGD. These agents promote gastric emptying and thus administration can improve visualization by evacuation of stomach contents (blood, clot, fluid).[22]

REFERENCES

1. Zhao Y, Encinosa W. *Hospitalizations for gastrointestinal bleeding in 1998 and 2006: HCUP statistical brief #65.* http://www.hcup-es.ahrq.gov/reports/statbriefs/sb65.pdf. Accessed December 10, 2010.
2. Lanas A, Garcia-Rodriguez LA, Polo-Tomas M, et al. Time trends and impact of upper and lower gastrointestinal bleeding and perforation in clinical practice. *Am J Gastroenterol.* 2009;104:1633–1641.
3. Laine L. Upper gastrointestinal bleeding. *ASGE Clin Update.* 2007;14:1–4.
4. Laine L, Peterson WL. Bleeding peptic ulcer. *N Engl J Med.* 1994;331:717–727.
5. Garcia-Tsao G, Bosch J. Management of varices and variceal hemorrhage in cirrhosis. *N Engl J Med.* 2010;362:823–832.

6. Garcia-Tsao G, Abraldes JG, Berzigotti A, et al. Portal hypertensive bleeding in cirrhosis: risk stratification, diagnosis, and management: 2016 practice guidance by the American Association for the study of liver diseases. *Hepatology.* 2017;65:310–335.
7. Perini RF, Camara PR, Ferraz JG. Pathogenesis of portal hypertensive gastropathy: translating basic research into clinical practice. *Nat Clin Pract Gastroenterol Hepatol.* 2009;6:150–158.
8. Esrailian E, Gralnek I. Nonvariceal upper gastrointestinal bleeding: epidemiology and diagnosis. *Gastroenterol Clin North Am.* 2005;34:589–605.
9. Strate LL, Naumann CR. The role of colonoscopy and radiological procedures in the management of acute lower intestinal bleeding. *Clin Gastroenterol Hepatol.* 2010;8:333–343.
10. Strate LL. Lower GI bleeding: epidemiology and diagnosis. *Gastroenterol Clin North Am.* 2005;34:643–664.
11. Davila RE, Rajan E, Adler DG, et al. ASGE guideline: the role of endoscopy in the patient with lower-GI bleeding. *Gastrointest Endosc.* 2005;62:656–660.
12. Rockey DC. Gastrointestinal bleeding. *Gastroenterol Clin North Am.* 2005;34:581–588.
13. Bindewald H. Indikationen und treffsicherheit der rektoskopie. *MMW Much Med Wochenschr.* 1976;118:1271–1272.
14. Ahmad A, Bruno JM, Boynton R, et al. Nasogastric aspirates frequently lead to erroneous results and delay of therapy in patients with suspected UGI bleeding. *Gastrointest Endosc.* 2004;59:163.
15. Strate LL, Gralnek IM. ACG clinical guideline: management of patients with acute lower gastrointestinal bleeding. *Am J Gastroenterol.* 2016;111:459–474.
16. Enns RA, Hookey L, Armstrong D, et al. Clinical practice guidelines for the use of video capsule endoscopy. *Gastroenterology.* 2017;152:497–514.
17. Villanueva C, Colomo A, Bosch A. Transfusion strategies for acute upper gastrointestinal bleeding. *N Engl J Med.* 2013;368:11–21.
18. Leontiadis GI, Sharma VK, Howden CW. WITHDRAWN: proton pump inhibitor treatment for acute peptic ulcer bleeding. *Cochrane Database Syst Rev.* 2010;12(5):CD002094.
19. Lanza FL, Chan FKL, Quigley EM; Practice Parameters Committee of the American College of Gastroenterology. Guidelines for prevention of NSAID-related ulcer complications. *Am J Gastroenterol.* 2009;104:728–738.
20. Bhatt DL, Cryer BL, Contant CF, et al. Clopidogrel with or without omeprazole in coronary artery disease. *N Engl J Med.* 2010;363:1909–1917.
21. Garcia-Tsao G, Lim J. Members of the Veterans Affairs Hepatitis C Resource Center Program. Management and treatment of patients with cirrhosis and portal hypertension: recommendations from the Department of Veterans Affairs Hepatitis C Resource Center Program and the National Hepatitis C Program. *Am J Gastroenterol.* 2009;104:1802–1829.
22. Cappell MS. Therapeutic endoscopy for acute upper gastrointestinal bleeding. *Nat Rev Gastroenterol Hepatol.* 2010;7:214–229.
23. Laine L. Multipolar electrocoagulation in the treatment of active upper gastrointestinal tract hemorrhage: a prospective controlled trial. *N Engl J Med.* 1987;316:1613–1617.
24. Laine L. Multipolar electrocoagulation in the treatment of peptic ulcers with nonbleeding visible vessels: a prospective, controlled trial. *Ann Intern Med.* 1989;110:510–514.
25. Cheung FKY, Lau JYW. Management of massive peptic ulcer bleeding. *Gastroenterol Clin North Am.* 2009;38:231–243.
26. Green BT, Rockey DC. Lower gastrointestinal bleeding-management. *Gastroenterol Clin North Am.* 2005;34:665–678.

7

Obscure Gastrointestinal Bleeding

Chien-Huan Chen

GENERAL PRINCIPLES

- Persistent gastrointestinal (GI) bleeding with unsuccessful diagnosis on initial endoscopy ranks among the most common reasons for gastroenterology referral to a tertiary care center. It can often present challenges in management causing frustration to patients and physicians. In these cases, the pretest probability of diagnostic modalities and clinical significance of the most likely bleeding etiologies play a major role in determining the optimal course of action.
- The American College of Gastroenterology has published guidelines[1] recommending that a diagnosis of "suspected small bowel bleeding" be made in place of what was previously defined as an "obscure GI bleed." Furthermore, suspected small bowel bleeding now includes the unobserved or "occult GI bleed" as well.

Definition

- **Suspected small bowel bleeding** refers to GI bleeding that persists or recurs with no identifiable origin after initial upper and lower endoscopic evaluation.[1]
- **Obscure GI bleeding** consists of blood loss from the GI tract, the etiology of which remains elusive in spite of endoscopic and radiologic investigation of the entire gut including the small bowel.
- **Occult GI bleeding** is defined as anemia, usually with iron deficiency, accompanied by a positive test for blood in the stool to pinpoint the GI tract as the most likely source of blood loss.[2]
  - The term "obscure overt" defines obscure bleeding that is visible to the patient.
  - The term "obscure occult" defines occult bleeding that is undiagnosed following investigation of the GI system.

Etiologies

For patients with overt or occult bleeding and a negative upper and lower endoscopic evaluation, the majority of bleeding sources ultimately are detected in the small bowel.[3] Nonetheless, because missed lesions in the upper and lower GI tract remain frequent, the list of potential etiologies of suspected small bowel bleeding is exhaustive (see Table 7-1).[4,5]

DIAGNOSIS

Clinical Presentation

Patients presenting with suspected small bowel bleeding can present with a range of symptoms similar to those with upper and lower GI bleeding.

- Hematemesis reliably localizes bleeding proximal to the second portion of the duodenum while bright red blood per rectum indicates lower GI bleeding except in the instance of a massive GI bleed.[6]
- Other signs and symptoms, however, may carry questionable clinical utility. Regardless, a careful history and physical examination should be undertaken in each situation, and

TABLE 7-1 POTENTIAL SOURCES OF SUSPECTED SMALL BOWEL BLEEDING

Upper Gut
Esophagitis
Gastritis
  Helicobacter pylori gastritis
  Autoimmune gastritis
NSAID enteropathy
Peptic ulcer disease
Angiodysplasia
Gastric antral vascular ectasia
Dieulafoy lesion
Hemobilia
Hemosuccus pancreaticus
Sarcoidosis
Aortoenteric fistula
Neoplasia/Lymphoma

Small Bowel
Andiodysplasia
Crohn disease

Celiac disease
Meckel diverticulum
Neoplasia/Lymphoma
Ischemia
HIV-related causes
Bacterial infection

Colorectal
Colitis
  Ischemic colitis
  Infectious colitis
  Inflammatory bowel disease
Angiodysplasia
Diverticulosis
Neoplasia/Lymphoma
Endometriosis
Amyloidosis
Radiation proctopathy
Rectal ulcer

---

attention should be paid to the medical history to identify independent predictors for various bleeding etiologies.[4,7,8]

- Occult GI bleeding by definition carries no signs of overt bleeding and may be diagnosed incidentally or after the patient has presented with symptomatic anemia in the form of exertional fatigue, shortness of breath, or light-headedness.

- Because the degree of anemia can vary widely in the setting of occult GI bleeding, the primary goal in evaluation should be to rule out insidious causes such as celiac disease, inflammatory bowel disease, and GI neoplasia.

- For occult GI bleeding, evaluation should begin with confirmation of the gut as the source of bleed prior to proceeding to endoscopic evaluation in a fashion similar to that of obscure overt GI bleeding.

  Fecal occult blood tests (FOBTs), although useful for initial screening, may not always denote GI bleeding even if positive. False-positive results can occur because of diet, medications, or trauma while obtaining a sample. In fact, physiologic bleeding of up to 1.5 mL/day can occur in healthy patients.

  The commonly used FOBT tests are as follows[6,9]:

  - **Guaiac (hemoccult) tests** are widely available, simple, and inexpensive, but are qualitative tests and provide little quantitative information. Guaiac is a colorless compound obtained from tree bark that turns blue with peroxidase-like substances. This detects free circulating heme molecules or heme bound to its apoprotein (e.g., globin, myoglobin, and certain cytochromes). Heme degradation products that may form with more proximal (upper GI) bleeding are not detected. Because guaiac reacts with any peroxidase substance, the test can give false-positive results with red meats or blood-containing foods, as well as plant peroxidases such as that found in radish. Iron, however, does not cause false-positive results. Vitamin C can cause a false-negative result.

  - **Fecal immunochemical tests** (FIT) use antibodies against human hemoglobin. They do not react with free heme and thus, require no dietary restrictions before the test. Some of these tests may also provide quantitative information. Because these antibodies interact with the globin chain, they are only useful for colorectal bleeding, as globin from upper GI sources are degraded in the small bowel.

- For overt GI bleeding, the following studies are worth considering after the preceding upper and lower endoscopies have been nondiagnostic:

    Second-look endoscopy specific to the clinical presentation remains the next recommended step in the evaluation of suspected small bowel bleeding. Prior studies have demonstrated a 35–75% diagnostic yield for missed bleeding lesions in cases of repeat upper or lower endoscopy.[2,6,9-11] During any second-look colonoscopy, it is critical to examine the terminal ileum where blood, if found, can suggest a more proximal source in the small intestine. If repeat endoscopic studies give negative results, several other diagnostic modalities exist to help determine the source of bleeding.

    Push enteroscopy allows direct visual examination of the proximal small bowel, using a longer endoscope. Push enteroscopy involves advancing a pediatric colonoscope, which is longer than the typical upper endoscope, into the small bowel. This technique allows visualization of up to 50 cm of the small bowel beyond the ligament of Treitz and is increasingly performed instead of the standard second-look upper endoscopy.

    Deep enteroscopy evaluates more extensive portions of the small bowel and can be performed by a variety of techniques. By utilizing both the oral (antegrade) and anal (retrograde) approaches, deep enteroscopy may allow evaluation of the entire small bowel. In addition to its expanded diagnostic ability, deep enteroscopy also allows for interventions such as hemostasis, biopsy, polypectomy, and dilation.[12,13] Lesions identified on endoscopy that are not amenable to conventional endoscopic therapies can also be marked using mucosal tattoos or hemoclips near the bleeding source. Such localization often significantly facilitates any radiologic or surgical attempts at hemostasis to follow.

    - **Single-balloon enteroscopy (SBE)** and **double-balloon enteroscopy (DBE)**[12] utilize an enteroscope with a balloon attached toward the distal end of an overtube, but DBE adds a second balloon at the tip of the enteroscope itself. Patients with latex allergy should receive SBE because balloons of DBE are made of latex. The balloon system serves as an anchor by gripping on to the intestinal wall to allow further advancement of the endoscope.

    - **Spiral enteroscopy** uses an enteroscope through an overtube with a soft-raised helix at its distal end. Spiral enteroscopy requires two operators to perform.[14]

    Video capsule endoscopy (VCE) has become the standard for initial examination of the small bowel once second-look endoscopy has returned without a diagnosis.

    - VCE involves ingestion of a capsule containing a small camera that sends images to a recorder worn on the patient's belt. Images are typically recorded at a rate of two to six frames per second, although newer models can surpass this.[5,10,15,16]

    - Because VCE is noninvasive and can examine the entire small intestine, VCE is frequently used before deep enteroscopy to guide further intervention.

    - Unfortunately, VCE has no therapeutic capability, provides no real-time data, demonstrates limited visualization of the duodenum and proximal jejunum, and can miss small bowel masses.[17,18] Given these limitations, VCE should be in concert with other modalities including enteroscopy and CT enterography (CTE; see below) given the context of the clinical presentation.

    - Of note, VCE studies can be incomplete if the cecum is not traversed within the battery life of the capsule (typically 8–12 hours). Capsule retention, particularly in patients with strictures or diverticuli, remains the major risk at 0–2% in the general population and 4–8% for patients with suspected or established inflammatory bowel disease.[19] Retained capsules can often be retrieved by deep enteroscopy, and surgical extraction is seldom required.[5,7]

Tagged red blood cell nuclear scans, formally described as technetium 99m–labeled erythrocyte scans, can help identify the origin of obscure bleeding when other modalities fail to reveal a source.

- The test, however, must be performed during episodes of active bleeding at a rate exceeding 0.1–0.4 mL/min. This often restricts its use to the setting of brisk GI bleeding as the first next test of choice following a negative upper endoscopy and before the patient can safely receive a bowel preparation to allow for colonoscopy.
- False localization of bleeding sites is a well-known limitation of this procedure.
- A specific scan with technetium 99m pertechnetate, termed **Meckel scan**, which has an affinity for ectopic gastric mucosa can be used to identify the presence of Meckel diverticulum, one of the causes of small bowel bleeding in younger patients. This compound is taken up by heterotrophic gastric mucosa within the Meckel diverticulum and can be found on a radionuclide scan.

Computed tomography angiography (CTA) represents an alternative to the tagged red blood cell scan, usually in the setting of brisk GI bleeding. Institutional preference may dictate which of the two is recommended by radiology prior to selective angiography.

- As a noninvasive test, CTA can be rapidly deployed, and has higher specificity than a tagged red blood cell scan for site of bleeding when positive. On the other hand, it requires an active bleed of at least 0.3 mL/min. Care should be taken to evaluate for contrast allergies or renal insufficiency.
- Highly vascular lesions such as angiodysplasias and neoplasms can sometimes be identified during angiography by demonstrating typical vascular patterns, even if active bleeding is not manifest.

Selective angiography and embolization is the invasive, therapeutic correlate to radiologic evaluation for GI bleeding, usually of the brisk variety requiring bleeding of 0.5–1.0 mL/min for detection. Patients who receive this intervention must be clinically stable enough to tolerate conscious sedation just as they would for an endoscopic procedure, and such cases almost always proceed from a positive tagged red cell scan or CTA. Once a culprit vessel with intraluminal extravasation of contrast is identified, therapeutic interventions can be attempted. Depending on the extent of embolization performed, bowel ischemia is the primary adverse effect against which hemostasis must be weighed.

CT enterography (CTE) has been proposed as a potential alternative to VCE following negative endoscopic evaluation.[20] It employs traditional CT techniques with additional mucosal enhancement via ingestion of a nonabsorbable contrast dye, typically 1 hour prior to the procedure. Performed in multiple phases (arterial, enteric, and delayed) based on the timing of intravenous contrast administration, CTE may detect not only small bowel masses but also vascular lesions as potential sources of obscure bleeding.[21] Of the limited comparison studies available, however, CTE demonstrated an overall decreased diagnostic yield relative to VCE.[22,23] We propose considering CTE when the suspicion for mass lesions is suitably high.

Intraoperative enteroscopy has largely been overtaken by less invasive means of small bowel investigation for recurrent GI bleeding. In certain refractory situations, however, it may yet have utility as the most accurate study for identifying suspected bleeding sources over the full extent of small bowel. This is also used in situations where the intended therapy for hemostasis is surgical resection of the bleeding source. The risks of continued bleeding should also be carefully evaluated and must outweigh the surgical risks of laparotomy.[24]

TREATMENT

Treatment of small bowel bleeding should be directed at the primary disorder leading to the bleeding.[5,7] The treatment modalities generally fall into four main categories:

- **Endoscopic therapy**
  - The basis for endoscopic therapy of small bowel bleeding is accurate identification of the bleeding source. Upper endoscopy and colonoscopy represent the initial screening tests of choice with push enteroscopy reserved for the second-look endoscopy. The time-consuming deep enteroscopies are typically employed following a positive diagnosis made by capsule endoscopy or other radiologic procedure, although enteroscopy is indicated in spite of negative prior studies if clinical suspicion is high.
  - Endoscopic techniques utilized include epinephrine injection, thermal therapy with a heater probe, bipolar cautery, argon plasma coagulation, endoscopic mucosal resection, and band ligation depending on the lesion identified.
- **Angiographic therapy**
  - Infusion of vasopressin into the bleeding vessel can induce spasm and allow hemostasis. This is possible when the bleeding lesion is identified on angiography. Alternatively, Gelfoam or coils can be used to embolize and occlude the bleeding vessel. The risk of ischemic changes in the affected bowel segment is greatly reduced with superselective catheterization of bleeding vessels.
- **Pharmacologic therapy**
  - Depending on the lesion identified, simple measures may include acid suppression, avoidance of NSAIDs, and careful downtitration of anticoagulation medications in patients who must receive them. Misoprostol can sometimes be used for mucosal protection in patients requiring NSAID therapy—there is some evidence that misoprostol may provide mucosal protection extending into the small bowel, whereas proton pump inhibitors provide benefit that is limited to the gastroduodenum under similar circumstances.[7,25]
  - If extensive evaluation fails to yield a diagnosis, generalized supportive care including periodic iron supplementation, optimization of coagulation status, and transfusions, if necessary, should be continued.
- **Surgery**
  - Depending on the lesion identified, surgical resection may sometimes be necessary, especially with stromal tumors and other neoplastic lesions. Rapid bleeding isolated to a limited bowel segment may require intraoperative endoscopy for precise localization; some of these procedures are followed by resection of the bleeding segment.

ANGIODYSPLASTIC LESIONS

- Angiodysplastic lesions are frequent causes of suspected small bowel bleeding and can be notoriously difficult to manage, with bleeding recurrence rates of 30–40% with or without endoscopic identification and treatment of an actively bleeding lesion.[21,26]
- There is a high prevalence of concurrent lesions (40–60%)[27] undetected during the index episode of bleeding. Persisting underlying pathophysiology predisposes the patient to the future formation of lesions, but the pathophysiology is not well defined.
- Comorbidities highly associated with angiodysplastic lesions are listed in Table 7-2.
- A current theory is that mechanical shearing of large von Willebrand multimers results in a state of acquired von Willebrand disease which then produces bleeding from angiodysplastic lesions which may have otherwise resolved spontaneously without event.[28] A contributing theory is that angiodysplastic lesions, as dilated and dysplastic thin-walled blood vessels at the surface of the submucosa, may be predisposed to formation through chronic low-grade venous obstruction and increased tension in the ectatic vessel wall.[29]

TABLE 7-2 CONDITIONS ASSOCIATED WITH BLEEDING ANGIODYSPLASTIC LESIONS AND PROPOSED UNDERLYING MECHANISMS

Clinical Conditions
Age >60-yr old
Von Willebrand disease
End-stage renal disease
Aortic stenosis
Cardiac valve replacement
Left ventricular assist device placement

Potential Mechanisms
Acquired von Willebrand syndrome
Chronic low-grade venous obstruction
Uremic platelet dysfunction
Use of antiplatelet or anticoagulant medication

- Bleeding angiodysplastic lesions may be identified in any portion of the GI tract and produce symptoms relative to the location in which bleeding arises. Initial management should follow protocols for upper, lower, or suspected small bowel bleeding until angiodysplastic lesions are diagnosed. Angiodysplastic lesions cannot be presumed until they are found on imaging or endoscopy, as even patients predisposed to this condition, such as those with left ventricular assist device placement have been found to have bleeding due to peptic ulcer disease at an equal frequency.[30]

- When identified in the setting of GI bleeding, obscure, or occult, an initial attempt at endoscopic treatment should be undertaken with the technique most likely to be able to access the site of bleed.

- When angiodysplastic lesions are diagnosed on VCA, CTA, or CTE but are not identified on subsequent endoscopy, the initial approach is to maintain a stable blood count with intermittent transfusions, discontinue all anticoagulant and antiplatelet agents when possible, and replete iron, either orally or parenterally. Although recurrent bleeding rates are high, index bleeds which go untreated often resolve spontaneously with supportive care alone.

- Incidentally observed angiodysplasia in nonbleeding settings are not treated because such lesions are frequently found in patients without anemia undergoing endoscopy for other purposes and may never be symptomatic.[31]

- Refractory recurrent bleeding requiring frequent hospitalization and high utilization of healthcare resources is a rare but known complication of angiodysplasia-related GI bleeding. In this context, some pharmacologic interventions are worth considering but remain outside of the standard of care due to a lack of data supporting their use. Previous enthusiasm for hormonal therapies was proven unfounded in a large clinical trial and is no longer considered an option in management of recurrent GI bleeding.[26]

  - **Octreotide** can be administered as a long-acting release intramuscular injection just prior to discharge following an admission for recurrent GI bleeding. Although the effects of this medication are thought to last only 90 days, published studies have demonstrated significant declines in the rebleeding rate and transfusion requirements over the subsequent year. Of note, none of these studies included placebo comparison arms, and only two employed external or historical control groups.[32,33]

  - **Thalidomide** is a vascular endothelial growth factor inhibitor used primarily in the treatment of multiple myeloma. Because of its antiangiogenic properties, interest has grown of late for its utility in angiodysplasia-related bleeding. An initial case series showed dramatic improvement in patients who remained on the medication, and this was confirmed by a randomized controlled trial demonstrating 71% rate of resolution of rebleeding for patients who remained on the medication versus 4% who received the iron supplementation placebo.[34,35] The primary question surrounding thalidomide is not one of efficacy but rather tolerability. Seventy percent of patients in the large trial reported significant adverse symptoms including fatigue, somnolence, peripheral edema, abdominal pain, constipation, and in rarer instances leukopenia or thrombocytopenia. Due to the notorious teratogenicity of thalidomide, all patients who are placed on the medication must have pregnancy ruled out and remain on birth control for the duration of therapy. Interest in newer agents with similar antiangiogenic properties but improved tolerance profiles is ongoing.

REFERENCES

1. Gerson LB, Fidler JL, Cave DR, et al. ACG clinical guideline: diagnosis and management of small bowel bleeding. *Am J Gastroenterol.* 2015;110(9):1265–1287.
2. Concha R, Amaro R, Barkin JS. Obscure gastrointestinal bleeding: diagnostic and therapeutic approach. *J Clin Gastroenterol.* 2007;41(3):242–251.
3. Tee HP, Kaffes AJ. Non-small-bowel lesions encountered during double-balloon enteroscopy performed for obscure gastrointestinal bleeding. *World J Gastroenterol.* 2010;16(15):1185–1189.
4. Raju GS, Gerson L, Das A, et al. American Gastroenterological Association (AGA) Institute medical position on obscure gastrointestinal bleeding. *Gastroenterology.* 2007;133:1694–1696.
5. Pasha AF, Hara AK, Leighton JA. Diagnostic evaluation and management of obscure gastrointestinal bleeding: a changing paradigm. *Gastroenterol Hepatol (NY).* 2009;5(12):839–850.
6. Zuckerman GR, Prakash C, Askin M, et al. AGA medical position statement: evaluation and management of occult and obscure gastrointestinal bleeding. *Gastroenterology.* 2000;118(1):197–201.
7. ASGE Standards of Practice Committee; Fisher L, Lee Krinsky M, Anderson MA, et al. The role of endoscopy in the management of obscure GI bleeding. *Gastrointest Endosc.* 2010;72(3):471–479.
8. Lepere C, Cuillerier E, Van Gossum A, et al. Predictive factors of positive findings in patients explored by push enteroscopy for unexplained GI bleeding. *Gastrointest Endosc.* 2005;61(6):709–714.
9. Rockey DC, Koch J, Cello JP, et al. Relative frequency of upper gastrointestinal and colonic lesions in patients with positive fecal occult blood tests. *N Engl J Med.* 1998;339(3):153–159.
10. Adler DG, Knipshield M, Gostout C. A prospective comparison of capsule endoscopy and push enteroscopy in patients with GI bleeding of obscure origin. *Gastrointest Endosc.* 2004;59(4):492–498.
11. Gerson LB. Small bowel bleeding: updated algorithm and outcomes. *Gastrointest Endosc Clin N Am.* 2017;27(1):171–180.
12. Gerson LB, Flodin JT, Miyabayashi K. Balloon-assisted enteroscopy: technology and troubleshooting. *Gastrointest Endosc.* 2008;68(6):1158–1167.
13. Bresci G. Occult and obscure gastrointestinal bleeding: causes and diagnostic approach in 2009. *World J Gastrointest Endosc.* 2009;1(1):3–6.
14. Rockey DC, Cello JP. Evaluation of the gastrointestinal tract in patients with iron deficiency anemia. *N Engl J Med.* 1993;329(23):1691–1695.
15. Fireman Z. Capsule endoscopy: future horizons. *World J Gastrointest Endosc.* 2010;2(9):305–307.
16. Leighton JA. The role of endoscopic imaging of the small bowel in clinical practice. *Am J Gastroenterol.* 2011;106(1):27–36.
17. Huprich JE, Fletcher JG, McCollough CH, et al. Prospective blinded comparison of wireless capsule endoscopy and multiphase CT enterography in obscure gastrointestinal bleeding. *Radiology.* 2011;260(3):744–751.
18. Clarke JO, Giday SA, Mullin GE, et al. How good is capsule endoscopy for detection of periampullary lesions? Results of a tertiary referral center. *Gastrointest Endosc.* 2008;68(2):267–272.
19. Rezapour M, Amadi C, Gerson LB. Retention associated with video capsule endoscopy: systematic review and meta-analysis. *Gastrointest Endosc.* 2017;85(6):1157–1168.e2.
20. Lee SS, Oh TS, Ha HK, et al. Obscure gastrointestinal bleeding: diagnostic performance of multidetector CT enterography. *Radiology.* 2011;259(3):739–748.
21. Huprich JE, Barlow JM, Hansel SL, et al. Multiphase CT enterography evaluation of small-bowel vascular lesions. *AJR Am J Roentgenol.* 2013;201(1):65–72.
22. Wang Z, Chen JQ, Huang Y, et al. CT enterography in obscure gastrointestinal bleeding: a systematic review and meta-analysis. *J Med Imaging Radiat Oncol.* 2013;57(3):263–273.

23. He B, Gong S, Ji Y. Obscure gastrointestinal bleeding: diagnostic performance of 64-section multiphase CT enterography and CT angiography compared with capsule endoscopy. *Br J Radiol.* 2014;87(1043):20140229.

24. Somsouk M, Gralnek IM, Inadomi JM. Managements of obscure occult gastrointestinal bleeding: a cost-minimization analysis. *Clin Gastroenterol Hepatol.* 2008;6(3):661–670.

25. Fujimori S, Seo T, Sakamoto C, et al. Prevention of nonsteroidal anti-inflammatory drug-induced small-intestinal injury by prostaglandin: a pilot randomized controlled trial evaluated by capsule endoscopy. *Gastrointest Endosc.* 2009;69(7):1339–1346.

26. Junquera F, Feu F, Papo M, et al. A multicenter, randomized, clinical trial of hormonal therapy in the prevention of rebleeding from gastrointestinal angiodysplasia. *Gastroenterology.* 2001;121(5):1073–1079. (Used to show conservative management results in spontaneous cessation of bleeding 30–40% of the time.)

27. Clouse RE, Costigan DJ, Mills BA, et al. Angiodysplasia as a cause of upper gastrointestinal bleeding. *Arch Intern Med.* 1985;145(3):458–461.

28. Vincentelli A, Susen S, Jude B, et al. Acquired von Willebrand syndrome in aortic stenosis. *N Engl J Med.* 2003;349(4):343–349.

29. Boley SJ, Sammartano R, Sprayregen S, et al. Degenerative lesions of aging. *Gastroenterology.* 1977;72(4 Pt 1):650–660.

30. Kushnir VM, Sharma S, Gyawali CP, et al. Evaluation of GI bleeding after implantation of left ventricular assist device. *Gastrointest Endosc.* 2012;75(5):973–979.

31. Pasha SF, Leighton JA, Das A, et al. American Gastroenterological Association (AGA) Institute technical review on obscure gastrointestinal bleeding. *Gastroenterology.* 2007;133(5):1697–1717.

32. Junquera F, Sapreras E, Videla S, et al. Long-term efficacy of octreotide in the prevention of recurrent bleeding from gastrointestinal angiodysplasia. *Am J Gastroenterol.* 2007;102(2):254–260.

33. Shah KB, Gunda S, Smallfield GB, et al. Multicenter evaluation of octreotide as secondary prophylaxis in patients with left ventricular assist devices and gastrointestinal bleeding. *Circ Heart Fail.* 2017;10(11):e004500.

34. Kamalaporn P, Saravanan R, Cirocco M, et al. Thalidomide for the treatment of chronic gastrointestinal bleeding from angiodysplasias: a case series. *Eur J Gastroenterol Hepatol.* 2009;21(12):1347–1350.

35. Ge ZZ, Chen HM, Gao YJ, et al. Efficacy of thalidomide for refractory gastrointestinal bleeding from vascular malformation. *Gastroenterology.* 2011;141(5):1629–1637.

Jaundice

Surachai Amornsawadwattana

8

GENERAL PRINCIPLES

Jaundice is a common condition encountered in both inpatient and outpatient settings, with a broad spectrum of causes, ranging from benign to life threatening. An in-depth understanding of the presentation and pathophysiology of jaundice is essential for appropriate investigation and accurate diagnosis.

Definition

- Jaundice is defined as a yellow discoloration of skin, sclera, and mucous membranes caused by accumulation of bilirubin, a by-product of heme metabolism.
- The upper limit of normal for total serum bilirubin is 1.0–1.5 mg/dL, of which conjugated bilirubin constitutes <0.3 mg/dL.[1] Hyperbilirubinemia (total serum bilirubin >1.5 mg/dL) may be present without overt jaundice, but it nevertheless represents an abnormal condition.
- Jaundice typically becomes apparent when the serum total bilirubin concentration reaches 2.5–3.0 mg/dL. Increased bilirubin levels may be caused by a defect at any site along the bilirubin metabolic pathway, from increased bilirubin production, decreased bilirubin clearance, or a combination of factors.[1]

Classification

There are two approaches to the classification of jaundice.
- Jaundice can be classified according to location of the defect in the bilirubin pathway as prehepatic, intrahepatic, or posthepatic.
    - *Prehepatic* jaundice may be due to overproduction of bilirubin.
    - *Intrahepatic* jaundice can be caused by abnormalities in bilirubin transport, conjugation, or excretion.
    - *Posthepatic* jaundice is due to biliary obstruction.
- Jaundice can also be classified by the predominant type of bilirubin in the blood as primarily unconjugated bilirubin, conjugated bilirubin, or both.[2,3]
    - *Unconjugated bilirubin* is mostly water insoluble, and reversibly binds to albumin in the blood. Unconjugated hyperbilirubinemia may be due to bilirubin overproduction, impaired uptake, decreased storage, or abnormal bilirubin conjugation.
    - *Conjugated bilirubin* is conjugated with glucuronic acid, becomes water soluble, and is subsequently excreted in the stool and urine.
        - The half-life of conjugated bilirubin bound to albumin is approximately 17 days, thus explaining the slow recovery from jaundice even after resolution of the illness.
        - Conjugated hyperbilirubinemia may be due to decreased bilirubin excretion, hepatocyte dysfunction, or biliary obstruction.
    - *Combination hyperbilirubinemia* can also be seen in hepatocellular disease, biliary obstruction, and decreased canalicular excretion.

Etiology

- **Unconjugated hyperbilirubinemia**
  - **Bilirubin overproduction**
    - **Hemolysis** and **ineffective erythropoiesis** are seen with sickle cell anemia, thalassemia, G6PD deficiency, pyruvate kinase deficiency, malaria, ABO blood group mismatch, and lead toxicity.
      - Bilirubin is usually <3–5 mg/dL, and overt jaundice is uncommon in the absence of severe hemolysis or concomitant liver disease.
      - Hemolysis can be evaluated with measurement of lactate dehydrogenase (LDH), haptoglobin, reticulocyte count, and a peripheral smear.
    - Resorption of **large hematomas** results in bilirubin overproduction and subsequent unconjugated hyperbilirubinemia.
  - **Impaired hepatic bilirubin uptake**
    - **Decreased hepatic blood flow** can result in impaired hepatic bilirubin uptake and is caused by cirrhosis, portocaval shunts, or congestive heart failure.
    - **Drugs** that can cause impaired bilirubin uptake include rifampin, probenecid, sulfonamides, aspirin, nonsteroidal anti-inflammatory drugs, and contrast dye.
  - **Impaired conjugation of bilirubin**
    - Inherited uridine diphosphate glucuronyl transferase (UGT) deficiencies include Gilbert syndrome and Crigler–Najjar syndrome.
      - **Gilbert syndrome** affects 3–7% of the US population,[3] predominantly men, and presents with intermittent jaundice often precipitated by illness, stress, fatigue, or fasting. It is the most common cause of unconjugated hyperbilirubinemia and is benign with no deleterious long-term consequences.
      - **Crigler–Najjar** syndrome is less common and can be of two types: type I with complete deficiency of UGT-1A1 and type II with partial inactivation of the enzyme.
    - **Neonatal jaundice** can be due to physiologic jaundice from an initial relatively low activity of UGT and is usually seen between 5 and 14 days in full-term infants.
      - On the other hand, **breast milk jaundice** is seen later in life and is due to an inhibitor of UGT activity in breast milk.
      - Unconjugated hyperbilirubinemia in newborns can also be caused by ABO incompatibility, G6PD deficiency, hypothyroidism, and so forth.
      - Newborns with severe elevations of unconjugated bilirubin are often treated to prevent kernicterus, which manifests as hypotonia, lethargy, and seizures.
- **Conjugated hyperbilirubinemia**
  - **Intrahepatic cholestasis**
    - **Hepatitis** including alcoholic hepatitis, hepatitis B, hepatitis C, Epstein–Barr virus, and Cytomegalovirus can present with cholestatic hepatitis.
    - **Primary biliary cholangitis (primary biliary cirrhosis)** is an autoimmune liver disease commonly seen in middle-aged women. Antimitochondrial antibody is usually positive.
    - **Primary sclerosing cholangitis (PSC)** is a chronic liver disease with scarring of the bile ducts ("beads on a string" appearance) and is commonly associated with inflammatory bowel disease.
    - **Postoperative cholestasis** may have many causes including hemolysis, ischemia, anesthetics, and so forth.
    - **Total parenteral nutrition (TPN)** can cause intrahepatic as well as extrahepatic cholestasis from gallstones formation.[4]
    - **Cholestasis of pregnancy** may be due to morbid pregnancy-related conditions such as HELLP syndrome (hemolysis, elevated liver enzymes, and low platelet count) and acute fatty liver of pregnancy or the more common, but benign, intrahepatic cholestasis of pregnancy (the cause of 30–50% of jaundice in pregnancy).

- *Infiltrative disorders:* granulomatous disease (sarcoidosis, lymphoma, mycobacterial infection, granulomatosis with polyangiitis [Wegener granulomatosis]), amyloidosis, and malignancy (paraneoplastic syndrome: renal cell carcinoma).
- *Infections* such as bacterial, sepsis, fungal, or parasitic.
- *Vascular* causes such as hepatic vein thrombosis (Budd–Chiari syndrome) or shock liver.
- *Stem cell transplant related* such as sinusoidal obstruction syndrome (veno-occlusive disease), graft-versus-host disease, or chemotherapy-induced hepatitis.
- *Drugs* that cause a predominantly cholestatic picture (elevated alkaline phosphatase [AP] and total bilirubin) include anabolic steroids, oral contraceptives, estrogens, amoxicillin–clavulanic acid, chlorpromazine, clopidogrel, erythromycin, irbesartan, mirtazapine, phenothiazines, terbinafine, and tricyclics.

Extrahepatic cholestasis
- *Choledocholithiasis* which is the presence of gallstones in the common bile duct (CBD).
- *PSC* can also have dominant extrahepatic biliary strictures.
- *AIDS cholangiopathy* has an appearance similar to PSC, presents with elevated AP, and is caused by opportunistic infections of the biliary tree.
- *Malignancy* such as hepatocellular carcinoma (manifest as intraluminal with tumor thrombus or fragments, extraluminal tumor, or hemobilia), cholangiocarcinoma, pancreatic cancer, and ampullary tumors.[5]
- *Pancreatitis* (acute, chronic, or autoimmune) can be associated with cholestasis.
- *Mirizzi syndrome* caused by gallstones compressing the common hepatic duct.
- *Postsurgical strictures* may cause obstruction resulting in extrahepatic cholestasis.
- *Choledochal cystic disorders* including Caroli disease and choledochal cysts.
- *Vascular enlargement* from aneurysms or portal cavernoma.
- **Congenital and familial causes of cholestasis:** Rotor syndrome; Dubin Johnson syndrome; progressive familial intrahepatic cholestasis: PFIC-1 (Byler disease), PFIC-2 (BSEP mutation), and PFIC-3 (MDR-3 mutation); benign recurrent intrahepatic cholestasis (BRIC).

- **Mixed conjugated and unconjugated hyperbilirubinemia**
  - A mixed pattern of hyperbilirubinemia may be seen in hepatocellular disorders. A combination of unconjugated hyperbilirubinemia and parenchymal liver disease can also result in a mixed pattern of hyperbilirubinemia.
  - **Hepatocellular disorders:** Viral hepatitis, alcoholic liver disease, Wilson disease, Reye syndrome, hemochromatosis, autoimmune hepatitis, α_1-antitrypsin deficiency, celiac sprue, nonalcoholic steatohepatitis, pregnancy related (acute fatty liver of pregnancy and preeclampsia).
  - **Drugs:** Amoxicillin–clavulanic acid, anabolic steroids, azathioprine, carbamazepine, clindamycin, enalapril, erythromycin, nitrofurantoin, phenytoin, sulfonamides, trazodone, verapamil.[6]

Pathophysiology

- Bilirubin is the end product of degradation of the heme moiety of hemoproteins, including hemoglobin; please see Figure 8-1.
  - Hemoglobin from senescent red blood cells accounts for 80–90% of the daily bilirubin production, with the remainder coming from ineffective erythropoiesis and degradation of heme-containing proteins (cytochrome P450, peroxidase, and catalase).
  - Normal daily bilirubin production averages 4 mg/kg of body weight (approximately 300 mg). The reticuloendothelial system has the capacity to metabolize up to 1500 mg daily, so hemolysis rarely causes jaundice by itself, unless this ceiling is exceeded or the hemolysis is associated with liver disease.

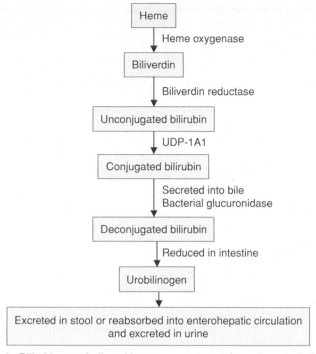

Figure 8-1. Bilirubin metabolism. Heme oxygenase catalyzes the rate-limiting step within the reticuloendothelial system. Unconjugated bilirubin is transported bound primarily to albumin, at which point it is taken up by the hepatocyte and undergoes glucuronidation by uridine diphosphate glucuronyl transferase (UGT-1A1). It is then secreted in the water-soluble conjugated form into the canaliculi (70–90% diglucuronide and 5–25% monoglucuronide). Within the intestine, it is deconjugated and reduced by bacterial β-glucuronide to urobilinogen, which is either excreted in stool or reabsorbed into the enterohepatic circulation. A defect at or before glucuronidation results in primarily unconjugated hyperbilirubinemia, whereas problems after this step cause conjugated hyperbilirubinemia.

- Unconjugated or indirect hyperbilirubinemia is present when >80–85% of the total bilirubin is unconjugated. Defects proximal to, and including, the conjugation step result in primarily unconjugated hyperbilirubinemia. Defects after the glucuronidation step within the hepatocyte result in primarily conjugated hyperbilirubinemia. Conjugated or direct hyperbilirubinemia is present when >30% of the total bilirubin is in the conjugated form.

DIAGNOSIS

The history, physical examination, and initial laboratory evaluation should be directed at answering the following questions:
- Is the process acute or chronic?
- Is the hyperbilirubinemia unconjugated, conjugated, or mixed?

- If there is unconjugated hyperbilirubinemia, is it caused by increased production, decreased uptake, or impaired conjugation?
- If there is conjugated hyperbilirubinemia, is it caused by intrahepatic or extrahepatic cholestasis?

Clinical Presentation

History

A detailed history is important for developing a differential diagnosis and identifying the cause of the patient's jaundice. Factors that can provide clues to the diagnosis include the following[7]:

- **Age:** Patients younger than 30 years are more likely to have acute parenchymal disease, including acute viral hepatitis, biliary tract disease, alcoholic liver disease, and autoimmune hepatitis, whereas those older than 65 years are more likely to have gallstones, malignancy, or drug-induced hepatotoxicity in the setting of polypharmacy. Autoimmune disease can have a second peak in the elderly.
- **Gender:** In male patients, consider alcohol, pancreatic cancer, hepatocellular carcinoma, and hemochromatosis. In female patients, gallstones, primary biliary cholangitis, and autoimmune hepatitis are more common.
- **Acute versus chronic** jaundice can be differentiated by a thorough history, physical examination, and laboratory tests. Xanthelasma, spider angioma, presence of ascites, and hepatosplenomegaly are indicative of a chronic process. Similarly, hypoalbuminemia, thrombocytopenia, and prolonged prothrombin time (PT) are mostly seen in the setting of chronic jaundice.[7] Fever, chills, right upper quadrant abdominal pain, leukocytosis, and hypotension are not only indicative of an acute cause, but suggest ascending cholangitis and require urgent intervention. Asterixis, confusion, or stupor could represent fulminant hepatic failure and require immediate therapy.
- Patients with **viral hepatitis** often give a history of a viral prodrome, including anorexia, malaise, and myalgia. Infectious sexual exposures, intravenous drug use, and prior blood transfusions also support a diagnosis of viral hepatitis. Essential are a careful travel history and human immunodeficiency virus status, as well as alcohol and drug history, including over-the-counter and herbal remedies, because a multitude of drugs can cause jaundice by diverse mechanisms, including hemolysis, hepatocellular damage, and cholestasis.
- **Pruritus** suggests a longer duration of disease and can be seen in both intrahepatic cholestasis and biliary obstruction. Increased urine urobilinogen may represent increased bilirubin production and subsequent enterohepatic circulation or decreased hepatic clearance of urobilinogen and, therefore, does not distinguish between hemolysis and liver disease. In the presence of cholestasis, however, conjugated bilirubin is filtered in the urine. Bilirubin in the urine is a definitive indicator of conjugated hyperbilirubinemia. Abdominal pain with radiation to the back can suggest pancreatic disease, whereas a right upper quadrant aching pain is frequently seen in patients with viral hepatitis.

Physical Examination

The physical examination can reveal evidence of chronic liver disease and may also provide evidence of less common forms of liver disease.

- **Chronic liver disease** is manifested by muscle wasting, cachexia, palmar erythema, Dupuytren contracture, parotid enlargement, leukonychia, gynecomastia, and testicular atrophy.[7]
- **Cirrhosis** is suggested by the findings of spider angiomata, palmar erythema, and caput medusae (or dilated veins).
- **Liver size and consistency** should also be evaluated. A shrunken and nodular liver would suggest cirrhosis, whereas a palpable mass can be indicative of a malignancy or

an abscess. An enlarged liver with a span of >15 cm may be seen in nonalcoholic fatty liver disease, infiltrative disease, or congestive hepatopathy.

- **Ascites** is typically seen in advanced cirrhosis but may also be seen with severe viral and alcoholic hepatitis. The presence of ascites usually indicates an evidence of portal hypertension.
- **Asterixis** is usually indicated the sign of hepatic encephalopathy.
- Other useful findings include hyperpigmentation (**hemochromatosis**), xanthomas (**primary biliary cholangitis**), and Kayser–Fleischer rings (**Wilson disease**).

Diagnostic Testing
Laboratory Testing

- Essential initial laboratory tests should include levels of direct and indirect bilirubin, transaminases (aspartate aminotransferase and alanine aminotransferase), AP, total protein, albumin, and PT. If available, results of prior liver biochemical test are essential to evaluate the trend of changes.
- If laboratory results are consistent with **unconjugated hyperbilirubinemia**, a hemolysis workup should be initiated (reticulocyte count, LDH, haptoglobin, Coombs test, and peripheral smear). In the absence of hemolysis, most asymptomatic healthy patients with isolated unconjugated hyperbilirubinemia have Gilbert disease and require no further evaluation.[1]
- If laboratory results demonstrate **conjugated hyperbilirubinemia** or are indeterminate, then additional workup is required.
  - Patients with transaminases elevated out of proportion to the AP most likely have a hepatocellular disorder. Levels of transaminases <300 IU/mL are seen in alcoholic hepatitis, drug-induced liver injury, chronic liver disease, and obstruction. Levels >1000 IU/mL are indicative of acute hepatitis, drug-induced hepatotoxicity (acetaminophen toxicity), and shock liver.
  - If AP is elevated (usually more than three times upper limit of normal) out of proportion to the transaminases, this suggests intrahepatic cholestasis or extrahepatic obstruction. An increased γ-glutamyl transferase (GGT), 5'-nucleotidase, or leucine aminopeptidase confirms the hepatic origin of an elevated AP.
  - Disproportionate elevation of AP compared with bilirubin could be seen in partial biliary obstruction or in early intrahepatic cholestasis (primary biliary cholangitis and PSC). High levels of AP and bilirubin may; however, indicate presence of a CBD stone.
  - High levels of GGT could be seen in many other medical conditions other than biliary disease, including congestive heart failure, alcohol intake, pancreatitis, chronic lung disease, renal failure, diabetes, and as a result of use of many drugs.
- The presence of **low albumin** or **prolonged PT** suggests chronic liver disease with impaired synthetic function.
  - In cirrhotic patients, high levels of globulins and low albumin levels are frequently seen.
  - Prolonged PT may, however, also be seen in obstructive jaundice. Of note, administration of vitamin K corrects the coagulopathy in patients with obstructive jaundice, but not hepatocellular disease.
  - Testing for urinary bilirubin or urobilinogen may be of some use, because clinical jaundice may lag behind bilirubinuria.
  - High cholesterol levels are seen in patients with cholestasis.
- If the initial evaluation does not reveal an obvious etiology (alcohol, drugs, infections), then **specific biochemical studies** should be ordered, including viral hepatitis serologies, antinuclear antibody, antimitochondrial antibody, antismooth muscle antibody, serum quantitative immunoglobulins, ferritin, iron studies, ceruloplasmin, and α_1-antitrypsin levels. If the cause still remains unclear, then liver biopsy should be considered. Figure 8-2 is helpful in planning the evaluation of the patient with jaundice.

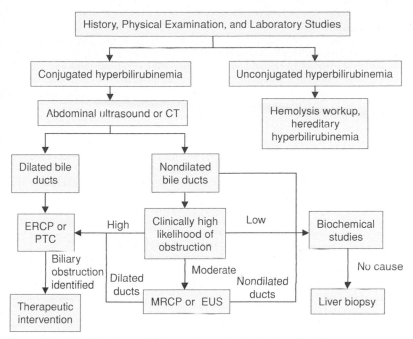

Figure 8-2. Algorithm for evaluation of the patient with jaundice. See comments in text regarding selection of appropriate imaging study when given a choice in the algorithm. ERCP, endoscopic retrograde cholangiopancreatography; EUS, endoscopic ultrasound; MRCP, magnetic resonance cholangiopancreatography; PTC, percutaneous transhepatic cholangiography.

- The evaluation of **conjugated hyperbilirubinemia** requires careful selection of the appropriate imaging procedure, because many of these studies are expensive or invasive.
  - If the initial evaluation suggests a possible vascular cause (Budd–Chiari syndrome or shock liver), then ultrasound with Doppler should be the initial study to evaluate patency of the hepatic and portal veins and hepatic artery.
  - Increased transaminases should prompt a search for hepatocellular disorders.
  - If the history and examination cause concern for malignancy, then an abdominal computed tomographic (CT) scan should be ordered, followed by ultrasound- or CT-guided liver biopsy, if appropriate. Tumor markers have limited role in terms of making the diagnosis of cancer.
- Patients with **increased AP** should be evaluated for causes of cholestatic jaundice.
  - Ultrasound should be the initial study to evaluate for evidence of biliary ductal dilatation. Abdominal CT can also be used to evaluate for ductal dilatation, but it has limitations.
  - If ductal dilatation is present or if the suspicion for obstruction remains high despite a normal study finding, then endoscopic retrograde cholangiopancreatography (ERCP) or percutaneous transhepatic cholangiography (PTC) should be performed. Of note, a mild dilatation of CBD can be a normal feature in patients who have had prior cholecystectomy or in elderly.
  - If ductal dilatation is not seen and the suspicion for obstruction is low, then biochemical studies should be ordered as above to look for parenchymal disease.
  - Again, liver biopsy should be considered if no etiology can be identified.

Imaging

- **Ultrasound**
  - Ultrasound is the best initial study for detection of biliary obstruction as evidenced by ductal dilatation. This has a sensitivity of 77% and specificity of 83–95% for identification of bile duct dilation. Advantages are portability, noninvasiveness, and relatively low cost. Disadvantages include operator-dependent nature, decreased image quality in obese patients or in those with overlying bowel gas, and poor visualization of distal ducts in 30–50% of patients.
  - Nondilated ducts, especially in the setting of acute or intermittent obstructions, cannot definitively rule out biliary obstruction, however. Therefore, additional studies are required if a high suspicion of obstruction remains.
  - Ultrasound can also identify hepatic parenchymal lesions, gallbladder disease, cholelithiasis, and occasionally choledocholithiasis.
- **Abdominal CT** is a first-line study for evaluation of hepatic parenchymal lesions; it is also an alternative to ultrasound for identifying biliary obstruction. Its advantages are a less operator-dependent nature and improved images in obese patients. Limitations include higher cost, lack of portability, inability to detect noncalcified gallstones, radiation exposure, and requirement of radiocontrast dye.
- **Magnetic resonance imaging** is a useful test for assessing liver parenchyma, specifically focal and malignant lesions. This is also sensitive in assessment of liver fat and iron. Magnetic resonance cholangiopancreatography (MRCP) is a special technique used to visualize the biliary tract. Advantages include its noninvasive nature and ability to accurately identify various liver lesions. Unlike ERCP, MRCP does not have therapeutic capabilities.
- **Hepatic iminodiacetic acid (HIDA) scan**
  The test of choice, if acute cholecystitis with cystic duct obstruction or biliary leakage is suspected, is a HIDA scan. False-negative results should be expected, however, in the setting of TPN use or with fasting serum bilirubin concentrations >5 mg/dL.

Diagnostic Procedures

- **Endoscopic retrograde cholangiopancreatography** (ERCP) provides direct visualization of the biliary and pancreatic ducts and identifies the site of obstruction in >90% of patients. Advantages include high accuracy in locating the site of obstruction, as well as the ability to perform therapeutic interventions (sphincterotomy, stone extraction, stent placement, cytology, and brushing and direct visualization using SpyGlass). Disadvantages include expense, invasiveness, difficulty after certain surgeries (Roux-en-Y), and morbidity. Complications of perforation, bleeding, cholangitis, and pancreatitis are uncommon but can be serious (2–3% overall morbidity rate).
- **Endoscopic ultrasound** can detect small CBD stones with similar accuracy to ERCP without a risk of post-ERCP pancreatitis. It can detect small (<3 cm) pancreatic tumors that are usually not discovered by CT scans. Choledocholithiasis cannot be removed by endoscopic ultrasound, which is a major disadvantage to ERCP, although therapeutic endoscopic ultrasound has been increasingly utilized nowadays.
- **Percutaneous transhepatic cholangiography (PTC)**
  - PTC is also an excellent test for evaluating biliary obstruction, with accuracy similar to ERCP (up to 90–100%) in identifying the site of biliary obstruction if the ducts are dilated. Advantages include lower cost and therapeutic capabilities (decompression of biliary system).
  - This test is less accurate than ERCP; however, if there are nondilated ducts, and several passes into the liver may be required to access the biliary tree. Aside from limited usefulness with nondilated ducts, other problems include inability to perform the test in the presence of coagulopathy or ascites, as well as complication risks (bleeding, arteriovenous fistulas, sepsis, pneumothorax, peritonitis). The decision of

whether to perform ERCP or PTC should be based partially on local expertise of the gastroenterologists and radiologists.

- *Liver biopsy*
  - If imaging studies are inconclusive and a hepatocellular process is suspected, a liver biopsy may be useful. It is an invasive procedure, however, and a complication rate of 0.1–3% is expected. Complications include pain, hemobilia, hemoperitoneum, arteriovenous fistula, pneumothorax, or hemothorax. Ultrasound guidance may decrease some of the risks. In patients with thrombocytopenia, coagulopathy, or ascites, a transjugular approach is recommended.

TREATMENT

Management of jaundice should be directed at the underlying cause. These management options are discussed in detail elsewhere in this handbook.

- Watchful waiting can be appropriate for acute viral hepatitis, where recovery is expected in most instances. Hepatitis B and C have chronic phases that require monitoring and management with antiviral agents as described in Chapter 20. Liver transplant may be an option for end-stage liver disease with decompensation.
- Discontinuation of offending medications or toxins is recommended for drug- or toxin-induced jaundice. Specific treatment with *N*-acetyl cysteine is available for acetaminophen-induced liver damage but is effective only in early disease course.
- Management of chronic autoimmune liver diseases causing jaundice may include use of corticosteroids, immunomodulators, or liver transplantation. See Chapter 20 for further details.
- The goal of treating a patient with bile duct obstruction is to drain the bile to decrease the risk of complications and to provide symptom relief. In patients with choledocholithiasis, a laparoscopic cholecystectomy with CBD exploration using intraoperative or postoperative ERCP is recommended. In many cases of CBD stones, an ERCP with sphincterotomy and stone extraction would be the appropriate therapeutic procedure. In elderly or frail patients who cannot undergo surgery, externally inserted drains into the gallbladder or main hepatic ducts would be suggested to overcome malignant strictures or for temporary relief of symptoms. EUS-guided drainage is also a promising approach.

SPECIAL CONSIDERATIONS

- **Pregnancy**
  - In pregnant patients, jaundice could be caused by disorders that are unique to pregnancy or coincident with, or exacerbated by, pregnancy (hepatitis E, herpes simplex virus, Budd–Chiari syndrome, choledocholithiasis).
  - Low serum albumin, and hemoglobin level and high AP, and α-fetoprotein (up to two to four times normal from placenta) can be parts of expected pregnancy-related changes. Levels of transaminases, bilirubin, PT/INR, 5′-nucleotidase, and GGT do not change with pregnancy; however, abnormal levels need to be further investigated.[8]
  - Liver diseases associated with pregnancy occur at special time points.[8,9] Chronic hepatitis, autoimmune liver disease, Wilson disease, and primary biliary cholangitis may be exacerbated during pregnancy as well. Gallstone disease can occur at anytime.
    - **Hyperemesis gravidarum** may cause mild elevations of AP, bilirubin, and transaminases during the first trimester.
    - **Intrahepatic cholestasis of pregnancy** normally presents with intense itching in the third trimester (up to 100 times increase in total serum bile acids).
    - **Dubin–Johnson syndrome** can be exacerbated by pregnancy. Jaundice develops in the second or third trimester.

- **Acute fatty liver of pregnancy** (with marked elevations of transaminases), **pre-eclampsia** or **eclampsia**, and **HELLP** (hemolysis, elevated liver enzymes, and low platelet count) syndrome could present with jaundice, usually late in the pregnancy. When jaundice occurs late in the course of these hepatocellular diseases, it indicates severe hepatic dysfunction.
- **Critically ill patients**
  - Jaundice is commonly seen in patients in the intensive care unit, where it is usually nonobstructive and multifactorial.[10] Bilirubin overproduction caused by hemolysis of transfused blood (10% of red blood cells in a transfused unit are hemolyzed within 24 hours), drug-induced hemolysis, and prosthetic valves are most common explanation of this finding. Hepatocellular dysfunction secondary to ischemia (shock liver), right-sided heart failure, drug-induced liver injury, sepsis with multisystem organ failure, viral hepatitis, and TPN should also be considered in the differential diagnosis of nonobstructive jaundice.[11]
  - Obstructive jaundice seen in critically ill patients is usually due to choledocholithiasis, cholangitis, biliary tract tumors, or bile duct stricture. Acalculous cholecystitis causes jaundice, especially after trauma, shock, recent surgery, and burns. Injuries of the biliary tract are commonly seen in patients who have recently undergone cholecystectomy or other upper abdominal surgeries.[11,12]
- **Liver transplantation**
  - **Biliary strictures** are a major source of morbidity after liver transplantation. The incidence has been reported as 5–15% after deceased donor liver transplant, and 28–32% after living donor right lobe transplant. Strictures can often be managed endoscopically with a success rate of more than 70% for anastomotic strictures, and 50–70% for nonanastomotic strictures.[13]
  - **Cholestasis after liver transplantation** can be related to early or late complications (using an approximate cutoff of a 6-month period). Early complications include acute rejection, ischemia-reperfusion injury (cold and rewarming ischemia), primary graft nonfunction, acute rejection, bacterial or viral infections, and drug-induced cholestasis. Late complications are predominantly related to chronic rejection, and recurrence of the original disease.[14]

COMPLICATIONS

Complications of jaundice will depend on the primary cause and severity of the jaundice:

- **Kernicterus** caused by deposition of bilirubin in the brain can result in irreversible motor and cortical impairment. This is seen in infants when levels of total bilirubin are >20 mg/dL.
- **Mechanical obstruction of the extrahepatic ducts** can predispose to life-threatening complications, including cholangitis, secondary biliary cirrhosis, and hepatic abscess formation.
- **Other long-term complications** include hepatic osteodystrophy, malabsorption of fat and fat-soluble vitamins, and pruritus.

ADDITIONAL RESOURCES

- ACG Guidelines: Evaluation of Abnormal Liver Chemistries. https://journals.lww.com/ajg/Fulltext/2017/01000/ACG_Clinical_Guideline__Evaluation_of_Abnormal.13.aspx (last accessed 11/5/19)
- AGA Technical Review on the Evaluation of Liver Chemistry Tests. http://www.gastrojournal.org/article/S0016-5085(02)00241-X/fulltext (last accessed 11/5/19).
- American Association for the Study of Liver Diseases (AASLD) Practice Guidelines. https://www.aasld.org/publications/practice-guidelines-0 (last accessed 11/5/19)

REFERENCES

1. Qayed E, Srinivasan S, Shahnavaz N. *Sleisenger and Fordtran's Gastrointestinal and Liver Disease. Review and Assessment*. 10th ed. Philadelphia, PA: Elsevier; 2017.
2. Green RM, Flamm S. AGA technical review on the evaluation of liver chemistry tests. *Gastroenterology*. 2002;123:1367–1384.
3. Kwo PY, Cohen SM, Lim JK. ACG clinical guideline: evaluation of abnormal liver chemistries. *Am J Gastroenterol*. 2017;112:18–35.
4. Podolsky DK. *Yamada's Textbook of Gastroenterology*. 6th ed. Chichester, West Sussex; Hoboken, NJ: John Wiley & Sons Inc.; 2016.
5. Qin LX, Tang ZY. Hepatocellular carcinoma with obstructive jaundice: diagnosis, treatment and prognosis. *World J Gastroenterol*. 2003;9:385–391.
6. Leise MD, Poterucha JJ, Talwalkar JA. Drug-induced liver injury. *Mayo Clin Proc*. 2014;89:95–106.
7. Schiff ER, Sorrell MF, Maddrey WC. *Schiff's Diseases of the Liver*. 10th ed. Philadelphia, PA: Lippincott Williams & Wilkins; 2007.
8. Tran TT, Ahn J, Reau NS. ACG clinical guideline: liver disease and pregnancy. *Am J Gastroenterol*. 2016;111:176–194; quiz 196.
9. Westbrook RH, Dusheiko G, Williamson C. Pregnancy and liver disease. *J Hepatol*. 2016;64: 933–945.
10. Bansal V, Schuchert VD. Jaundice in the intensive care unit. *Surg Clin North Am*. 2006;86: 1495–1502.
11. Chand N, Sanyal AJ. Sepsis-induced cholestasis. *Hepatology*. 2007;45:230–241.
12. Huffman JL, Schenker S. Acute acalculous cholecystitis: a review. *Clin Gastroenterol Hepatol*. 2010;8:15–22.
13. Kochhar G, Parungao JM, Hanouneh IA, et al. Biliary complications following liver transplantation. *World J Gastroenterol*. 2013;19:2841–2846.
14. Corbani A, Burroughs AK. Intrahepatic cholestasis after liver transplantation. *Clin Liver Dis*. 2008;12:111–129, ix.

Abnormal Liver Chemistries

9

Claire Meyer

GENERAL PRINCIPLES

- Elevations in serum markers of liver function or injury may be found in routine laboratory evaluation of asymptomatic patients, or as an initial step in the evaluation of patients with symptoms of suspected hepatobiliary origin, and persistent liver test abnormalities warrant further evaluation.
- The pattern of liver chemistries, along with a thorough history and physical examination, can help direct additional testing to arrive at a diagnosis.
- Liver chemistries are commonly referred to as **liver function tests**, although only the bilirubin, albumin, and prothrombin time (PT) actually reflect liver function; the liver enzymes (aminotransferases, alkaline phosphatase, and γ-glutamyltransferase [GGT]) are better thought of as markers of liver injury.
- Liver function tests are considered to be abnormal when these blood tests are consistently elevated. However, none of these tests are completely sensitive and specific; they may be abnormal in the absence of a primary hepatic disease, or normal even in the presence of significant liver fibrosis.
    - **Aminotransferases (also called transaminases).** Aspartate aminotransferase (**AST**, previously called SGOT) and alanine aminotransferase (**ALT**, previously called SGPT) are markers of hepatocellular injury, when there is translocation of these enzymes across the disrupted cell membranes and a subsequent rise in serum levels. ALT is a more specific indicator of liver damage because it is found primarily in the liver, while AST may be elevated due to injury to other tissues, such as cardiac or skeletal muscle.[1]
    - **Alkaline phosphatase.** Alkaline phosphatase is an enzyme found in the hepatocyte canalicular membranes (the hepatocyte cell membrane through which bile is secreted into the bile canaliculi). Elevated alkaline phosphatase levels commonly arise from the liver and/or bones, but the enzyme is also found in other tissues, including placenta and intestines. The source of an elevated alkaline phosphatase can be distinguished by measuring alkaline phosphatase isoenzymes (which quantifies the different forms of the enzyme associated with different organs), or by measurement of **GGT** or **5′-nucleotidase** (which are expected to be elevated if the liver is the source of elevated alkaline phosphatase).
    - **Bilirubin.** Bilirubin is a degradation product of heme metabolism. Breakdown of red blood cells produces unconjugated (indirect) bilirubin, which is taken up into hepatocytes and converted into conjugated (direct) bilirubin and secreted into bile. Measurement of the direct bilirubin (in addition to total bilirubin) is important to distinguish whether hyperbilirubinemia is primarily conjugated or unconjugated. Both forms of hyperbilirubinemia manifest as jaundice; usually a serum bilirubin concentration of around 3 mg/dL is required for jaundice to become clinically apparent. A complete discussion of the pathophysiology and differential diagnosis of jaundice can be found in Chapter 8.
    - **Prothrombin time (PT) and international normalized ratio (INR).** Many of the proteins involved in hemostasis are produced by the liver. When there is significant

hepatocellular injury, synthesis of clotting factors can be decreased, leading to a prolonged PT and elevated INR. In addition, several of the clotting factors require vitamin K in order to function normally, and impaired secretion of bile can result in decreased absorption of this fat-soluble vitamin; in this way, significant cholestasis can also lead to a prolonged PT and elevated INR. Coagulopathy due to cholestasis should respond to parenteral supplementation of vitamin K, while the coagulopathy due to hepatic synthetic dysfunction will not.

Albumin. The serum albumin concentration is often decreased in chronic liver disease, reflecting decreased synthesis. Levels may be normal in acute liver disease because the half-life of albumin is approximately 20 days. In addition, a decreased albumin concentration is not specific to liver disease. In particular, albumin is considered a negative acute phase protein, so levels can be decreased due to inflammation of a variety of causes.

DIAGNOSIS

A series of laboratory tests alone rarely leads to a diagnosis in a patient suspected of having hepatobiliary disease. Instead, the clinical context must be considered and tests carefully chosen; disease-specific laboratory tests and other appropriate studies are necessary to arrive at a diagnosis.

Clinical Presentation

History

A thorough history is essential to the evaluation of a patient with abnormal liver chemistries. Particular attention should be given to:

- History of prior hepatobiliary disease or liver test abnormalities
- Symptoms that may result from liver disease, such as jaundice, pruritus, right upper quadrant abdominal pain, unintentional weight loss, poor appetite, fever, nausea, and vomiting
- Medical conditions that suggest risk for specific liver diseases such as nonalcoholic fatty liver disease (diabetes, obesity, hypertension, hyperlipidemia) and autoimmune liver disease (inflammatory bowel disease and other autoimmune diseases)
- Whether the patient is pregnant and/or has a history of any liver abnormalities during prior pregnancies (if applicable)
- Medications and supplements, including any history of prior antibiotics, immunosuppressants, and chemotherapy. Table 9-1 lists some of the drugs which may be associated with abnormal liver tests. The NIH's LiverTox website provides a searchable database of information on drug-induced liver injury.[2]
- Extent and duration of alcohol consumption (more than 14 drinks/week for women or 21 drinks/week for men is considered significant), drug use, risk factors for viral hepatitis (intravenous and intranasal drug use, tattoos, piercings, sexual history, transfusions), and any significant dietary or environmental exposures
- Family history of liver disease or autoimmune disease

Physical Examination

The physical examination should **focus on stigmata of liver disease** as well as **signs suggestive of systemic diseases** that commonly affect the liver. This includes jaundice, palmar erythema, temporal wasting, spider nevi, caput medusa, gynecomastia, ascites, hepatosplenomegaly, abdominal tenderness, and encephalopathy. Certain liver diseases can also have particular findings on physical examination such as the Kayser–Fleischer rings of Wilson disease and xanthelasmas (fatty nodules around the eyes) in primary biliary cholangitis.

TABLE 9-1 SELECTED DRUGS ASSOCIATED WITH LIVER TEST ABNORMALITIES

Antiarrhythmics	Amiodarone
Analgesics	Acetaminophen, nonsteroidal anti-inflammatory drugs
Antibiotics	Isoniazid, amoxicillin/clavulanate, nitrofurantoin, ketoconazole, fluconazole, macrolides, fluoroquinolones
Antihypertensives	Methyldopa, labetalol
Antiepileptics	Valproate, phenytoin, carbamazepine, lamotrigine
Drugs of abuse	Anabolic steroids, cocaine, amphetamines
Herbs and supplements	Green tea extract, vitamin A
HMG-CoA inhibitors	Atorvastatin, pravastatin, lovastatin, simvastatin
Immunosuppressants	Methotrexate, azathioprine

Differential Diagnosis

- A **nonhepatic source** should be considered in any patient with abnormal liver chemistries. When a **hepatic source** is suspected, categorizing the **pattern of liver test abnormalities** can help to determine more and less likely causes. Elevated liver enzymes can be classified as hepatocellular (aminotransferase predominant), cholestatic (alkaline phosphatase predominant), or mixed. In drug-induced liver injury, this can be quantified using the R ratio[3] which is calculated as follows:

  R ratio = (measured ALT/upper limit of normal ALT)/
  (measured alkaline phosphatase/upper limit of normal alkaline phosphatase)

  R ratio >5 indicates a hepatocellular pattern and R ratio <2 a cholestatic pattern; if the R ratio is 2–5, it is considered a mixed pattern.
- **Hepatocellular pattern.** Hepatocellular injury typically manifests with modest to profound elevations in serum aminotransferases. Alkaline phosphatase and bilirubin may or may not be elevated, depending on the nature and severity of the injury. The degree and pattern of transaminase elevations offers additional clues to the etiology. As a general rule, the highest elevations in transaminases (>10,000 U/L) are seen with ischemic and acute viral hepatitis (including herpes simplex hepatitis; see also Chapter 19). AST and ALT >1000 U/L are seen primarily in acute viral, toxin-induced (i.e., acetaminophen), or ischemic hepatitis; these can also be encountered in autoimmune hepatitis, bile duct obstruction, acute Budd–Chiari syndrome, and Wilson disease, among other causes. Alcohol-induced liver injury is classically associated with AST:ALT ratio ≥2:1, and transaminases of 300 U/L or less. Table 9-2 lists some of the common causes of hepatocellular injury.
- **Cholestatic pattern.** Cholestatic processes typically produce moderate to profound elevations in alkaline phosphatase, often with hyperbilirubinemia. Depending on the underlying condition, serum transaminases may or may not be elevated. After confirming a hepatic source of elevated alkaline phosphatase, hepatobiliary imaging can determine whether there is evidence of bile duct obstruction and/or liver masses. If there are no imaging findings to explain the liver test abnormalities, consideration should be given to causes of intrahepatic cholestasis, microscopic bile duct injury (such as drug-induced liver injury and primary biliary cholangitis), and infiltrative processes (such as sarcoidosis); see Table 9-3.

TABLE 9-2 SELECTED CAUSES OF HEPATOCELLULAR INJURY PATTERN OF LIVER CHEMISTRIES

Viral hepatitis
Hepatitis A, B, C, D, E, and other viruses (Cytomegalovirus, Epstein–Barr virus, herpes simplex virus)

Drugs and toxins
Alcoholic liver disease, medications, herbs/supplements, and drugs of abuse

Metabolic syndrome
Nonalcoholic fatty liver disease

Autoimmune
Autoimmune hepatitis, thyroid disorders, celiac disease

Vascular
Budd–Chiari syndrome, ischemia and shock liver (hypotension), congestive hepatopathy, veno-occlusive disease

Hereditary
Hemochromatosis, Wilson disease, α_1-antitrypsin deficiency

Pregnancy associated
Acute fatty liver of pregnancy, preeclampsia, eclampsia, HELLP syndrome

HELLP, hemolysis, elevated liver enzymes, low platelet count.

- **Elevated bilirubin** is a feature of many of the conditions that result in hepatocellular and cholestatic patterns of injury, and may also occur without liver enzymes abnormalities (isolated hyperbilirubinemia). Distinguishing between predominantly conjugated or unconjugated hyperbilirubinemia helps to narrow the differential diagnosis; unconjugated hyperbilirubinemia is commonly seen in hemolysis, hematoma resorption, and Gilbert syndrome, while conjugated hyperbilirubinemia suggests some form of liver

TABLE 9-3 SELECTED CAUSES OF A CHOLESTATIC INJURY PATTERN OF LIVER CHEMISTRIES

Biliary
Biliary stricture, choledocholithiasis

Inflammatory/Autoimmune
Primary biliary cholangitis, primary sclerosing cholangitis, sarcoidosis, IgG4 cholangiopathy

Infectious
Sepsis, liver abscesses, tuberculosis, viral hepatitis, histoplasmosis

Malignancy
Primary hepatobiliary tumors, liver metastases, lymphoma

Medications

Pregnancy associated
Intrahepatic cholestasis of pregnancy

dysfunction or injury (including cirrhosis, biliary obstruction, and congestive hepatopathy related to heart failure).

Diagnostic Testing

Diagnostic testing should be directed towards the most likely causes of the abnormal liver chemistries on the based on the overall clinical presentation. The urgency of diagnostic testing is largely determined by the acuity and severity of the patient's symptoms and laboratory findings.

Laboratory Testing

Laboratory tests for the more common causes of abnormal liver chemistries are outlined in Table 9-4. In the majority of cases, an abnormal result on initial testing may suggest a particular diagnosis, but requires further testing to confirm. For example, a positive antismooth muscle antibody at a high titer suggests the possibility of autoimmune hepatitis, but a liver biopsy is required for diagnosis; positive antismooth muscle antibody at a low titer is not specific for autoimmune hepatitis and, depending on the clinical setting, may or may not warrant further evaluation. Similarly, elevated iron indexes or low ceruloplasmin can be seen in a variety of conditions, and are not by themselves diagnostic of inherited liver disease.

Imaging

The choice of imaging to evaluate the cause of abnormal liver chemistries depends on the most likely causes as determined by the history, physical examination, and initial laboratory investigation. It is often reasonable to start with an **abdominal ultrasound** to evaluate for abnormalities of the liver parenchyma, masses, and evidence of biliary obstruction. The addition of Dopplers to the ultrasound examination can evaluate for Budd–Chiari syndrome or portal vein thrombosis. Ultrasound has the advantage of being relatively inexpensive and safe (no ionizing radiation or intravenous contrast); disadvantages include being operator dependent and visualization can be limited by obesity and bowel gas. An **abdominal computed tomographic (CT) scan** also evaluates the hepatic parenchyma and biliary tree, but is not operator dependent or as limited by bowel gas or obesity; use of intravenous contrast is needed to evaluate for malignancy. When there is concern for hepatocellular carcinoma, a triple-phase contrast CT may be diagnostic. However, **magnetic resonance imaging (MRI)** is often the most informative imaging technique for evaluation of the liver parenchyma (for steatosis, iron deposition, and evidence of cirrhosis) and characterizing liver masses. **MRCP** sequences (three-dimensional reconstructions of the biliary and pancreatic ducts) allow for detection of biliary strictures or stones. Both CT and MRI are limited by cost and the need for intravenous contrast in most cases.

Diagnostic Procedures

Liver biopsy should be considered when the results will change management and provide information that cannot be obtained by noninvasive testing—for example, to confirm the diagnosis of autoimmune hepatitis, or when there are significant, persistent unexplained liver test abnormalities. The decision must be individualized, taking into account the patient's overall clinical presentation, age, and comorbidities. Assessment of fibrosis often does not require a liver biopsy, given the availability of noninvasive measures of liver stiffness (such as ultrasound- or MR-based elastography).[4]

TREATMENT

Treatment of abnormal liver chemistries is directed toward the suspected or confirmed cause of the abnormalities. In suspected **drug-induced liver injury**, the initial step is to discontinue the suspected medication(s); in select cases where there is evidence for

TABLE 9-4 LABORATORY EVALUATION FOR SOME OF THE MORE COMMON CAUSES OF ABNORMAL LIVER CHEMISTRIES

Cause of Abnormal Liver Chemistries	Initial Test(s)	Confirmatory Test(s)
Hepatitis A	HAV IgM (if acute hepatitis suspected)	
Hepatitis B	HBV surface antigen HBV core IgM (if acute hepatitis suspected) HBV core total antibody and HBV surface antibody (to assess for prior exposure, immunity)	HBV PCR
Hepatitis C	HCV antibody	HCV PCR
Biliary obstruction	Liver ultrasound	+/− MRCP
Liver mass lesions	Liver ultrasound	CT or MRI, with IV contrast
Autoimmune hepatitis	Antismooth muscle antibody Antinuclear antibody Quantitative IgG	Liver biopsy
Primary biliary cholangitis	Antimitochondrial antibody	+/− liver biopsy
Primary sclerosing cholangitis	MRCP	
Budd–Chiari syndrome	Liver Dopplers	
Hereditary hemochromatosis	Ferritin and transferrin saturation	HFE gene mutation testing +/− liver biopsy
α_1-Antitrypsin deficiency	α_1-Antitrypsin proteotype	
Wilson disease	Ceruloplasmin	24-hr urine copper Slit lamp eye examination Serum copper +/− liver biopsy
Thyroid disease	TSH	Free T3 and T4
Celiac disease	Tissue transglutaminase IgA Total IgA	Duodenal biopsy

HAV, hepatitis A virus; HBV, hepatitis B virus; HCV, hepatitis C virus; HFE, human homeostatic iron regulator protein; MRCP, magnetic resonance cholangiopancreatography; PCR, polymerase chain reaction.

autoimmune-type injury, steroids may be considered. If **viral hepatitis** is identified, treatment decisions depend on whether the patient has acute or chronic disease and whether or not the patient has developed hepatic fibrosis or cirrhosis. Patients with suspected **nonalcoholic fatty liver disease** should optimize management of metabolic risk factors such as diabetes and hypertension, and those who are overweight should aim for weight loss of 5–10% of their body weight. When **alcoholic liver disease** is suspected on the basis of history, labs, and other studies, complete alcohol avoidance should be recommended and supportive services such as Alcoholics Anonymous or one-on-one counseling should be offered. In patients with chronic liver disease, immunization against hepatitis A and B should be offered. Further details on the treatment of acute and chronic liver diseases can be found in Chapters 19–21.

REFERENCES

1. Green RM, Flamm S. AGA technical review on the evaluation of liver chemistry tests. *Gastroenterology.* 2002;123:1367–1384.
2. *NIH Livertox database.* Available at https://livertox.nih.gov/. Accessed May 11, 2019.
3. Chalasani NP, Hayashi PH, Bonkovsky HL, et al.; Practice Parameters Committee of the American College of Gastroenterology. ACG clinical guideline: the diagnosis and management of idiosyncratic drug-induced liver injury. *Am J Gastroenterol.* 2014;109(7):950–966.
4. Tapper EB, Lok AS. Use of liver imaging and biopsy in clinical practice. *N Engl J Med.* 2017;377(8):756–768.

Ascites

Scott A. McHenry

10

GENERAL PRINCIPLES

- Ascites refers to an increased volume of fluid in the peritoneal cavity. This must be differentiated from other causes of abdominal distension such as anasarca or obesity.
- A confident clinical diagnosis of cirrhosis can be made in approximately 85% of patients with ascites,[1] which can usually be diagnosed without the need of a liver biopsy.
- As the most common form of decompensation in cirrhosis, ascites will develop at a rate of 7–10% per year.[2] The presence of ascites is an important milestone in the natural history of cirrhosis as it increases the 1-year mortality rate from approximately 1% to 20%.[2]

Pathophysiology

- When the low-resistance, high-capacitance portal circulation is altered (e.g., fibrosis, nodularity, mechanical obstruction to flow), the influx of fluid into the hepatic parenchyma is increased in accordance with Starling forces.
- Ascites will form when the lymphatics can no longer compensate for this influx. In cirrhosis, this requires an 8–12 mm Hg hepatic venous pressure gradient (HVPG).[3]
- Portal hypertension facilitates bacterial translocation across the bowel wall, which stimulates splanchnic and systemic vasodilation. This leads to a decrease in effective arterial volume and ultimately triggers compensatory sodium and water retention.[4]
- Other factors in the pathophysiology of ascites include altered oncotic pressure, decreased lymphatic drainage, and increased endothelial permeability.

DIAGNOSIS

- See Figure 10-1 for diagnostic approach to ascites.
- Ascites is divided functionally by the presence or absence of portal hypertension (see Tables 10-1 and 10-2). This is done by measuring the serum-ascites albumin gradient (SAAG), the numeric difference between serum albumin level and ascites albumin level.
- Ascites fluid due to portal hypertension will be characterized by a high SAAG to balance the hydrostatic pressure gradient. A threshold of 1.1 g/dL is 97% accurate in making this important clinical differentiation.[1]
- Several vascular disorders will result in portal hypertension by either increasing total blood flow or increasing resistance to flow through the portal venous system. Noncirrhotic portal hypertension is divided anatomically into prehepatic, hepatic (including presinusoidal, sinusoidal, and postsinusoidal), or posthepatic.[5]
- Myxedema is a rare condition that is an exception to the rule that high SAAG is synonymous with portal hypertension.[6]

Clinical Presentation

The major roles of the history and physical examination for patients with ascites are:

1. Confirming that abdominal distension is truly ascites,
2. Determining the likelihood of cirrhosis,

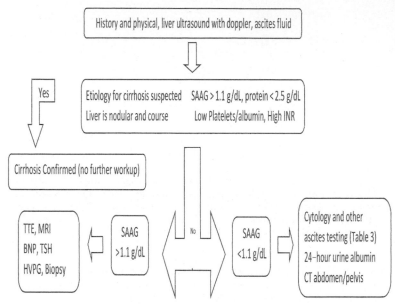

Figure 10-1. Diagnostic approach to new onset ascites. BNP, brain natriuretic peptide; CT, computed tomography; HVPG, hepatic venous pressure gradient; INR, international normalized ratio; MRI, magnetic resonance imaging; SAAG, serum-ascites albumin gradient; TSH, thyroid-stimulating hormone; TTE, transthoracic echocardiography.

3. Raising suspicion for noncirrhotic causes (e.g., heart failure, malignancy), and
4. Ruling out comorbid infections.

History

• For ascites of unknown etiology, symptoms of and risk factors for chronic liver disease (see Chapters 20 and 21) and heart failure (e.g., presence of orthopnea, paroxysmal nocturnal dyspnea) should be the focus of the history.

TABLE 10-1 CAUSES OF NON-CIRRHOTIC PORTAL HYPERTENSION

Prehepatic	Hepatic	Posthepatic
Portal vein thrombosis	Polycystic liver disease	Pulmonary hypertension
Splenic vein thrombosis	Congenital hepatic fibrosis	Constrictive pericarditis
Splanchnic AV fistula	Methotrexate, amiodarone	Restrictive cardiomyopathy
Extrahepatic portal vein obstruction	Sarcoidosis, amyloidosis	IVC web/obstruction
Massive splenomegaly (e.g., lymphoma)	Sinusoidal obstructive syndrome	Hepatic vein thrombosis

AV, arteriovenous; IVC inferior vena cava.

TABLE 10-2 CAUSES OF ASCITES NOT ASSOCIATED WITH PORTAL HYPERTENSION

Peritonitis	Cancer/Chylous	Fluid Leaks	Oncotic Disorders
Bacterial, fungal Tuberculosis, chlamydia Chemical (e.g., barium) Vasculitis (e.g., SLE)	Peritoneal carcinomatosis Malignant chylous Lymphatic injury Lymphangiectasia	Pancreatitis (pancreatic duct) Biloma (bile duct) Nephrogenous (ureter or bladder)	Myxedema Severe malnutrition Nephrotic syndrome Protein-losing enteropathy

SLE, systemic lupus erythematosus.

- Patients with known cirrhosis presenting with new onset or more difficult to control ascites should be questioned to determine adherence to therapy and symptoms consistent with a superimposed infection such as spontaneous bacterial peritonitis (SBP).

Physical Examination
- Though dependent on the patient's sex and body habitus, approximately 1500 cc of ascites is required to be detectable on physical examination.[7]
- Several physical examination maneuvers are used to determine the presence of equivocal volumes of ascites. These include flank dullness, shifting dullness, and a fluid wave.[8]
- Signs of chronic liver disease (see Chapters 20 and 21) and heart failure (e.g., jugular venous distention, hepatojugular reflex, pulsatile liver) should also be ascertained.
- A firm umbilical nodule, hepatic artery bruit, or left supraclavicular lymphadenopathy should raise concern for malignant ascites or hepatocellular carcinoma (HCC).

Diagnostic Testing

- **Ascites Fluid Analysis, please see Table 10-3.**
  Routinely testing for cell count and albumin allows for early diagnosis of portal hypertension and SBP (SAAG of >1.1 g/dL and polymorphonuclear [PMN] count >250 cells/cc, respectively). As approximately 12% of patients will have SBP at time of presentation to the hospital[9] and a 12-hour delay of SBP diagnosis[10] is associated with an increased inhospital mortality, all patients with ascites should have their fluid tested regardless of their chief complaint.

TABLE 10-3 ASCITES FLUID LABORATORY ANALYSIS BY CLINICAL SUSPICION

Routine	Infectious Peritonitis	Chylous/ Malignant	Traumatic or Surgical Leaks
Cell count with differential Albumin Total protein Routine cultures	Blood culture bottles LDH, glucose ADA (if tuberculosis suspected)	Cytology Triglycerides Chylomicrons	Amylase (pancreatic duct) Bilirubin (bile duct or gallbladder) Urea, creatinine (ureter or bladder)

ADA, adenosine deaminase; LDH, lactate dehydrogenase.

○ When SBP is suspected clinically, inoculating ascites directly into blood culture bottles increases the microbiologic yield by approximately 30%.[11] In cases of secondary bacterial peritonitis, ascites glucose should be <50 mg/dL and LDH > ULN. These findings should prompt cross-sectional imaging as nonsurgical management is almost universally fatal.

○ The transition from a cirrhotic with a typical high SAAG ascites to a low SAAG/high-protein ascites should prompt an evaluation for malignancy. Ascites fluid should be sent for cytology and sensitive liver imaging (e.g., MR w/wo contrast) obtained.

○ The combination of high triglycerides (>200 mg/dL), high protein, and the presence of chylomicrons is diagnostic of a primary chylous ascites.[12] In equivocal cases, a 72-hour NPO trial can be used to differentiate this from cirrhosis as the volume of ascites will not improve and the ascites color will become more amber in the later.

○ Though uncommon, peritoneal tuberculosis remains overrepresented in alcoholic cirrhotics and HIV patients. Though highly specific, an elevated ascites adenosine deaminase level is only approximately 60% sensitive for tuberculous peritonitis in patients who have cirrhosis.[13]

- **Liver Ultrasound and Doppler Examination**
  ○ Ultrasonography is first line in patients suspected to have ascites due to its high sensitivity, specificity, and portability. The amount of ascites that can be detected by ultrasound is approximately 150 cc.[14]

  ○ Doppler examination (as opposed to 2D gray-scale only) is more sensitive for portal vein thrombosis (PVT) or hepatic vein obstruction (i.e., Budd–Chiari syndrome).

  ○ Congestive hepatopathy is suspected by the presence of a dilated IVC with reversal of hepatic venous flow.[15] Decreased portal vein velocity, reversal of portal venous flow, and increased portal vein diameter are more suggestive of cirrhosis.[16]

  ○ A noncirrhotic liver can appear radiographically nodular with coarse architecture if congested, highlighting that these findings are not pathognomonic for cirrhosis.

- **Miscellaneous Diagnostic Testing**
  ○ A urinalysis is a useful screen for renal disorders (e.g., nephrotic syndrome) or a urinary tract infection that prompts decompensation of ascites. Myxedema can be screened for with serum thyroid-stimulating hormone (TSH) level.

  ○ Transthoracic echocardiography (TTE) is used to evaluate for pulmonary hypertension and heart failure. The presence of pulmonary hypertension and ascites is not sufficient to diagnose congestive hepatopathy due to the possibility of portopulmonary hypertension or simply comorbid liver and cardiopulmonary disease.

  ○ In equivocal cases, additional information can be obtained by a transjugular liver biopsy with hemodynamic measurements (see Table 10-4).

  ○ A normal HPVG (<5 mm Hg) is useful in ruling out hepatic causes of portal hypertension. The presence of a free hepatic-right atrial pressure gradient raises

TABLE 10-4	HEMODYNAMIC MEASUREMENTS OBTAINED AT TIME OF TRANSJUGULAR LIVER BIOPSY		
	Right Atrial Pressure	Free Hepatic Pressure	HPVG
Cirrhosis	Normal	Normal	Elevated (>5 mm Hg)
Congestive hepatopathy	Elevated	Elevated	Normal
Budd–Chiari syndrome	Normal	Elevated	Normal
Portal vein thrombosis	Normal	Normal	Normal

concern for Budd–Chiari syndrome and should prompt venography. However, normal hemodynamic measurements do not rule out a prehepatic cause of portal hypertension.

TREATMENT

- Please see Figure 10-2 for overview of treatment.
- Initial treatment for tense ascites should be a large-volume paracentesis (LVP). This achieves both rapid improvement of symptoms and provides ascites fluid for analysis. Subsequent treatment should be tailored to the underlying pathophysiology.
- The following points will focus on managing the cirrhotic patient with ascites. These strategies are also applicable for most other causes of a high SAAG ascites due to the shared pathophysiology of portal hypertension. The exception is ascites due to myxedema, which will respond to thyroid hormone supplementation.

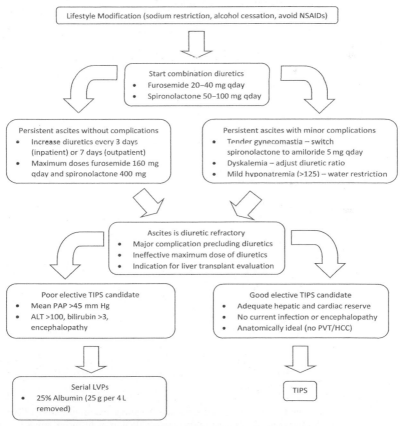

Figure 10-2. Treatment of ascites associated with portal hypertension. ALT, alanine aminotransferase; HCC, hepatocellular carcinoma; NSAIDs, nonsteroidal anti-inflammatory drugs; PAP, pulmonary artery pressure; PVT, portal vein thrombosis; TIPS, transjugular intrahepatic portosystemic shunt.

- **Lifestyle Modification**
  - Sodium restriction to less than <2000 mg (78 mEq) per day is the cornerstone of ascites treatment. This is based on the principal that the concentration of sodium is 3 g/L of ascites (120 mEq),[17] and a negative sodium balance will lead to reabsorption.
  - In alcoholic cirrhosis, complete abstinence from alcohol can lead to marked improvement in ascites severity.[18] Nephrotoxic agents such as NSAIDs should also be avoided.
  - Fluid restriction is not a treatment for ascites per se and should be reserved only for patients with hyponatremia (Na <130 mEq/L).
  - It is important to be aware of saline-containing fluids. This is especially true in the postoperative period when poor ascites control can lead to surgical site complications.
- **Diuretics**
  - Upfront combination therapy with both a potassium sparing and a potassium wasting diuretic (as opposed to sequential therapy) leads to fewer complications and lower failure rates.[19] Therefore, a starting regimen consists of furosemide and spironolactone in a ratio of 20 mg/50 mg.
  - The goal of diuretic therapy should be to lose 0.5 kg/day as ascites fluid resorption will be rate limiting. More aggressive diuresis (e.g., 1 kg/day) can be used if there is edema as this will act as a protective buffer against iatrogenic intravascular volume depletion.
  - With inpatient monitoring, the diuretic dose can be increased every 3 days, while diuretic titration an outpatient is at weekly intervals (i.e., time until pharmacologic steady state). The maximum daily dose of furosemide is 160 mg and spironolactone 400 mg.
  - Side effects (e.g., acute kidney injury, dyskalemia, hyponatremia, hypotension) may limit the ability to achieve maximum doses. Diuretic therapy should not be started or continued when the creatinine is unstable because of the risk of precipitating hepatorenal syndrome (HRS).
  - If tender gynecomastia results from the use of spironolactone, amiloride (starting dose 5 mg daily) or triamterene (starting dose 50 mg daily) can be substituted.
  - Due to its vasodilatory properties and risk of HRS, intravenous diuretics should generally be avoided in cirrhotic patients unless required for pulmonary edema.
  - In situations where bioavailability or intrinsic renal disease is felt to make furosemide ineffective, the use of bumetanide or torsemide can be considered.[20,21] Though cumbersome and costly to implement, weekly albumin infusions have been shown to increase the efficacy of furosemide therapy in cirrhosis.[22]
- **Refractory Ascites**
  - Once ascites begins to quickly recur despite maximum doses of diuretics and sodium restriction (diuretic resistant) or develop side effects precluding diuretic use (diuretic intractable),[23] the 1-year mortality rate increases to 70% per year.[24] This is an indication for liver transplant evaluation.
  - If in doubt, a 24-hour urine sodium measurement (>78 mEq) or a spot sodium/potassium ratio (>2.5) can be used to demonstrate nonadherence to sodium restriction.[25]
  - Compared to serial LVPs, transjugular intrahepatic portosystemic shunt (TIPS) is now the preferred treatment for refractory ascites as it improves transplant-free survival in carefully selected patients.[26]
- **TIPS**
  - The modern method to mechanically decompress the portal venous system is a TIPS. Surgical approaches (e.g., splenorenal shunt) are mostly of only historical value.
  - In the setting of diuretic-resistant ascites, there is a 70% complete response rate for TIPS.
  - The technical success of a TIPS placement requires an open venous inflow and outflow. Imaging (e.g., US/Doppler, MRI) is required for procedural planning.

Techniques for overcoming prior limitations (PVT, HCC) have been developed and should prompt consultation with the interventional radiologist in otherwise good TIPS candidates.

After a TIPS, the increased right heart filling pressures can precipitate heart failure. A TTE should be obtained as part of the workup with the goal of demonstrating a hyperdynamic LVEF and a PASP <45 mm Hg.

In patients with poor hepatic reserve, the liver is more dependent on portal blood supply for oxygenation and will experience a relative ischemia after a TIPS. Several factors predict which patients are at higher risk of hepatic decompensation: MELD >17, presence of encephalopathy, bilirubin >3, or ALT >100.[27] These are not absolute contraindications especially when a patient can be rescued with a liver transplant.

- **Serial LVP**
  Serial LVPs are typically performed on a 1–2-week schedule for symptomatic relief. If consistently needed more frequently, infection/malignancy should be ruled out and adherence to sodium restriction should be stressed since even in the absence of any sodium excretion, 2 g of sodium per day should yield only 9 L of ascites after 2 weeks.

  Paracentesis-induced circulatory dysfunction (PICD) occurs in up to 80% of all LVPs and is defined by a sustained increase in renin–angiotensin–aldosterone system activity. This is felt to be a function of splanchnic vasodilation due to relief of intraperitoneal pressure rather than loss of intravascular fluid into the peritoneal cavity.[28]

  The use of volume expansion with 25% albumin (25 g/4 L ascites removed) decreases the rate of PICD to approximately 10%[29]; however, when <5 L of ascites is removed, albumin is not effective in further lowering the risk of PICD. Extrapolating this data, when LVPs are required for patients with renal or hemodynamic instability, a limit of 5 L is reasonable.

  When less than all ascites fluid is removed, there is a predisposition for the ascites to leak from the paracentesis site. When one anticipates not removing all the ascites, one should avoid dilating the needle tract and should use a Z-track technique.

  Ascites leaks can be quite frustrating to treat as persistent flow through the tract will delay closure. Treatment options include pressure dressing, purse-string sutures, cyanoacrylate glue, and temporary use of an ostomy bag while in the lateral decubitus position (leak side up), while the dependent side is drained of the remaining ascites.

- **Treatment of Ascites Without Portal Hypertension**
  As low SAAG ascites has a different pathophysiology, sodium restriction and diuretics should not be used with the goal of improving ascites control.

  Symptomatic malignant ascites can be treated with serial LVPs (if relatively infrequent) or an indwelling catheter (e.g., Tenckhoff catheter). It is important to rule out a symptomatic partial small bowel obstruction in this setting with on oral contrast study (e.g., small bowel follow-through, CT with oral contrast).

  Chylous ascites is treated by a low-fat diet and medium-chain triglycerides supplements.

ASSOCIATED CONDITIONS

- **Spontaneous Bacterial Peritonitis (SBP) (see Chapter 20)**
  SBP is a monomicrobial infection of the ascites fluid that is not due to bowel perforation. It is felt to be a function of the ascites being seeded by transient gut-microbial bacteremia and decreased opsonization capacity of the ascites fluid itself.

  The diagnosis of SBP is made with >250/mL PMN cells in the ascites with ascites culture growth. The term neutrocytic ascites refers to when the clinical picture and the PMNs are diagnostic of SBP but the culture results are negative.

In patients that have had prior episodes of SBP, the use of antibiotics for secondary prophylaxis dramatically decreases rates of SBP and is cost effective.[30] Additionally, in those with advanced liver disease and a low protein (<1 g/dL) ascites, primary prophylaxis appears to improve short-term mortality.[31] Prophylaxis regimens include ciprofloxacin, trimethoprim-sulfamethoxazole, and rifaximin.

- **Hepatohydrothorax (HH)**
  - HH refers to the phenomena of ascites tracking into the pleural space (usually the right hemithorax). This is felt to be a function of microscopic pores in the diaphragm and a vacuum phenomenon due to the negative intrathoracic pressure.
  - The diagnosis is established by ruling out other etiologies of pleural effusions in a patient with cirrhosis and requires a diagnostic thoracentesis demonstrating a serous transudate.
  - Treatment approaches are identical to ascites (sodium restriction, diuretics, TIPS).
  - For symptomatic pleural effusions, therapeutic thoracentesis should be performed. As the morbidity of serial thoracentesis is higher than for paracentesis, the use of percutaneous drains (e.g., PleurX catheter) can be considered despite the infection risk.
- **Hepatorenal Syndrome (HRS)**
  - HRS is associated with ascites due to the shared pathophysiology of peripheral vasodilation from portal hypertension eventually leading to renal artery vasoconstriction.
  - The clinical picture is typically gross volume overload (ascites, lower extremity edema), intravascular volume depletion resistant to 72 hours of albumin (e.g., hyponatremia, hypotension, dry mucous membranes), and the absence of a causative intrinsic renal disorder (e.g., normal urinalysis and urine sodium <20 mmol).

REFERENCES

1. Runyon BA, Montano AA, Akriviadis EA, et al. The serum-ascites albumin gradient is superior to the exudate-transudate concept in the differential diagnosis of ascites. *Ann Intern Med*. 1992;117(3):215–220.
2. D'Amico G, Garcia-Tsao G, Pagliaro L. Natural history and prognostic indicators of survival in cirrhosis: a systematic review of 118 studies. *Int J Hepatol*. 2006;44(1):217–231.
3. Morali GA, Sniderman KW, Deitel KM, et al. Is sinusoidal portal hypertension a necessary factor for the development of hepatic ascites? *Int J Hepatol*. 1992;16(1–2):249–250.
4. Salerno F, Guervara M, Bernardi M, et al. Refractory ascites: pathogenesis, definition and therapy of a severe complication in patients with cirrhosis. *Liver Int*. 2010;30(7):937–947.
5. Khanna R, Sarin SK. Non-cirrhotic portal hypertension—diagnosis and management. *Int J Hepatol*. 2014;60(2):421–441.
6. Ji JS, Chae HS, Cho YS, et al. Myxedema ascites: case report and literature review. *J Korean Med Sci*. 2006;21(4):761–764.
7. Cattau EL Jr, Benjamin SB, Knuff TE, et al. The accuracy of the physical examination in the diagnosis of suspected ascites. *JAMA*. 1982;247(8):1164–1166.
8. Williams JW, Simel DL. The rational clinical examination. Does this patient have ascites? How to divine fluid in the abdomen. *JAMA*. 1992;267(19):2645–2648.
9. Cadranel JF, Nousbaum JB, Bessaquet C, et al. Low incidence of spontaneous bacterial peritonitis in asymptomatic cirrhotic outpatients. *World J Hepatol*. 2013;5(3):104–108.
10. Kim JJ, Tsukamoto MM, Mathur AK, et al. Delayed paracentesis is associated with increased in-hospital mortality in patients with spontaneous bacterial peritonitis. *Am J Gastroenerol*. 2014; 109(9):1436–1442.
11. Runyon BA, Antillon MR, Akriviadis EA, et al. Bedside inoculation of blood culture bottles with ascetic fluid is superior to delayed inoculation in the detection of spontaneous bacterial peritonitis. *J Clin Microbiol*. 1990;28(12):2811–2812.
12. Campisi C, Bellini C, Eretta C, et al. Diagnosis and management of primary chylous ascites. *J Vasc Surg*. 2006;43(6):1244–1248.
13. Hillebrand DJ, Runyon BA, Yasmineh WG, et al. Ascites fluid adenosine deaminase insensitivity in detecting tuberculous peritonitis in the United States. *Hepatology*. 1996;24(6):1408–1412.

14. Von Kuenssberg Jehle D, Stiller G, Wagner D. Sensitivity in detecting free intraperitoneal fluid with the pelvic views of the FAST exam. *Am J Emerg Med.* 2003;21(6):476–478.

15. Wells ML, Fenstad ER, Poterucha JT, et al. Imaging findings of congestive hepatopathy. *Radiographics.* 2016;36(4):1024–1037.

16. Iranpour P, Lall C, Houshyar R, et al. Altered Doppler flow patterns in cirrhosis patients: an overview. *Ultrasonography.* 2016;35(1):3–12.

17. Eisenmenger WJ, Blondheim SH, Bongiovanni AM, et al. Electrolyte studies on patients with cirrhosis of the liver. *J Clin Invest.* 1950;29(11):1491–1499.

18. Capone RR, Buhac I, Kohberger RC, et al. Resistant ascites in alcoholic liver cirrhosis: course and prognosis. *Am J Dig Dis.* 1978;23(10):867–871.

19. Angeli P, Fasolato S, Mazza E, et al. Combined versus sequential diuretic treatment of ascites in non-azotaemic patients with cirrhosis: results of an open randomized clinical trial. *Gut.* 2010; 59(1):98–104.

20. Sarin SK, Sachdev G, Mishra SP, et al. Bumetanide, spironolactone and a combination of the two, in the treatment of ascites due to liver disease. A prospective, controlled, randomized trial. *Digestion.* 1988;41(2):101–107.

21. Abecasis R, Guevara M, Miguez C, et al. Long-term efficacy of torsemide compared with furosemide in cirrhotic patients with ascites. *Scand J Gastroenterol.* 2001;36(3):309–313.

22. Gentilini P, Casini-Raggi V, Di Fiore G, et al. Albumin improves the response to diuretics in patients with cirrhosis and ascites: results of a randomized controlled trial. *J Hepatol.* 1999;30(4):639–645.

23. Arroyo V, Gines P, Gerbes AL, et al. Definition and diagnostic criteria of refractory ascites and hepatorenal syndrome in cirrhosis. International Ascites Club. *Hepatology.* 1996;23(1):164–176.

24. Planas R, Montoliu S, Balleste B, et al. Natural history of patients hospitalized for management of cirrhotic ascites. *Clin Gastroenterol Hepatol.* 2006;4(11):1385–1394.

25. El-Bokl MA, Senousy BE, El-Karmouty KZ, et al. Spot urinary sodium for assessing dietary sodium restriction in cirrhotic ascites. *World J Gastroenterol.* 2009;15(29):3631–3635.

26. Salerno F, Camma C, Enea M, et al. Transjugular intrahepatic portosystemic shunt for refractory ascites: a meta-analysis of individual patient data. *Gastroenterology.* 2007;133(3):825–834.

27. Boyer TD, Haskal ZJ; American Association for the Study of Liver Diseases. The Role of Transjugular Intrahepatic Portosystemic Shunt (TIPS) in the management of portal hypertension: update 2009. *Hepatology.* 2010;51(1):306.

28. Sola-Vera J, Such J. Understanding the mechanisms of paracentesis-induced circulatory dysfunction. *Eur J Gastroenterol Hepatol.* 2004;16(3):295–298.

29. Sola-Vera J, Minana J, Ricart E, et al. Randomized trial comparing albumin and saline in the prevention of paracentesis-induced circulatory dysfunction in cirrhotic patients with ascites. *Hepatology.* 2003;37(5):1147–1153.

30. Inadomi J, Sonnenberg A. Cost-analysis of prophylactic antibiotics in spontaneous bacterial peritonitis. *Gastroenterology.* 1997;113(4):1289–1294.

31. Saab S, Hernandez JC, Chi AC, et al. Oral antibiotic prophylaxis reduces spontaneous bacterial peritonitis occurrence and improves short-term survival in cirrhosis: a meta-analysis. *Am J Gastroenterol.* 2009;104(4):993–1001.

Malnutrition

Osama Altayar and Dominic N. Reeds

11

GENERAL PRINCIPLES

- Assessment of nutritional status is an important aspect in the care of all patients. Nutritional status represents effectiveness of nutrient intake in maintaining body composition and meeting metabolic demands.
- The best overall approach to evaluating nutritional status involves a thorough clinical and physical examination, a nutritional history, and appropriate laboratory studies.
- To effectively manage a patient's nutritional status, familiarity with the basic principles of clinical nutrition is imperative.

Definition

A state of over- or undernutrition can be called malnutrition. For the purposes of this chapter, malnutrition will refer to the state of undernutrition, where nutrient intake is not adequate to meet the body's metabolic demands.

Epidemiology

- Undernutrition is prevalent in hospitalized patients, occurring in 5–50% of patients at admission or during hospital course. In the outpatient setting, malnutrition is encountered in up to 15% of the elderly in addition to 40% being at risk for malnutrition.
- Malnutrition is frequently underdiagnosed. The diagnosis of malnutrition may be missed in up to 40% of patients at the time of admission.[1,2]

Pathophysiology

- Body composition encompasses **lean body mass** (LBM), and **fat mass**.
  - LBM represents total body mass and includes muscle, vital organs, fluid, and bone mass.
  - Fat, in the form of adipose tissue triglyceride, is the body's major fuel reserve.
  - In times of metabolic stress, the body tries to preserve LBM; however, as fat stores run out, visceral protein mass is mobilized to meet metabolic needs, which include acting as gluconeogenic precursors, wound healing, and maintenance of circulating proteins.
- Multiple changes occur in the body as a result of negative energy balance.
  - Initially, there is a modest decrease in resting energy expenditure (REE).
  - There is also a decrease in whole-body protein synthesis, particularly in persons with comorbid disease. This impaired protein synthesis can lead to a decrease in intestinal cell mass and gut mucosal atrophy. Even sustained inanition produces only minor reductions in gut mass, however.
- In most cases, malnutrition is multifactorial. Nutritional disturbance in hospitalized patients typically results from reduced food intake (prescribed by physicians, interruptions around tests or medical procedures, critical illness, dysphagia) and increased metabolic demands (burns, inflammation, fluids lost through drains). Unintentional weight loss is also commonly caused by malignancy, chronic infection/inflammation, gastrointestinal (GI), endocrine, cardiovascular (e.g., cardiac cachexia), and pulmonary disorders such as chronic obstructive pulmonary disease (COPD).

Associated Conditions

- Malnutrition adversely affects many outcomes in hospitalized patients. Increased length of hospital stay, mortality, morbidity, complications during hospitalization, perioperative complications, impaired wound healing, increased frequency of decubitus ulcers, risk to infections, readmission rates, and healthcare cost.
- As little as 5% unintentional weight loss in 1 month can be clinically significant and a weight loss of ≥10% over a 6-month period is associated with worse inhospital outcomes.[3–5]

DIAGNOSIS

- Multiple tools have been developed to assist in nutritional assessment, including the Subjective Global Assessment, Mini Nutritional Assessment, Nutrition Risk Score, Nutrition Risk Index, and Geriatric Risk Index. Studies have been done to validate these tools in assessing for malnutrition, but no gold standard exists. It is important that screening for malnutrition is performed at the time of admission and periodically throughout the hospital course.
- The best overall approach involves a thorough nutritional history and physical examination.
- Two or more of the following should be identified to make the diagnosis of malnutrition: insufficient energy intake, weight loss, loss of muscle mass, loss of subcutaneous fat, localized or generalized fluid accumulation, and/or diminished functional status.[6]
- The current recommended approach is to identify patients at high nutritional risk based on disease severity and nutritional status using specific scoring systems such as NRS-2002 and NUTRIC score. These patients are more likely to have clinical improvement when they receive early nutritional interventions.[7,8]

Clinical Presentation

History

Nutritional assessment includes the following[9]:
- Identification of pre-existing malnutrition before the acute presentation
  - The presence of mild (<5%), moderate (5–10%), or severe (>10%) unintentional weight loss in the last 6 months should be determined. Unintentional weight loss of >10% is associated with a poor clinical outcome.
- Relevant medical and surgical history
- Medications
- Social habits (e.g., alcohol, recreational drug use, who buys the food in the house, etc.)
- Focused dietary history (should assess changes in diet and, if present, the reasons for the changes)

Physical Examination

- Physical examination should include an assessment of the following[9]:
  - Hair, skin, eyes, mouth, dentition, and extremities
  - Fluid status
  - Stigmata of protein calorie malnutrition or vitamin and mineral deficiencies: Temporal muscle wasting, sunken supraclavicular fossae, and decreased adipose stores are easily recognized signs of malnutrition.
- Calculate body mass index (BMI) (BMI = weight in kilograms/height in meters squared) with a weight obtained in the hospital; please see Table 11-1.[9]

Diagnostic Testing

Historically, concentrations of several plasma proteins (e.g., albumin, transferrin, prealbumin) and total lymphocyte count have been used to determine the degree of protein

TABLE 11-1	BODY MASS INDEX–BASED ENERGY REQUIREMENTS FOR HOSPITALIZED PATIENTS
BMI (kg/m^2)	Energy Requirements (kcal/kg/day)
<15	36–45
15–19	31–35
20–29	26–30
>30	15–25

BMI, body mass index.
Adapted from Klein S. A primer of nutritional support for gastroenterologists. *Gastroenterology.* 2002;122(6):1677–1687.

malnutrition and to predict clinical outcomes. However, in many cases, inflammation and injury, not malnutrition, are responsible for low levels of these markers and for the increased incidence of morbidity and mortality. The use of such parameters should be avoided.[7]

TREATMENT

- **Calculating the nutrient requirement**
  - Nutritional requirements are determined by the body's energy demands or **total energy expenditure (TEE)**.
    - TEE = REE (~70% TEE) + thermal effect of food (related to digestion, ~10% TEE) + physical activity (~20% TEE)
    - At times of illness or trauma, the resting energy requirement can increase by as much as 50%. Although it is often not feasible to measure energy expenditure directly in hospitalized patients, a number of predictive equations have been devised to estimate macronutrient requirements.
  - The simplest approach to estimating the caloric needs of a hospitalized patient is based on BMI (Table 11-1).[9]
    - The general rule is that caloric requirement is inversely proportional to BMI, because LBM (which includes organ mass) is the main determinant of energy expenditure. Because organs do not significantly hypertrophy with increasing adiposity, energy expenditure per kilogram body mass progressively declines with increasing adiposity but increases with lower body weights.
    - In critically ill, insulin-resistant patients, a lower-energy dose should be used initially to avoid the deleterious effects of hyperglycemia.
    - In overweight patients, an adjusted body weight (see the following formula) should be used to avoid overfeeding. Adjusted body weight = ideal body weight (IBW) + 0.25 (actual body weight – IBW)
  - Individual protein requirement depends on multiple factors, including the overall nutritional state, energy requirement, and nonprotein caloric intake.[7–9]
    - The recommended protein intake is 0.8 g/kg/day in healthy adults.
    - Normal weight medically ill patients require 1.2–2.0 g/kg/day of protein; however, patients experiencing large protein losses from burns, multitrauma and wounds, or fistulas, might have higher requirements.
    - Where relevant (e.g., surgical drains, nephrotic syndrome), protein losses should be calculated. Both hemo- and peritoneal dialysis increase protein losses and such patients require 1.2–1.4 g/kg IBW/day and 1.3–1.5 g/kg IBW/day, respectively. Patients receiving continuous venovenous hemodialysis have protein requirements approximating 2g/kg IBW/day.

- An ongoing assessment of adequacy of protein provision should be performed.
- In patients with obesity, permissive underfeeding may be employed during acute illness. This may improve glycemic control and reduce infection risk.

- **Nutritional support**
  - Nutritional support (NS) is the provision of nutrients, enteral or parenteral, to treat or prevent malnutrition.
  - NS is indicated in patients in whom volitional, enteral feeding is not possible for a prolonged period of time to prevent the adverse effects of malnutrition.
  - Loss of LBM is tightly associated with mortality and therefore a key goal of NS is to prevent significant weight loss and preserve LBM until recovery from the underlying illness has been achieved.[9]
  - Patients most likely to benefit from early NS are those with baseline malnutrition in whom a protracted period of inadequate nutritional intake is anticipated.
  - A careful assessment of the patient's clinical condition and expected outcome help to determine the need for NS. These factors include baseline nutritional status, disease severity, comorbid conditions, ability to maintain volitional intake, function of GI tract, and risk of aspiration.
  - Individuals who are at high nutritional risk require early NS, whereas patients at low nutritional risk can tolerate longer periods without significant nutritional intake.
  - In general, low nutritional risk hospitalized patients may not require NS for the first week of hospitalization, whereas high nutritional risk patients should be considered for NS within the first 24 hours of admission.
  - Low nutritional risk patients should be assessed daily. The decision to initiate NS must be individualized and the type of support carefully chosen.[7,8]

- **Enteral nutrition**
  - Enteral nutrition is the preferred form of nutrition support because it is safer, more physiologic, and less expensive than parenteral nutrition.
  - Absolute contraindications to enteral feeding include mechanical obstruction, uncontrolled peritonitis, and ischemic bowel.
  - Relative contraindication for enteral feeding include ileus, open abdomen, recent gut anastomoses, GI bleeding, bowel wall edema, and use of vasopressors.[7]

- **Methods of enteral nutrition**
  - For short-term support (<4 weeks), nasogastric or nasoenteric tubes are preferred.
  - Gastrostomy or jejunostomy tubes are indicated if the duration is expected to be >4 weeks. Underlying condition and local expertise should dictate percutaneous, radiologic, or surgically placed gastrostomy tubes.[7]
  - Gastric tube feeds can be given as boluses or continuous pump-controlled infusion depending on tolerance. Small bowel feeds should always be given as continuous infusion to avoid distention, abdominal pain, and dumping syndrome.[9]
  - Boluses should be started at a low dose (150–200 mL) every 4–6 hours and increased by 50–100 mL each feeding until the feeding goal is reached. Each feeding should be followed by a water flush. The amount of water flush depends on the patient's volume status. Pill fragments or thick medications can clog the tube and should be avoided.[2]
  - Patients' upper body should remain upright or elevated by at least at 30 degrees during bolus tube feeds and for 2 hours after to avoid aspiration.[10]
  - Tube feeding should be advanced to goal within 48–72 hours in the absence of intolerance. If reduced tolerance is present, the goal should be reached with caution over 5–7 days.
  - Intolerance can present as vomiting, abdominal distention or discomfort, high gastric residual volumes (GRVs), diarrhea, reduced bowel movements or flatus, or abnormal radiographs.

GRVs should not be used routinely. If used, automatic cessation of gastric feeding in the absence of other signs of intolerance for GRVs <500 mL should be avoided and measures to reduce the risk of aspiration should be implemented.[7,8]

- **Postpyloric or small bowel feeding**
  - Small-caliber nasojejunal feeding tubes can be placed past the ligament of Treitz for short-term postpyloric or small bowel feeding and percutaneous, surgical, or radiographic jejunostomy tubes can be placed for long-term feeding.[10]
  - Small bowel feeds are associated with a decreased risk of aspiration, better tolerated by patients with impaired motility, and have less pancreatic stimulation. They are often used in the setting of severe acute pancreatitis, intolerance of gastric feeding, or patient with high risk of aspiration.
  - Small bowel feeds are given as a continuous infusion and typically start with 10–30 mL/hr and are increased in small increments (10 mL/hr every 8–12 hours) until the feeding goal is reached. Again, these tubes should be flushed with water every 4 hours to avoid tube occlusion.[9]
  - Bolus feeds should not be used with small bowel feeding tubes to prevent fluid shifts, abdominal distension, and diarrhea.[10]
- **Choosing an enteral formula**
  - Standard, intact-protein tube feeding formulas (e.g., Ensure[TM]) are sufficient for most patients.
    - They are free of gluten and lactose and are isotonic.
    - They contain 1.0 cal/mL, and intake of 1500 to 2000 mL/day provides 100% of carbohydrates, protein, fat, vitamins, and minerals.
  - Monomeric (e.g., Vivonex[TM]) and oligomeric (e.g., Peptamen[TM]) formulas consist of shorter, partially or completely, digested protein fragments and shorter chain glucose polymers which theoretically enhance absorption. They can be used in patients with malabsorption such as patients with pancreatic insufficiency or short gut syndrome. However, the use of these formulas is controversial because they are more expensive than standard formulas and only few studies have shown they may confer an advantage over intact formulas. They are also hyperosmotic and may cause osmotic diarrhea.[9]
- **Parenteral nutrition**
  - Total parenteral nutrition (TPN) is the infusion of a nutritional liquid formulation through a central venous catheter that can provide complete nutritional requirements. Partial parenteral nutrition (PPN) is an intravenous solution that is less concentrated than TPN and can therefore be infused through a peripheral venous catheter. However, PPN is not able to meet nutritional needs and generally causes venous thrombosis of the catheterized vein within a short timespan; this method of nutrition support should generally be avoided.
  - TPN is indicated if the GI tract is functionally (e.g. ileus) or physically obstructed distal to the site of enteral feeding (e.g., short gut syndrome, or malabsorptive process). In previously well-nourished patients, TPN may be indicated if enteral feeding is incapable of meeting caloric or macronutrient needs after 7–10 days. In malnourished patients, in whom enteral feeding is unlikely to be possible for a prolonged period of time, early institution of TPN should be considered.[7,8]
  - TPN-dependent patients who are hospitalized should be restarted on TPN as soon as possible in the absence of evidence of bacteremia.
  - Due to the hyperosmolality of TPN, it requires central venous access. The optimal location of the tip of the central venous catheter is at the junction of the superior vena cava and the right atrium. In patients in whom TPN is likely to be prolonged (>6 months) or lifelong, a tunneled central venous catheter should be placed as these are more durable. In appropriate catheters, an alcohol-lock technique may be applied to reduce infection risk.[11,12]

- **Composition and administration of TPN**
  - TPN solution can be purchased commercially or can be made by the hospital pharmacy.
  - Total number of calories and amount of protein are determined using the guidelines described in the Calculating the Nutrient Requirement section earlier in this chapter.
  - Lipid content of TPN ideally provides 20–30% of the daily calories; a 20% lipid emulsion yields 2.0 kcal/mL. The carbohydrate component is dextrose and provides the remainder of the calories; it contains 3.4 kcal/g.[9,12]
  - Electrolytes, minerals, trace elements, and a multivitamin preparation are generally added to the parenteral solution. Note that iron is not generally part of the standard additives.
  - TPN should be initiated at one-half to two-thirds of the total volume over the first 24 hours to avoid large fluid shifts and hyperglycemia. The volume is then advanced as tolerated. Once the volume goal has been reached, the rate of infusion can be increased and TPN can be infused over 10–14 hours.
  - Cyclic (rather than continuous) infusion of TPN improves quality of life and decreases incidence of hepatobiliary complications. Shortened infusion time, however, can lead to periods of hyperglycemia.
  - During initiation of nutrition support, **close monitoring is indicated**, with frequent measurement of vital signs, daily weights, intake and output, as well as the following:
    - Blood glucose checks every 6–8 hours.
    - Comprehensive metabolic panel should be checked daily until feeds are at goal and then twice weekly.
    - Complete blood cell count may be checked once weekly.

COMPLICATIONS

- **Complications of tube feedings**
  - Enteral feeding is a relatively safe procedure, and complications usually can be avoided or adequately managed. Tubes placed nasally must be avoided in patients with the potential for basilar skull fracture or recent cranial surgery. Perforation of the esophagus or small bowel may occur in patients with severe underlying bowel disease such as ischemia.
  - In addition to the complications of percutaneous tube placement (infection, bleeding, inadvertent colonic placement), patients may experience the following complications[9,10]:
    - **Aspiration.** To limit the risk of aspiration, the head of the patient's bed should be raised ≥30 degrees during feeding and for 2 hours afterward. Intermittent or continuous feeding regimens, rather than the rapid bolus method, should be used. All patients should be observed for signs of feeding intolerance. Small bowel access is helpful either in patients with recurrent tube feeding aspiration (not oropharyngeal) or in patients unable to tolerate gastric feeding.
    - **Diarrhea.** Evaluation for the presence of diarrhea versus incontinence, and common etiologies should be performed. This includes checking for antibiotic-associated diarrhea and to look for sorbitol in other orally administered medications. To minimize the incidence of diarrhea related to tube feeding, it is advisable to use an isosmotic, lactose-free formula and to advance tube feeds slowly. Decreasing the rate of the feeds, switching to continuous tube feeds, and adding fiber to the formula can be helpful. If these measures fail and infectious causes have been ruled out, an antidiarrheal agent may be appropriate.
    - **Hyperglycemia.** Adequate blood glucose monitoring is necessary when starting enteral nutrition. Initially, sliding-scale regular insulin can be used to control blood glucose concentrations. Once the feedings have reached 1000 kcal/day, scheduled, short-acting insulin given every 4 hours can be used for blood glucose control.

- **Small bowel necrosis.** Patients who require pressor support to maintain an adequate blood pressure are at risk for small bowel necrosis with small bowel feeds. The early signs of bowel ischemia are not specific and include bloating, loss of bowel sounds, abdominal pain, and ileus. If enteral nutrition is necessary in a patient with hypotension, he or she should be carefully monitored for any signs of early bowel ischemia.

- **Complications of parenteral nutrition**
  - Mechanical complications
    - **Central line placement.** Complications related to central line placement include pneumothorax, brachial plexus injury, subclavian or carotid artery puncture, hemothorax, and chylothorax.
    - **Thrombosis or pulmonary embolism.** This can occur secondary to central venous catheter use. Radiologically evident subclavian vein thrombosis occurs commonly (25–50%), but clinically significant manifestations (e.g., upper extremity edema, superior vena cava syndrome, or pulmonary embolus) are rare. Inline filters should be used with all TPN solutions.
    - **Infectious.** Complications are most commonly caused by *Staphylococcus epidermidis* or *Staphylococcus aureus* and fungal species. In immunocompromised patients, gram-negative rods and *Candida* species are also a major concern.
  - Metabolic complications
    - **Hyperglycemia.** In patients with type 2 diabetes mellitus (T2DM) and blood glucose levels <200 mg/dL, consideration should be made of using 1 unit insulin for every 10 g of carbohydrate in the TPN container. In patients with T2DM or receiving high-dose steroids with blood glucose >200 mg/dL, an insulin:carbohydrate ratio of 1:5 may be necessary. Blood glucose levels should be checked frequently and sliding-scale insulin (SSI) used to control hyperglycemia. If blood glucose levels remain elevated despite SSI, additional insulin should be added to the TPN solution, equal to 50% of the SSI from the previous 24 hours. If this fails, an intravenous insulin drip or further reduction in TPN carbohydrate dose may be required. Protocol-based empiric insulin therapy improves glycemic control more rapidly than an ad hoc method.[9,13]
    - **Hypertriglyceridemia.** Triglyceride levels >500 mg/dL can cause or exacerbate acute pancreatitis and have been associated with thrombocytopenia. The levels should be checked at baseline and at least once during lipid emulsion infusion to ensure adequate clearance. Most practitioners reduce or eliminate lipids in the emulsion with serum triglyceride levels >400 mg/dL. The sedative propofol is administered in a 10% (1.1 kcal/mL) lipid emulsion and should be counted as part of the lipid calories. Hyperglycemia is a reversible cause of hypertriglyceridemia in patients receiving TPN.
    - **Hepatobiliary.** Complications include elevated levels of serum transaminases and alkaline phosphatase. In addition, steatosis, steatohepatitis, lipidosis, cholestasis, fibrosis, and cirrhosis can occur. Although these abnormalities are usually benign and transient, more serious and progressive disease can develop in a small subset of patients, usually after 16 weeks of TPN. Biliary complications typically occur with TPN administered for longer than 3 weeks and include acalculous cholecystitis, gallbladder sludge, and cholelithiasis.
    - **Metabolic bone disease.** Osteomalacia or osteopenia may be seen with long-term (>3 months) total TPN.

- **Refeeding syndrome**
  - Refeeding syndrome refers to the massive fluid and electrolytes shifts that can occur when a severely malnourished patient is initiated on NS, leading to volume overload, cardiovascular collapse, and death.[9,14]
  - **Electrolyte depletion** is the most dangerous complication of initial refeeding.

- With the administration of a carbohydrate load, serum levels of phosphorous, potassium, and magnesium rapidly fall, because of insulin-mediated transcellular shifts in the face of whole-body electrolyte depletion.
- Hypophosphatemia can lead to respiratory muscle paralysis and cardiovascular collapse.
- The rapid fall in potassium and magnesium levels can lead to cardiac dysfunction and arrhythmias.
- **Volume overload** (secondary to fluid administered with the nutritional supplement and insulin-mediated sodium retention) is the characteristic of refeeding syndrome and may progress quickly to congestive heart failure.
- **Cardiac abnormalities** include prolongation of the QT interval, which, combined with plasma electrolyte abnormalities, lead to an increased risk of ventricular arrhythmias and sudden cardiac death during the first week of refeeding.
- **Thiamine deficiency** can lead to acute beriberi, which, in turn, can lead to lactic acidosis, edema, and heart failure.
- The best approach to refeeding syndrome is prevention by starting feeds slowly and aggressively supplementing potassium, magnesium, and phosphate in patients with normal renal function.
  - Initial feeding should start at 15 kcal/kg/day and can advance slowly as tolerated.
  - Serum levels of potassium, magnesium, and phosphorus should be checked every 12 hours until at goal feeds with stable electrolytes.
  - Thiamine should be supplemented intravenously at 500 mg/day for 3 days.
  - To prevent fluid overload, initial fluid intake and sodium should be limited, and patient weight should be monitored daily. Weight gain in excess of 0.25 kg/day or 1.5 kg/wk should be treated as volume overload; fluid intake should be reduced, and diuretics used as necessary.
  - Electrocardiogram should be obtained at baseline, and patients should be monitored on telemetry during early refeeding.

REFERENCES

1. Norman K, Pichard C, Lochs H, et al. Prognostic impact of disease-related malnutrition. *Clin Nutr.* 2008;27(1):5–15.
2. Win AZ, Ceresa C, Arnold K, et al. High prevalence of malnutrition among elderly veterans in home based primary care. *J Nutr Health Aging.* 2017;21(6):610–613.
3. Kirkland LL, Shaughnessy E. Recognition and prevention of nosocomial malnutrition: a review and a call to action! *Am J Med.* 2017;130(12):1345–1350.
4. Linn BS. Outcomes of older and younger malnourished and well-nourished patients one year after hospitalization. *Am J Clin Nutr.* 1984;39(1):66–73.
5. Dewys WD, Begg C, Lavin PT, et al. Prognostic effect of weight loss prior to chemotherapy in cancer patients. Eastern Cooperative Oncology Group. *Am J Med.* 1980;69(4):491–497.
6. White JV, Guenter P, Jensen G, et al. Consensus statement: Academy of Nutrition and Dietetics and American Society for Parenteral and Enteral Nutrition: characteristics recommended for the identification and documentation of adult malnutrition (undernutrition). *JPEN J Parenter Enteral Nutr.* 2012;36(3):275–283.
7. McClave SA, DiBaise JK, Mullin GE, et al. ACG clinical guideline: nutrition therapy in the adult hospitalized patient. *Am J Gastroenterol.* 2016;111(3):315-334; quiz 335.
8. McClave SA, Taylor BE, Martindale RG, et al. Guidelines for the Provision and Assessment of Nutrition Support Therapy in the adult critically ill patient: Society of Critical Care Medicine (SCCM) and American Society for Parenteral and Enteral Nutrition (A.S.P.E.N.). *JPEN J Parenter Enteral Nutr.* 2016;40(2):159–211.
9. Klein S. A primer of nutritional support for gastroenterologists. *Gastroenterology.* 2002;122(6):1677–1687.
10. Kirby DF, Delegge MH, Fleming CR. American Gastroenterological Association technical review on tube feeding for enteral nutrition. *Gastroenterology.* 1995;108(4):1282–1301.

11. Abu-El-Haija M, Schultz J, Rahhal RM. Effects of 70% ethanol locks on rates of central line infection, thrombosis, breakage, and replacement in pediatric intestinal failure. *J Pediatr Gastroenterol Nutr*. 2014;58(6):703–708.
12. Koretz RL, Lipman TO, Klein S; American Gastroenterological Association. AGA technical review on parenteral nutrition. *Gastroenterology*. 2001;121(4):970–1001.
13. Jakoby MG, Nannapaneni N. An insulin protocol for management of hyperglycemia in patients receiving parenteral nutrition is superior to ad hoc management. *JPEN J Parenter Enteral Nutr*. 2012;36(2):183–188.
14. Kraft MD, Btaiche IF, Sacks GS. Review of the refeeding syndrome. *Nutr Clin Pract*. 2005;20(6):625–633.

Obesity

Michael C. Bennett and
Vladimir M. Kushnir

12

GENERAL PRINCIPLES

- Obesity is a chronic disease characterized by excess body fat. It is increasing in prevalence and is associated with many of the leading causes of morbidity and mortality in the United States and worldwide.
- Recognition of the complex pathophysiologic, environmental, and societal factors contributing to weight gain is important in the evaluation and management of the patient with obesity.
- An understanding of the impact of obesity on other disease states should inform clinical decision making.
- Treatment of obesity requires a multidisciplinary approach. Strategies include therapeutic lifestyle intervention, medications, and surgical or endoscopic therapy.

Definition

- Body mass index (BMI), or weight in kilograms divided by the square of height in meters, is used as a surrogate marker for body fat and is a useful screening tool. BMI of 18.5–25 is considered normal. BMI between 25 and 30 is considered overweight. Obesity is defined as a BMI over 30.
- Obesity is further subdivided into class 1 (BMI 30–35), class 2 (BMI 35–40), and class 3 or severe obesity (BMI above 40).
- Other measures of body fat composition include skinfold thickness measurement, bioelectrical impedance, underwater weighing, and dual energy x-ray absorptiometry.[1]

Epidemiology

- The prevalence of obesity in US adults is 39.8%. The rate of obesity is higher among Hispanic (47.0%) and non-Hispanic black (46.8%) adults compared with non-Hispanic white adults (37.9%).[2]
- The rates of obesity and severe obesity among US adults have been increasing since the 1980s. Between 2007 and 2016, the prevalence of obesity increased from 33.7 to 39.6%, and the prevalence of severe obesity increased from 5.7 to 7.7%.[3]

Etiology

- Changes in the food environment, eating behaviors, and physical activity level have contributed to the increased prevalence of obesity. Among these changes are increased availability and consumption of processed foods containing high sugar, salt, fat, and flavor additive content, less time spent preparing meals at home, larger portion sizes, and less occupational physical activity.[4]
- Complex genetic factors increase susceptibility to obesity, and the rate of heritability of BMI has been estimated to be between 40% and 70%. Obesity has been associated with abnormalities in multiple genes, including leptin, melanocortin-4, and fat mass and obesity related (FTO) gene, though these abnormalities account for only a small percentage of individual BMI variation.[5]

- Intrauterine and early childhood factors impact risk for obesity later in life. Maternal diabetes, smoking, and poor nutrition increase obesity risk. Children who breastfeed and those who get more sleep appear to have decreased obesity risk.[6]
- The intestinal microbiota has a complex role in the breakdown of nutrients and maintenance of gut barrier function, among other interactions with the host. Variations in microbiota composition have been associated with obesity and insulin resistance in humans, and causal relationships have been demonstrated in animal models.[7]
- Energy balance is regulated in part through hypothalamic and other brain pathways, which control food intake and energy expenditure. Creation of a negative energy balance by increasing activity or decreasing food intake produces compensatory mechanisms such as increased appetite signals; clinically, this may lead to weight regain in patients who have lost weight.[5]
- Obesity can occur as a result of other medical conditions, such as hypothyroidism, polycystic ovarian syndrome (PCOS), Cushing syndrome, and hypogonadism. Many medications can promote weight gain, including corticosteroids, insulin, and several antipsychotics and antidepressants. Psychological illness can be both a cause and consequence of obesity.

Pathophysiology

- Obesity is characterized by gradual accumulation of excess lipids, primarily triglycerides, which are distributed to subcutaneous and visceral adipose tissue.[5] This results in enlarged fat cells, which produce effect through increased fat mass and increased production of adipokines and other endocrine activity.[6]
- Increased fat mass can produce mechanical stress leading to multiple disease processes. Mechanical effect on pharyngeal tissue can cause obstructive sleep apnea, weight load on joints can lead to osteoarthritis, and increased intra-abdominal pressure can lead to gastroesophageal reflux disease (GERD) and its complications, Barrett esophagus, and esophageal adenocarcinoma.[5]
- Increased circulation of adipokines along with proinflammatory cytokines, produced by fat cells and associated macrophages and other inflammatory cells, lead to insulin resistance and type II diabetes. Insulin resistance and increased lipid production from adipocytes lead to nonalcoholic fatty liver disease (NAFLD) and its complications, steatohepatitis, and cirrhosis. Increased adiposity also activates the renin-angiotensin-aldosterone system and sympathetic nervous system, leading to systemic and pulmonary hypertension. These processes together can cause coronary artery disease, congestive heart failure, stroke, and chronic kidney disease.[5]

Associated Conditions

- All-cause mortality has a J-shaped relationship with BMI, with underweight individuals and those with BMI above 25 having increased risk of death that increases with BMI.[6]
- Obesity is associated with disorders of nearly all organ systems. Weight loss typically results in improvement in obesity-associated comorbidity, though the degree varies.
- Diabetes is strongly associated with obesity. BMI, waist circumference, and total body weight are predictors of type II diabetes development. Weight loss therapy has demonstrated benefit in hemoglobin A1c levels in multiple studies.[8]
- Obesity and in particular central adiposity correlate with dyslipidemia, or low HDL and high triglyceride and LDL levels.[6]
- Hypertension is more common in patients with obesity, and intentional weight loss decreases blood pressure—for every kilogram lost, systolic blood pressure drops by 1.2 mm Hg.[8]
- Cardiovascular disease, the leading cause of mortality in the United States, is increased in patients with obesity, in large part due to increased diabetes, dyslipidemia, and

hypertension. Risk for congestive heart failure, atrial fibrillation, and stroke are also increased with obesity.[6]

- NAFLD refers to the development of hepatic steatosis and hepatomegaly due to fat deposition, which progresses to steatohepatitis, fibrosis, cirrhosis, and hepatocellular carcinoma. NAFLD prevalence is around 30% in the overall population, and increases to 65–92% in patients with obesity class 2 or higher.[8]

- Gallstone disease occurs in patients with obesity at 2.5–3-fold higher rates than in the general population. Rapid weight loss, though, can also be associated with symptomatic cholelithiasis.[8]

- Obesity contributes to the development of pancreatitis through its association with gallstone disease, hypertriglyceridemia, and diabetes. Obesity may increase the severity of acute pancreatitis, in part related to visceral fat necrosis.[9]

- GERD increases with BMI, as do erosive esophagitis, Barrett esophagus, and esophageal adenocarcinoma. BMI above 25 confers an odds ratio of 1.4 for GERD compared to normal weight, and BMI over 30 increases the odds ratio to 1.9.[6] Risk for Barrett esophagus increases by approximately 35% for each 5-unit increase in BMI, and BMI over 40 confers an odds ratio of 4.76 for esophageal adenocarcinoma, compared with nonoverweight patients.[10]

- Higher BMI progressively increases risk for end-stage renal disease (ESRD) even correcting for common causes of ESRD including hypertension and diabetes.[6]

- Many types of cancers show increased prevalence in patients with obesity. Death rate from all cancers is higher with severe obesity, with a relative risk of 1.5–1.6 compared to normal weight. Stronger associations are demonstrated with colon, renal, pancreatic, esophageal adenocarcinoma, breast, and prostate cancers.[8]

- Pulmonary complications include obstructive sleep apnea and the related obesity hypoventilation syndrome, which can result in pulmonary hypertension. Pneumonia also appears to be more common with obesity.[6]

- Osteoarthritis and chronic back and joint pain are associated with obesity by a factor of three. Symptoms improve with weight loss.[8]

- Prevalence of obesity is higher in patients with several different mental illnesses, including depression, anxiety, bipolar disorder, and schizophrenia.[8]

- Social stigmatization of overweight and obesity can reduce quality of life and impact patients' interactions with physicians and other healthcare professionals.

DIAGNOSIS

Clinical Presentation

- Patients should be screened for overweight and obesity as part of a comprehensive annual physical examination. It is useful to consider BMI as a vital sign.[11]

- Patients with a BMI over 25 should be evaluated for risk factors for cardiovascular disease and other obesity-related comorbidities. This evaluation, along with an assessment of readiness to make lifestyle changes to achieve weight loss, should guide shared decision making with the patient regarding treatment modalities.[11]

- The patient's lifestyle and weight history should be reviewed. Age of onset of weight gain, prior weight loss attempts, dietary habits, physical activity level, psychosocial factors, smoking history, and family history of obesity and related diseases are important.

- Careful attention should be given to the patient's medication list. Medications associated with weight gain include: corticosteroids, insulin, sulfonylureas, antipsychotics, antiepileptic and mood stabilizing agents, antihistamines, antidepressants, hormonal agents, β-blockers, and α-blockers.[12]

- In addition to BMI, blood pressure should be measured in all patients, and waist circumference is a useful measurement in patients with a BMI between 25 and 35. Central adiposity as measured by waist circumference correlates with visceral adiposity, which increases the risk of complications such as diabetes and NAFLD. Abnormal waist circumference is >35 in (88 cm) in women and >40 in (102 cm) in men.[12]

- The physical examination should include assessment both for causes of secondary obesity and complications of obesity. Acne or hirsutism can suggest PCOS, acanthosis nigricans suggests insulin resistance, and purple striae may be seen with Cushing syndrome, along with proximal muscle weakness. Thyroid nodules or goiter point to hypothyroidism. Atrial fibrillation and congestive heart failure can be detected by irregular heart rhythm and S3 or S4 gallop, respectively. Peripheral edema may suggest venous stasis or pulmonary hypertension. Pseudotumor cerebri manifests with papilledema.[12]

Diagnostic Testing

- Laboratory testing should be performed in patients with obesity. This should include a hemoglobin A1c (or fasting glucose), fasting lipid panel, liver chemistries, and thyroid function testing.
- Additional diagnostic testing should be performed if the history, physical examination, or routine blood tests raise suspicion for an obesity-related comorbidity. These may include electrocardiography, echocardiography, overnight sleep study, right upper quadrant ultrasound for fatty liver or gallstone disease, or transvaginal ultrasound for ovarian cysts.[12]

TREATMENT

Lifestyle/Risk Modification

- Patients with a BMI over 30 or a BMI over 25 with risk factors for obesity-associated comorbidity and who are ready to make lifestyle changes should be offered comprehensive lifestyle intervention, which should be the foundation of any weight loss program. Components include diet, exercise, and behavior modification.
- Dietary intake should be reduced to attain a negative energy balance. For most adults, 1200–1500 kcal/day for women and 1500–1800 kcal/day for men[13] is appropriate.
- Sustained weight loss is more likely to be successful with an individualized, structured meal plan, which can be developed with the guidance of a registered dietician. There is little evidence supporting any particular macronutrient or elimination diet.[13] Very low–calorie diets (typically 800 kcal/day or less) result in short-term weight loss, but weight is often regained and complications may occur.
- Physical activity should be increased. Aerobic exercise for at least 150 minutes per week and a goal of 10,000 steps per day are recommended. For patients with limited mobility, assistance from a physical therapist may be needed to successfully begin such a program.
- Behavioral interventions are most successful with in-person, individual ,or group sessions with a trained interventionist. A high-intensity intervention should include at least 14 sessions in a 6-month period.[11] Behaviors to develop include self-monitoring, stimulus control, social support, and relapse prevention.
- After a period of intensive weight loss intervention, continued support should be provided to help the patient maintain a stable weight. Intermittent goal-setting and positive behavior reinforcement are needed. Patients who maintain increased physical activity levels and regularly monitor weight and food intake are less likely to regain weight.[11]

Medications

- Pharmacotherapy is an appropriate addition to lifestyle intervention in patients with a BMI >27 with weight-related comorbidity or in patients with a BMI >30.[11] Several medications have been approved by the U.S. Food and Drug Administration (FDA) for the treatment of obesity.

- In general, weight loss medications should be considered long-term therapy for a chronic relapsing illness. Discontinuation of medications often leads to regain of lost weight.

  ○ *Phentermine* is the most commonly prescribed weight loss medication in the United States. It is a sympathomimetic amine that likely reduces appetite by releasing cate-cholamines in the hypothalamus. In one study, patients achieved an average of 5.1% total body weight loss (TBWL) on phentermine compared with placebo. Side effects include elevations in heart rate and blood pressure, insomnia, irritability, and gastro-intestinal complaints. Treatment is not approved for long-term use, but off-label use may be appropriate in some cases.[14]

  ○ *Orlistat* impairs fat absorption by inhibiting pancreatic and gastric lipase. Around 3% TBWL average has been reported. Side effects include flatulence, oily stools, fecal urgency and incontinence, and risk of fat-soluble vitamin deficiencies.

  ○ *Phentermine/topiramate* is a combination pill that acts centrally to reduce appetite and improve satiety. Large randomized controlled trials showed TBWL of 6.6–8.6% compared to placebo. In addition to phentermine adverse effects, neurologic or men-tal status changes can occur.

  ○ *Lorcaserin* is a 5-hydroxytryptamine receptor 2C (5-HT2c) agonist that acts in the hypothalamus to promote satiety. 3.6% TBWL was reported in a randomized con-trolled trial. Older serotonin analogs were withdrawn due to cardiac valve disease, but lorcaserin did not have this effect due to its selectivity. Serotonergic overload is a risk if co-administered with other serotonin agents.

  ○ *Naltrexone/bupropion* is another combination pill that appears to work by activating satiety centers in the hypothalamus. 4.8% TBWL above placebo was reported in a randomized controlled trial. It should not be used in patients with seizure disorder, eating disorders, or addiction. Nausea is the most common side effect.

  ○ *Liraglutide* is a glucagon-like peptide 1 (GLP 1) receptor agonist, which may slow gastric emptying in addition to acting centrally. It is an injectable drug. Around 4.5% TBWL is average. Gastrointestinal side effects are most common, and hypoglycemia is a risk. It is contraindicated in patients with thyroid cancer history or multiple endocrine neoplasia.[14]

Surgical Management

- Adults with BMI over 40 or BMI over 35 with obesity-related comorbidity, motivation to lose weight, and prior unsuccessful response to behavioral treatment are candidates for bariatric surgery. Patients should be offered referral to an experienced bariatric sur-geon for evaluation.[11]

- Bariatric surgery should be offered as part of a comprehensive program including ther-apeutic lifestyle intervention, with involvement of experts in nutrition, mental health, medical weight management, and surgery.

- Weight loss surgery has demonstrated high efficacy in attaining substantial rapid and durable weight loss as well as improvement in comorbid conditions and survival.[15]

- Roux-en-Y gastric bypass (RYGB) works by restrictive and malabsorptive processes to induce weight loss. The stomach is divided to create a small gastric pouch, and the jejunum is divided distal to the ligament of Treitz. The gastric pouch is anastomosed to the distal jejunal ("roux") limb, such that the food stream bypasses the biliopancreatic limb. The two limbs are anastomosed into a common channel, usually about 100 cm distal to the gastrojejunal anastomosis.[15]

  ○ Expected weight loss with RYGB is between 25% and 35% TBWL, or 60–80% excess weight loss.[15,16] There is initial rapid weight loss followed by stabilization. Weight loss is durable over a decade or more in the majority of patients.

  ○ Short-term complications include bleeding, anastomotic leak, wound complications, and bowel obstruction. Serious complications occur in about 3.4% of patients.[15]

- Long-term complications include abdominal pain, marginal ulcer, internal hernia, nutritional deficiencies, and dumping syndrome (postprandial fluid shifts or hypoglycemia).
- Sleeve gastrectomy (SG) is a restrictive procedure in which the greater curvature of the stomach is resected, leaving a narrow gastric sleeve.
  - Most recent comparative studies have shown similar efficacy between RYGB and SG, though weight loss with SG was slightly lower in some studies.[15,16]
  - Complications include bleeding or leaking at the staple line. Nutritional deficiencies and dumping syndrome may occur. GERD may be worsened by SG.
- Gastric banding involves placement of an adjustable, inflated band around the proximal stomach, resulting in restriction. This procedure has declined in popularity due to long-term complication risk and frequent reoperation.
- Biliopancreatic diversion with duodenal switch is a more radical malabsorptive procedure than RYGB, involving a partial gastrectomy and Roux-en-Y gastroileostomy. It is highly efficacious but has considerable risk of complications including malnutrition and is not commonly performed, usually limited to patients with BMI over 50. In a head-to-head comparison, patients with BMI between 50 and 60 had an average BMI reduction of 22.1 with duodenal switch compared to 13.6 with RYGB.[15]
- **Endoscopic bariatric therapy** refers to the use of devices requiring flexible gastrointestinal endoscopy for placement and/or removal. These devices have been shown to have greater efficacy than lifestyle intervention alone. Reported weight loss is generally greater than that with pharmacotherapy and less than that with surgery, though with lower complication risk.[17]
  - Intragastric balloons (IGB) work by occupying space in the stomach and slowing gastric emptying. They are approved for use in patients with BMI between 30 and 40.
    - Fluid-filled IGBs are placed endoscopically, and gas-filled IGBs are swallowed in an encapsulated form and inflated in the stomach via an attached catheter. Both devices are removed endoscopically after 6 months.
    - Reported weight loss in randomized controlled trials is 6.6–10.2% TBWL.[17]
    - Common complications include abdominal pain, vomiting, and GERD, which can lead to early removal.
    - Serious complications (balloon migration, bowel perforation, GI bleeding) are very uncommon, occurring in <0.05% of patients.
  - Aspiration therapy involves endoscopic placement of a percutaneous gastrostomy tube that is used to remove a portion of gastric contents after a meal, reducing caloric absorption in the small bowel. In a randomized controlled trial, an average of 14.2% TBWL was reported.[17] Skin site complications are most common, including granulation tissue, irritation, and infection. Aspiration therapy is approved for use in patients with a BMI over 35.
  - Endoscopic sleeve gastroplasty (ESG) uses an endoscopic suturing device to place full-thickness sutures along the greater curvature of the stomach, reducing effective gastric volume. 16.2–19.8% TBWL has been reported in multicenter case series.[17] Complications include accommodative symptoms and rarely perigastric fluid collections. ESG is an appropriate procedure for patients with BMI over 30.

REFERENCES

1. Centers for Disease Control and Prevention. *Defining adult overweight and obesity.* 2017. Available at https://www.cdc.gov/obesity/adult/defining.html. Accessed August 11, 2019.
2. Hales CM, Carroll MD, Fryar CD, et al. Prevalence of obesity among adults and youth: United States, 2015–2016. *NCHS Data Brief.* 2017;288:1–8.
3. Hales CM, Fryar CD, Carroll MD, et al. Trends in obesity and severe obesity prevalence in US youth and adults by sex and age, 2007–2008 to 2015–2016. *JAMA.* 2018;319:1723–1725.

4. Hall KD. Did the food environment cause the obesity epidemic? *Obesity (Silver Spring)*. 2018;26:11–13.

5. Heymsfield SB, Wadden TA. Mechanisms, pathophysiology, and management of obesity. *N Engl J Med*. 2017;376:254–266.

6. Bray GA. Obesity. In: Feldman M, Friedman LS, Brandt LJ, eds. *Sleisenger and Fordtran's Gastrointestinal and Liver Disease*. Philadelphia, PA: Saunders Elsevier; 2016:102–118.

7. Bouter KE, van Raalte DH, Groen AK, et al. Role of the gut microbiome in the pathogenesis of obesity and obesity-related metabolic dysfunction. *Gastroenterology*. 2017;152:1671–1678.

8. Rueda-Clausen CF, Ogunleye AA, Sharma AM. Health benefits of long-term weight-loss maintenance. *Annu Rev Nutr*. 2015;35:475–516.

9. Khatua B, El-Kurdi B, Singh VP. Obesity and pancreatitis. *Curr Opin Gastroenterol*. 2017;33: 374–382.

10. Chang P, Friedenberg F. Obesity and GERD. *Gastroenterol Clin North Am*. 2014;43:161–173.

11. American College of Cardiology/American Heart Association Task Force on Practice Guidelines, Obesity Expert Panel, 2013. Executive summary: guidelines (2013) for the management of overweight and obesity in adults: a report of the American College of Cardiology/American Heart Association Task Force on Practice Guidelines and the Obesity Society published by the Obesity Society and American College of Cardiology/American Heart Association Task Force on Practice Guidelines. Based on a systematic review from the The Obesity Expert Panel, 2013. *Obesity (Silver Spring)*. 2014;22(Suppl 2):S5–S39.

12. Tsai AG, Wadden TA. In the clinic: obesity. *Ann Intern Med*. 2013;159:ITC3-1–ITC3-15; quiz ITC3-6.

13. Acosta A, Streett S, Kroh MD, et al. White Paper AGA: POWER—practice guide on obesity and weight management, education, and resources. *Clin Gastroenterol Hepatol*. 2017;15:631–649.e10.

14. Srivastava G, Apovian CM. Current pharmacotherapy for obesity. *Nat Rev Endocrinol*. 2018;14:12–24.

15. Nudel J, Sanchez VM. Surgical management of obesity. *Metabolism*. 2019;92:206–216.

16. Li J, Lai D, Wu D. Laparoscopic Roux-en-Y gastric bypass versus laparoscopic sleeve gastrectomy to treat morbid obesity-related comorbidities: a systematic review and meta-analysis. *Obes Surg*. 2016;26:429–442.

17. Sullivan S, Edmundowicz SA, Thompson CC. Endoscopic bariatric and metabolic therapies: new and emerging technologies. *Gastroenterology*. 2017;152:1791–1801.

Esophageal Disorders

Stephen Hasak and C. Prakash Gyawali

13

Gastroesophageal Reflux Disease

GENERAL PRINCIPLES

Definition

- The Montreal consensus defines gastroesophageal reflux disease (GERD) as "a condition which develops when the reflux of stomach contents causes troublesome symptoms and/or complications."
- Symptoms are "troublesome" if they are frequent and have an adverse effect on a patient's well-being.[1]

Epidemiology

- The true prevalence of GERD is difficult to ascertain because clinical diagnosis is relatively subjective, and not all patients with GERD undergo confirmatory testing.
- Various studies have estimated the prevalence of patients in the Western world with GERD to be as high as 20%, with 30–40% of the population reporting at least occasional symptoms consistent with GERD.[2]

Pathophysiology

- Several mechanisms underlie abnormal reflux, all of which result in the failure of the gastroesophageal junction to prevent gastric contents from entering the esophagus and/or poor clearance of refluxate.
- The gastroesophageal junction is composed of the lower esophageal sphincter (LES), the crural diaphragm, and the phrenoesophageal ligament.
- Under most circumstances, GERD is related to transient, inappropriate LES relaxations. Less frequently, the gastroesophageal junction may be mechanically compromised, with decreased LES resting tone, a hiatus hernia, or both.
- Regardless of the mechanism, the acid and enzymes present in gastric contents directly injure the lining of the esophagus. Significant mucosal damage can occur when the esophagus is exposed to a pH value <4 for a prolonged period of time, because the esophageal mucosa does not have protective mechanisms against acid and pepsin as in the stomach.[3]

Risk Factors

- Alcohol intake
- Caffeine intake
- Obesity
- Smoking
- Impaired esophageal peristalsis, including ineffective esophageal motility (IEM)
- Impaired salivation
- Poor gastric emptying
- Hypersecretion of gastric acid (as seen in Zollinger–Ellison syndrome)

DIAGNOSIS

Clinical Presentation

The evaluation of GERD has three important aspects:

- Any **alarm symptoms** should be elicited. These include dysphagia, weight loss, occult or overt gastrointestinal bleeding, symptoms lasting more than 5 years, symptoms unresponsive to proton pump inhibitors (PPI), and age more than 45 years.[3] Alarm symptoms indicate the need for invasive investigation, typically with upper endoscopy.
- The **severity** of GERD should be assessed.
- **Cardiac diseases** should be excluded, especially when chest pain is a presenting symptom.

History

- The duration, frequency, and severity of heartburn should be determined.
- Patients with GERD commonly report an "acidic" taste in the mouth and nocturnal wheezing or coughing.
- Symptoms can be characterized as typical or atypical:
  - Typical symptoms are heartburn and regurgitation, and are considered more specific for GERD than atypical symptoms.
  - Atypical symptoms include noncardiac chest pain, globus sensation, cough, and hoarseness.[4]
- GERD is also the proposed mechanism for a number of extraesophageal syndromes with varying levels of evidence to support causation. These include laryngitis, asthma, dental erosions, pharyngitis, chronic bronchitis, pulmonary fibrosis, chronic sinusitis, and recurrent aspiration pneumonia.[3,4]
- Behaviors that increase reflux should be sought, including smoking, caffeine use, large meals, and recumbency after eating.
- The presence of "alarm symptoms" should be determined.

Physical Examination

The physical examination should include an assessment of body habitus and presence of alarm findings such as anemia and occult gastrointestinal blood loss.

Diagnostic Testing

- Many clinicians advocate an **empiric trial of a PPI orally** as the initial step in suspected GERD. A symptomatic response to PPI confers a high degree of certainty of the diagnosis of GERD.
- In the presence of alarm symptoms, uncertainty of diagnosis, or inadequate response to PPI, further workup is necessary.

Laboratory Testing

A **complete blood count** (CBC) may reveal a microcytic anemia if bleeding occurs from esophagitis, cancer, or an erosion.

Imaging

Barium swallow is a low-yield examination in GERD. A barium swallow is not indicated for the diagnosis of GERD, and reflux seen on a barium study is neither sensitive nor specific for a diagnosis of GERD. Barium studies are best used for characterization of anatomic relationships at the gastroesophageal junction prior to antireflux surgery, especially for evaluating hiatus hernias and their relationship to the gastroesophageal junction and the diaphragmatic hiatus; other uses could include better definition of tight strictures, or detection of subtle strictures where a barium pill swallow may have value.

Diagnostic Procedures

- The sensitivity of **endoscopy** as a diagnostic test for GERD is low, as the likelihood of finding visible esophagitis is <50% in treatment-naïve patients. The likelihood of esophagitis is extremely low when patients have already received PPI therapy.
- **Esophageal ambulatory reflux monitoring studies** involve measurement of intraluminal esophageal pH or pH impedance over at least a 24-hour period.
  - Catheter-based pH studies consist of placement of a thin catheter through the nostril with the pH recording site 5 cm above the proximal margin of the LES. Recordings last 24 hours.
  - Wireless pH studies involve attachment of a pH capsule 6 cm above the squamocolumnar junction, which corresponds to 5 cm above the LES. Recordings can last 48 hours or longer.
  - Catheter-based pH-impedance studies are now available, which can detect both acidic and nonacidic reflux events.
  - Generally, an elevated total acid exposure time (AET) (pH <4 for >6% of the time) is considered abnormal, and conclusive of pathologic reflux exposure.
  - Patients are asked to record their symptoms during the study. The pH recording can then be analyzed to determine whether symptoms correlate with reflux events. Simple proportions of symptoms associated with reflux events to overall symptoms reported (symptom index) can be used as a tool to record symptom reflux correlation. Statistical tests that also take the time at risk for reflux, reflux events, and reflux events without symptoms into consideration may provide more robust designation of symptom association, called symptom association probability (SAP). SAP is considered positive if the likelihood of a chance association between reflux events and symptoms is <5%, correlating to p <0.05.[5]
  - AET and SAP can be used to categorize patients into clinical phenotypes based on level of evidence supporting GERD.[5] These phenotypes are:
    - Strong evidence (both abnormal AET and positive acid or impedance SAP)
    - Good evidence (abnormal AET but negative SAP)
    - Reflux hypersensitivity (RH; normal AET but positive SAP to pH or pH-impedance–detected reflux events)
    - No evidence or equivocal evidence (normal AET and negative SAP)
  - Testing is performed off PPI therapy when the diagnosis of reflux disease is in question. Adequacy of reflux control or assessment of ongoing symptoms despite adequate therapy in well-diagnosed GERD patients can be best determined with a pH impedance study while on maximal PPI therapy.

TREATMENT

The goal of treatment is to alleviate symptoms, heal esophageal damage, and prevent complications.

Medications

- **PPIs**, administered once daily, can heal erosive esophagitis and relieve heartburn.
  - All PPIs are more effective than H2 blockers or motility agents in healing esophagitis.
  - The PPI can be administered twice daily with improved therapeutic benefit if once daily dosing is unsuccessful in relieving the symptoms of GERD, or if patients have severe erosive esophagitis, strictures, or ulcers.
  - Typical GERD symptoms respond better to PPI than atypical symptoms.[6]
  - Common side effects of PPI therapy include headache, diarrhea, constipation, and abdominal pain.
  - Recently, long-term use of PPIs has been linked to various adverse events including gastrointestinal and pulmonary infections, osteoporosis, heart disease, kidney disease,

and dementia. However to date, there have been no well-designed prospective studies that conclusively establish the link between PPI and these adverse events.[7]

  Available evidence and expert opinion support PPI use in GERD with evidence of mucosal damage and typical symptoms. However, continued use should be reevaluated regularly and step-down approach should be trialed with H2-receptor blockers with improvement of symptoms on PPI.[8]

- **H2-receptor blockers** can be used to step down patients with minor or uncomplicated GERD, after effective symptom relief with PPI therapy. These agents are not recommended for patients with erosive esophagitis, Barrett esophagus, strictures, or severe symptomatic GERD. If symptoms recur with the step-down approach, management will need to be stepped back up to PPI use.[8]
- There is no evidence that adding a nocturnal H2 blocker to twice daily PPI therapy has any lasting clinical or histopathologic benefit.[9]
- **Antacids** are the most rapidly acting agents but are not an appropriate long-term management option in patients with GERD. **Alginates** can be used in combination with antacids to reduce the acid pocket and can reduce heartburn and AET.[10]
- **Baclofen** reduces transient LES relaxations and reduces reflux events. It can be used in patients whose symptoms persist despite maximal PPI therapy.[6]

Surgical Management

- Surgical management is reserved for patients with well-documented GERD who do not respond to maximal medical therapy or do not wish to remain on lifelong PPI.
- The surgical procedure most often performed is laparoscopic **Nissen fundoplication**. Partial fundoplication (Toupet, Dor) can be performed when esophageal hypomotility coexists.
- Surgery is as effective as properly dosed PPI with less incidence of pulmonary aspiration. However, it entails more morbidity and mortality.[11]
- Estimates suggest that 30% of patients resume PPI therapy within 5 years of undergoing antireflux surgery.[1]
- The most common complaints following surgery are an inability to belch, increase in flatulence, and increased bowel symptoms. New transit symptoms (dysphagia, regurgitation) can develop in a minority of patients; the risk seems highest when transit symptoms predate surgery.
- Roux-en-Y gastric bypass can reduce GERD symptoms and reflux burden, in addition to reducing weight in morbidly obese patients.[12]
- **Magnetic sphincter augmentation** (MSA) is a newer surgical option with 5 years of outcome data. In MSA, a bracelet of titanium-encased magnets is surgically implanted at the esophagogastric junction (EGJ) to augment the LES. The magnets separate to allow sphincter opening for food passage, but prevent retrograde movement of gastric content. In a meta-analysis, MSA showed comparable discontinuation of PPI and quality of life compared to antireflux surgery and was superior in preserving ability to belch and vomit.[13]
- Endoscopic therapies for GERD include radiofrequency ablation and transoral incisionless fundoplication. Data for these interventions are mixed, but these options could be considered alternatives to medical or surgical therapy in the right setting and in an experienced center.[6]

Lifestyle/Risk Modification

- Lifestyle modification is not recommended in isolation, but rather in conjunction with pharmacologic therapy.
- Patients are encouraged to decrease consumption of alcohol, caffeine, and acidic foods that aggravate symptoms, such as onions and tomatoes.

- Patients should avoid the use of medications that lower LES tone whenever possible, such as calcium channel blockers, β-blockers, nitrates, and anticholinergic drugs.
- Other recommendations include weight loss, smoking cessation, avoidance of meals within 3 hours of bedtime, and elevation of the head end of the bed while supine.

SPECIAL CONSIDERATIONS

- The American Gastroenterological Association, in a survey of more than 1000 patients on PPI therapy for GERD, found that 38% had residual symptoms and 47% of those with residual symptoms took additional medications to control their symptoms.[9]
- **Causes of PPI failure** include:
  - Incorrect diagnosis (patient does not have GERD)
  - Incorrect medication dose timing
  - Residual pathologic acid secretion
  - Rapid PPI metabolism
  - Hypersecretory state
  - Hiatus hernia
  - Defective esophageal mucosal barrier
  - Reflux of nonacid material from the stomach or duodenum
  - Underlying dysmotility
  - Underlying eosinophilic or infectious esophagitis
- Patients who fail twice daily PPI therapy should undergo upper endoscopy; persisting symptoms on PPI constitutes an alarm symptom. Random biopsies from the proximal and distal are recommended to exclude eosinophilic esophagitis (EoE).
- If the esophagogastroduodenoscopy (EGD) is normal, pH or pH/impedance testing can define and quantitate AET, and determine reflux-symptom association. Ideally, testing is performed off PPI therapy if the diagnosis of reflux disease is in question.
- If the EGD and pH/impedance testing are both normal, the patient likely does not have significant reflux disease. Alternate explanations for symptoms could include functional heartburn or chest pain.[9]

COMPLICATIONS

- Complications of long-standing or incompletely treated GERD include esophageal stricture, hemorrhage, Barrett esophagus, and adenocarcinoma. It is important to note that these complications can occur in asymptomatic patients.
- The risk of developing esophageal adenocarcinoma in Barrett esophagus is approximately 0.5% per year.[14] However, endoscopic monitoring of patients with chronic GERD symptoms may not necessarily reduce the risk of malignancy.[14]

Esophageal Malignancies

GENERAL PRINCIPLES

- **Squamous cell carcinoma** and **adenocarcinoma** represent the two most common neoplasms of the esophagus.
- **Barrett esophagus** predisposes to esophageal adenocarcinoma, and consists of intestinal metaplasia of squamous esophageal mucosa. Adenocarcinoma develops through stages of low- and high-grade dysplasia from nondysplastic-specialized intestinal metaplasia.

Epidemiology

- In the United States, squamous cell carcinoma is decreasing in incidence, but the risk remains elevated in African American men.[3]
- The incidence of adenocarcinoma has risen over the past 20 years.[15]
- Both diseases have a strong male predilection with a high mortality rate. Most patients have regional and distant lymph node metastases at the time of diagnosis.

Pathophysiology

- **Squamous cell carcinoma**
  - This develops from carcinogenic exposure in susceptible individuals.
  - The most common locations of disease are the proximal and distal esophagus.
- **Adenocarcinoma**
  - Adenocarcinoma develops as a consequence of accumulation of genetic mutations within dysplastic intestinal metaplasia.
  - Most cases develop near the gastroesophageal junction in the setting of Barrett esophagus.
- **Barrett esophagus**
  - Barrett esophagus consists of replacement of normal squamous distal esophageal mucosa with specialized intestinal type epithelium in genetically predisposed individuals with chronic reflux exposure.
  - Barrett esophagus occurs in approximately 10% of patients with GERD.[2]
  - Patients with Barrett esophagus have a risk of developing esophageal adenocarcinoma that is approximately 100 times higher compared to patients without this condition.[16]

Risk Factors

- **Squamous cell carcinoma**
  - Chronic tobacco use
  - Chronic alcohol use
  - History of mediastinal or breast irradiation
  - Human papillomavirus 16 *or* 18 infection
  - Chronic ingestion of hot liquids
  - Achalasia
- **Adenocarcinoma**
  - Male gender
  - Caucasian race
- **Barrett esophagus**
  - GERD
  - Obesity
  - Scleroderma

DIAGNOSIS

Clinical Presentation

- A thorough history and physical examination should be performed.
- Patients are questioned for a history of **dysphagia** or **unintentional weight loss**.
- **Risk factors**, especially the use of tobacco or alcohol, are queried.
- The physical examination is typically normal. **Cachexia** may develop from poor nutritional intake in advanced cancer.

Diagnostic Testing

Once malignancy is suspected, diagnostic testing must be initiated in a timely manner.

Laboratory Testing

- Laboratory tests provide little information to aid in the diagnosis of esophageal malignancies.
- A CBC may reveal a microcytic anemia if bleeding has occurred.
- A low albumin may suggest malnutrition related to chronic dysphagia.

Imaging

- A **barium swallow** may reveal a mass in the esophageal lumen or compression from adjacent structures. However, endoscopy is generally recommended as the first diagnostic test in new-onset dysphagia.
- If malignancy is diagnosed, **computed tomography (CT)** and **positron emission tomographic (PET) scanning** are often useful to evaluate for distant metastases.

Diagnostic Procedures

- **Upper endoscopy** (EGD) allows for the visualization of the esophageal lumen and biopsy of lesions suspicious for malignancy or Barrett esophagus.
- EGD with high-definition white light is the gold standard for diagnosis.
- **Endoscopic ultrasound** is used frequently for staging in patients being considered for endoscopic eradication therapy (EET) to evaluate for submucosal cancer and/or lymph node metastasis.[17]
- Pathology should be reviewed by an expert pathologist before proceeding with EET.[17]
- **Endoscopic mucosal resection** should be performed in patients with visible, nodular mucosa in Barrett esophagus as it has value in diagnosis and therapy.[14]

TREATMENT

- For both squamous cell carcinoma and adenocarcinoma of the esophagus, the standard of care with curative intent is surgery alone or in combination with radiation and chemotherapy.
- Mounting evidence suggests that adjuvant chemotherapy followed by surgery may be effective therapy.
- Severe dysphagia may be relieved with palliative beam radiation therapy or endoscopic stent placement.

MONITORING/FOLLOW-UP

- **Surveillance intervals**, once Barrett esophagus is diagnosed, depend on presence and degree of dysplasia found on initial EGD. If no dysplasia is noted on histopathology, further surveillance can be performed in 3–5 years' time.[14]
- If **low-grade dysplasia** is discovered, follow-up is recommended in 6–12 months. Management of low-grade dysplasia is controversial and current guidelines emphasize shared decision making with the patient and endoscopist. Surveillance can be continued or EET can be considered.[17] If **high-grade dysplasia** is found, the patient should be referred for EET. Techniques for EET include endoscopic mucosal resection, radiofrequency ablation, cryotherapy, and endoscopic submucosal dissection.[17]
- Most patients with high-grade dysplasia can be treated with EET, but esophagectomy can be considered in certain patients.[14] In patients with severe surgical risks or those declining invasive therapy, surveillance can be repeated in 3-month intervals.

OUTCOME/PROGNOSIS

- Five-year survival rates for both squamous cell carcinoma and adenocarcinoma of the esophagus remain poor at 10–15%.[3]

- However, a cure is possible with early diagnosis. This is the basis for endoscopic surveillance for high-grade dysplasia and carcinoma in situ in patients with Barrett esophagus.

Infectious Esophagitis

GENERAL PRINCIPLES

- Infectious esophagitis is **most commonly seen in the immunosuppressed patient**.
- Fungal and viral diseases are the most common agents in this patient population.
- There are rare instances where infectious esophagitis is encountered in immunocompetent hosts.

Epidemiology

- Since the recognition of acquired immunodeficiency syndrome (AIDS) in the 1980s, the incidence of infectious esophagitis has increased, and the causal organisms have shifted over the past 20 years.
- Approximately 30% of patients with HIV infection have symptoms of infectious esophagitis during the course of their disease.[18]

Etiology

- **Fungal esophagitis**
  - Candidiasis is the most common infectious disease of the esophagus in patients with HIV, accounting for 70% of cases.[18]
  - The most common species is *Candida albicans,* but other species of *Candida* have been implicated.
  - Other fungi, such as *Histoplasma capsulatum*, can cause esophagitis, but these infections are rare.
  - In patients with AIDS that present with multiple infectious pathogens simultaneously, *Candida* is almost always one of the causal organisms.
- **Viral esophagitis**
  - The most common viral cause of esophagitis in patients infected with HIV is Cytomegalovirus (CMV). The risk of infection with CMV is low in patients with CD4 counts >100.[8]
  - Varicella zoster virus (VZV) can cause a devastating esophagitis in severely immunocompromised hosts. VZV esophagitis is rare in immunocompetent patients but can be seen in children with chickenpox or adults with herpes zoster.
  - Herpes simplex virus (HSV) is an uncommon etiology of viral esophagitis in both immunosuppressed and immunocompetent patients.
  - Other viruses, such as human papillomavirus and Epstein–Barr virus, can infect the esophagus, but are extremely rare.
- **Bacterial esophagitis**
  - Bacterial infection of the esophagus in HIV patients is rare.
  - This is sometimes superimposed in the setting of esophageal mucosal ischemia, and can result in a black discoloration of the esophagus on EGD, termed **black esophagus**.
  - Causal organisms include *Mycobacterium avium* complex, *Mycobacterium tuberculosis, Nocardia, Actinomyces,* and *Lactobacillus.*
- **Idiopathic esophagitis**
  - Idiopathic esophageal ulceration (IEU) is common in patients with a CD4 count <50.[8]
  - The etiologic agent of this disease has not been determined, although HIV itself has been implicated.

Risk Factors

- HIV or AIDS
- Ongoing treatment with chemotherapy
- Immunosuppressive therapy following organ transplantation

DIAGNOSIS

Clinical Presentation

Clinical presentation often varies depending on the causal organism.

History

- **Candidiasis**
  - Dysphagia is the most common symptom.
  - Patients will often have thrush.
  - Odynophagia, fever, nausea, and vomiting are less common.
- **Cytomegalovirus**
  - Odynophagia and chest pain are the most common symptoms.
  - Dysphagia is uncommon.
  - Patients may also have a low-grade fever, nausea, and vomiting.
- **Herpes simplex virus**
  - Most commonly present with both dysphagia and odynophagia, as well as chest pain and fever.
- **Varicella zoster virus**
  - Presentation is similar to that of HSV.
  - The characteristic skin lesions of chickenpox in children and zoster in adults may be helpful in diagnosis.
- **Idiopathic esophageal ulceration**
  - Almost all patients with idiopathic esophageal ulceration present with severe odynophagia and, as a result, are malnourished and dehydrated at presentation.

Physical Examination

The patient's vital signs may reveal fever and orthostatic hypotension from dehydration.

Diagnostic Testing

Laboratory Testing

- An elevated **white blood cell (WBC) count** may suggest infection, although this finding is variable in patients with immunodeficiency.
- The **CD4 count** is useful in determining which causal pathogen is most likely involved in patients with AIDS (Table 13-1).

TABLE 13-1	ETIOLOGY OF INFECTIOUS ESOPHAGITIS IN HIV OR AIDS
CD4 Count	**Typical Organisms Involved**
>200	HSV, VZV
100–200	Candida, HSV
50–100	Candida, CMV, HSV
<50	Idiopathic esophageal ulceration[10]

CMV, Cytomegalovirus; HSV, herpes simplex virus; VZV, varicella zoster virus.

Diagnostic Procedures

- EGD is typically only recommended in *Candida* esophagitis if a patient fails empiric antifungal therapy or if symptoms include weight loss, dehydration, or fever.
- **EGD can distinguish between the types of esophageal infections** by gross or histologic appearance of the lesions:
  - **Candidiasis**—Multiple adherent, white or yellow, "cottage cheese" plaques are easily seen on endoscopy. Brushings or biopsies reveal yeast or budding hyphae.
  - **CMV**—Large, well-demarcated ulcers are visualized on gross examination and immunohistochemistry staining of biopsy specimens aids in the diagnosis.
  - **VZV**—Multiple vesicles and confluent ulcers are seen on EGD. Cytology is difficult to distinguish from HSV and often requires immunohistochemistry or culture.
  - **HSV**—Characterized by small, superficial ulcers in early disease and by diffuse esophagitis in later stages. Cytology reveals giant cells and ground glass nuclei.
  - **IEU**—Well-circumscribed, often large, ulcers are seen on gross examination. Biopsies are useful primarily to rule out other infectious etiologies.[19]

TREATMENT

- Treatment **focuses on eradicating the causal organism**.
- Many clinicians recommend an empiric course of fluconazole to treat *Candida* esophagitis in patients with AIDS and dysphagia, but without other symptoms.

Medications

- **Candidiasis**
  - The first-line agent is fluconazole 200 mg loading dose followed by 100 mg daily for 5–10 days.[19]
  - In patients with azole-resistant *Candida,* the oral dose of fluconazole may be increased, or treatment with intravenous (IV) amphotericin can be initiated.
  - Other therapies include itraconazole, voriconazole, and micafungin.
  - Severe refractory cases may not improve until treatment of HIV is undertaken to raise the CD4 count.
- **Cytomegalovirus**
  - First-line therapy is IV ganciclovir 5 mg/kg q12h if the patient is not pancytopenic.
  - Alternate therapy consists of IV foscarnet 60 mg/kg q8h or PO valganciclovir.
  - Regardless of the regimen, treatment continues until healing occurs, usually up to 1 month.
  - Approximately 30% of patients relapse.[20]
- **Herpes simplex virus**
  - First-line therapy is acyclovir 5 mg/kg IV q8h for 7–14 days or 400 mg by mouth 5 times a day for 14–21 days.[19]
  - Other effective agents include famciclovir, valacyclovir, and ganciclovir.
  - HSV infection in immunocompetent patients is generally self-limited with spontaneous resolution occurring in 1–2 weeks.[21]
- **Varicella zoster virus**
  - First-line therapy is acyclovir 5 mg/kg IV q8h for 7–14 days in the immunocompromised or valacyclovir 1000 mg PO q8h for 7–14 days in the immunocompetent host.[19]
- **Idiopathic esophageal ulceration**
  - The mainstay of treatment for idiopathic esophageal ulceration is corticosteroids.
  - If the patient cannot tolerate PO intake, then IV formulations are used.
  - Given that corticosteroids predispose patients to *Candida* infection, many clinicians prescribe fluconazole twice weekly for prophylaxis.
  - Thalidomide can be used in refractory cases.

SPECIAL CONSIDERATIONS

- Many of these diseases have high recurrence rates and warrant **prophylaxis**.
- Primary prophylaxis of *Candida* is not recommended. However, secondary prophylaxis with fluconazole 100 mg weekly is recommended in patients with multiple recurrences.
- Although primary prophylaxis of CMV is recommended in patients with CD4 <100, there is no evidence that it decreases the incidence of gastrointestinal disease.
- Primary prophylaxis for HSV is not recommended. However, secondary prophylaxis with acyclovir 600 mg daily by mouth is recommended in patients with a history of recurrent disease.[20]
- Thalidomide can be used in refractory cases.

Eosinophilic Esophagitis

GENERAL PRINCIPLES

- During the last few decades, there has been a sharp increase in the number of patients with esophageal eosinophilia who were thought to have GERD but did not respond to traditional medical or surgical management.
- A unique disease termed **eosinophilic esophagitis (EoE)** is identified in many of these patients.

Definition

- Although eosinophilic infiltration of the esophagus can be seen secondarily in association with other conditions such as GERD, EoE is now recognized as a primary diagnosis.
- EoE is a clinicopathologic disease characterized by:
  - Symptoms of food impaction and dysphagia in adults, and feeding intolerance or GERD in children.
  - More than 15 eosinophils/high power field on pathologic examination.
  - Exclusion of other disorders with similar clinical or pathologic findings, especially GERD.[22]

Epidemiology

- For unclear reasons, there seems to be an increasing incidence of EoE that is not solely accounted for by increasing recognition.
- Disease occurs in all age groups but symptoms usually appear either in early childhood, adolescence, or before the fourth decade of life.[23] Males comprise 70% of cases.[24]

Pathophysiology

- The pathogenesis of EoE is unknown.
- There is some thought that the disease process originates from an immune-mediated response to a swallowed allergen.[24]
- Once eosinophils have infiltrated the esophageal mucosa, their presence appears to trigger a self-sustaining cascade of inflammatory mediators.

Risk Factors

- There seems to be an increased incidence of EoE in pediatric patients with a history of asthma, allergic rhinitis, eczema, and food or environmental allergies. This association has not been fully studied in the adult population.
- There is also a reported association of EoE in adults with eosinophilic gastroenteritis and peripheral eosinophilia.

DIAGNOSIS

Clinical Presentation

- Questions regarding the risk factors listed above should be elicited.
- The most common presenting symptoms are dysphagia, heartburn, and chest pain.
- Less common presenting symptoms include a history of food impaction or symptoms consistent with esophageal dysmotility.
- Patients may carry a diagnosis of GERD in the past but may have failed high-dose PPI.

Diagnostic Criteria

The diagnosis is most often made on the basis of the presence of characteristic clinical features, the presence of eosinophils on biopsy, and exclusion of other possible diagnoses (e.g., GERD, parasitic and fungal infections, Crohn disease, allergic vasculitis, and other connective tissue diseases).

Differential Diagnosis

The differential diagnosis for esophageal eosinophilia includes:
- GERD
- EoE
- Eosinophilic gastroenteritis
- Crohn disease
- Connective tissue disease
- Hypereosinophilic syndrome
- Infection
- Graft-versus-host disease
- Vasculitis
- Achalasia
- Drug hypersensitivity response[22]

Diagnostic Testing

Typically, a thorough history and physical is not enough to make a definitive diagnosis and further evaluation is warranted.

Laboratory Testing

A **CBC** can be performed to evaluate for peripheral eosinophilia, although this is more frequently seen in the pediatric population.[22]

Imaging

A **barium swallow** may add further information regarding a patient's anatomy and assessing for dominant strictures, but is not required in the routine management of this disease.

Diagnostic Procedures

- **EGD with biopsies** from the proximal and distal esophagus should be performed to confirm the diagnosis of EoE.
- Gross mucosal abnormalities include longitudinal furrowing, friability, edema, longitudinal shearing, whitish exudates, raised white specks, "crepe paper mucosa," narrow caliber esophagus, rings, felinization, and transient or fixed rings.[22]
- The esophageal mucosa is grossly abnormal on endoscopy in more than half of patients.
- Biopsy specimens should be obtained regardless of the gross appearance of the esophageal mucosa. In a study of 381 children with EoE, 30% had a grossly normal esophagus.[22]
- Biopsies should be obtained in the stomach and duodenum to determine whether the disease is confined to the esophagus or is a manifestation of another process, such as eosinophilic gastroenteritis or inflammatory bowel disease.

- Patients will have normal pH monitoring of the distal esophagus in contrast to GERD.
- Although allergen skin testing is sometimes performed, the diagnostic yield is very low.

TREATMENT

Medications

Medications are the mainstay of the management for EoE.

First Line

- **Acid suppression** with PPI is used for diagnostic and therapeutic purposes in EoE as GERD and EoE have a close relationship. Eosinophils may persist on biopsy despite 2 months of PPI trial in EoE. However, up to one-third of patients with suspected EoE have good clinical response to PPI alone, suggesting GERD is responsible for their symptoms or that some EoE is acid sensitive.[25]
- Swallowed steroids are used at the onset in patients with more severe symptoms or with an inadequate response to acid suppression.
- Inhaled steroids such as fluticasone and budesonide are the primary preparations used to be swallowed, but viscous steroids meant for rectal use in IBD can also be mixed with more tasteful solutions and swallowed.[25]
- Relief of dysphagia was seen in all study participants within the initial week of treatment.[22]

Second Line

- **Systemic corticosteroids** have been shown to have significant benefit in pediatric patients.
- However, symptoms recur quickly on cessation and, given the deleterious side effects of long-term systemic corticosteroid use, this remains a poor treatment option.
- Systemic steroids are an option when urgent symptom relief is required (severe dysphagia, dehydration, weight loss, stricture, etc.).
- General antihistamines, leukotriene receptor antagonists, and cromolyn have not been shown to be effective in treating EoE.
- Anti-IL-5 antibodies were initially promising, but showed mixed results in further studies.[25]

Lifestyle/Risk Modification

- **Avoidance of known food and environmental allergens** may provide relief in patients with EoE.
- In one study, 26 of 35 patients showed significant improvement clinically and histologically after initiating a diet free of the 6 most common allergenic foods (dairy, eggs, wheat, soy, peanuts, fish/shellfish).
- **Elemental, amino acid–based formulas** have been shown to be extremely effective in the pediatric population (90%), but usually have to be administered by gastrostomy or nasogastric tubes and are quite costly.[25]

COMPLICATIONS

- Chronic inflammation from EoE can lead to proximal esophageal strictures as well as mucosal rings, esophageal ulceration, and esophageal polyps.
- Some patients with significant dysphagia due to rings or strictures require esophageal dilation to relieve symptoms.
- While there is a risk of perforation, this procedure is relatively safe and the dysphagia often resolves for several months.

OUTCOME/PROGNOSIS

- The prognosis of EoE is not well described although the consensus is that it does not appear to limit life expectancy.[22]
- Esophageal metaplasia or malignancy has not been reported in patients with EoE, even in adults with advanced disease.[22]

Esophageal Strictures

GENERAL PRINCIPLES

- Esophageal strictures often arise as complications of other disease processes.
- Any type of chronic inflammation can lead to esophageal strictures.

Etiology

- **Peptic strictures**
  - Peptic strictures are relatively common, occurring in approximately 10% of patients with GERD and in >25% of patients with Barrett esophagus.[26]
  - Stricturing occurs typically in the distal esophagus, often just proximal to the squamocolumnar junction.
- **Schatzki rings**
  - This process often occurs in the distal esophagus, at the squamocolumnar junction. By definition, Schatzki rings have squamous mucosa on the proximal aspect, and gastric columnar mucosa on the distal aspect.
  - Schatzki rings can be associated with GERD, pill esophagitis, and hiatus hernias.[27]
  - Intermittent, nonprogressive solid food dysphagia can occur, sometimes termed "steakhouse syndrome."
- **Plummer–Vinson syndrome**
  - Characterized by anemia, upper esophageal webs, and dysphagia.
  - Typically seen in middle-aged women.[28]
- **Other causes** of esophageal narrowing:
  - Caustic ingestion
  - After band ligation for varices
  - Esophageal infections
  - Repetitive vomiting
  - Esophageal neoplasms
  - Radiation therapy
  - Pill-induced esophageal inflammation ("pill esophagitis")
  - Esophageal trauma (e.g., instrumentation, NG tube)
  - Crohn disease

Risk Factors

- GERD
- History of esophageal infections
- Crohn disease

DIAGNOSIS

Clinical Presentation

- A careful history is crucial in the assessment of dysphagia.
- In addition to helping rule out diseases other than stricture, the type of dysphagia and regurgitation can often localize the sire and involvement of disease.

History

Key points of the history should include
- Onset and duration of symptoms
- Association of dysphagia with types of food
- Description of regurgitated material if present
- History of weight loss
- History of GERD
- Evaluation for other risk factors listed above

Physical Examination

Physical signs of weight loss, dehydration, and malnutrition help to assess severity of disease.

Diagnostic Testing

Strictures may be identified on barium radiography and endoscopy. In most instances, evaluation for strictures starts with endoscopy, as this allows esophageal inspection, biopsy to evaluate for EoE, as well as dilation as a mode of therapy.

Laboratory Testing
- Laboratory studies are **generally not useful** in the workup of stricture.
- Anemia may support the diagnosis of esophageal inflammation, neoplasia, Plummer–Vinson syndrome.[28]
- A low albumin concentration may reflect nutritional deficiency.

Imaging

Barium swallow is a useful test in the workup of suspected stricture, ring, or web, especially when the lesion is subtle and not recognized on an upper endoscopy.[26] Barium swallow is not recommended as the initial test in new-onset dysphagia, as endoscopy provides both definitive diagnosis and therapy of strictures. If radiologic findings demonstrate a narrowing of the esophagus, dilation at endoscopy is warranted.

Diagnostic Procedures

EGD permits the operator to directly visualize the stricture, web, or ring. Further, biopsies can be performed to further evaluate the etiology, and dilation allows therapy of the stricture.

TREATMENT

- **Peptic stricture**
  - Aggressive acid control with high-dose PPI can cause regression of the stricture.
  - Dilation is often required, and is performed endoscopically with through-the-scope (TTS) dilators or bougie dilators.
  - Steroids can also be injected into peptic strictures after dilation, and this can prolong the interval to symptom recurrence.[27]
  - Despite their appeal, clinical trials evaluating the use of esophageal stents for benign strictures have not shown significant benefit, and stent placement carries the risk of stent migration.[27] Therefore, stent placement is not recommended.
  - Rarely, dysphagia is not relieved by maximal medical therapy, and antireflux surgery is required.
- **Schatzki ring**
  - Patients with mild disease should be advised to chew their food carefully.
  - Patients with more severe disease are at an increased risk for food bolus impaction and benefit from endoscopic dilation.

- Additional therapeutic options include incisional therapy with needle knife, jumbo biopsy forceps bites, or argon plasma coagulation.[27]
- All patients with Schatzki rings should be evaluated for GERD and started on PPI therapy, if indicated.[27]
- Treatment with PPI may also provide benefit if there is underlying EoE, as Schatzki rings have been linked to EoE.[27]

MONITORING/FOLLOW-UP

- Patients with Plummer–Vinson syndrome have an increased risk of developing squamous cell carcinoma of the esophagus. It is unclear whether they should undergo screening EGD.[28]
- Patients with peptic strictures may need repeat endoscopy for stricture dilation. Barrett's screening and surveillance may be appropriate if this is identified.

Esophageal Motility Disorders

GENERAL PRINCIPLES

- Motility disorders of the esophagus can involve both the striated and smooth muscle of the esophagus.
- Motility disorders can result in significant morbidity for patients.

Definition

- Swallowing involves two phases of muscular activity:
  - Swallowing is initiated in the oropharynx, by neural impulses from the central nervous system, controlling voluntary, striated muscles of the oropharynx. The upper esophageal sphincter, a striated muscle, opens during the oropharyngeal component of swallowing.
  - Swallowing is completed by the coordinated, involuntary contraction of the smooth muscle of the esophagus. The LES, a smooth muscle, relaxes concurrent with esophageal peristalsis, thereby transmitting luminal content into the stomach.
- Dysfunction at either phase can cause dysphagia.

Etiology

- **Striated muscle dysfunction** can be affected by:
  - Cerebrovascular accident
  - Myasthenia gravis
  - Polymyositis
  - Parkinson disease
  - Amyotrophic lateral sclerosis
- Causes of **smooth muscle failure** include:
  - Neurologic (achalasia, diffuse esophageal spasm [DES], nutcracker esophagus)
  - Autoimmune (scleroderma)[29]
  - Infectious (Chagas disease)
  - Invasive cancer

Pathophysiology

- In **striated muscle**, neuromuscular dysregulation results in the loss of a coordinated swallow and can lead to oropharyngeal dysphagia, regurgitation, and pulmonary aspiration.

- **Smooth muscle dysfunction** is caused by the loss of inhibitory neurons in the esophagus leading to disorganized peristalsis (mainly in the form of loss of sequencing of peristalsis, simultaneous waves, exaggerated wave amplitude, and prolonged wave duration) and increased LES tone with abnormal sphincter relaxation during swallows.

DIAGNOSIS

Clinical Presentation

- The most common symptoms of esophageal motor disorders are dysphagia and chest pain.
- In contrast, patients with oropharyngeal dysphagia often present with drooling, regurgitation of food immediately after swallowing, and pulmonary aspiration.

History

- As with strictures, the **type, duration, and severity of dysphagia** are important to address with a good history.
- A **description of regurgitated contents** is useful in differentiating esophageal versus oropharyngeal causes.
- Patients with DES or hypercontractile esophagus often present with **intermittent chest pain** exacerbated by hot or cold items. Given that the chest pain sometimes radiates to locations similar to cardiac disease, it is important to rule our myocardial ischemia in this population.
- The history should focus on **conditions that can cause motility disorders**, such as cerebrovascular accident, amyotrophic lateral sclerosis, and myasthenia gravis.
- A **history of travel** to Central and South American countries may warrant workup for Chagas disease.

Physical Examination

The physical examination should include a thorough **neurologic examination** as well as assessment of **nutritional status**.

Diagnostic Testing

Barium swallow and esophageal manometry are very useful in diagnosing esophageal motility disorders. Well-defined motor disorders such as achalasia can also be identified on endoscopy.

Imaging

- **Barium swallow**
  - In patients with achalasia, barium swallow often reveals a characteristic "bird's beak" tapered distal esophagus with proximal dilatation. This appearance can also occur with neoplastic compression of the lower esophagus (pseudoachalasia).[29]
  - In patients with DES, barium swallow demonstrates the typical "corkscrew" or "rosary bead" appearance.[29]
  - Jackhammer esophagus often appears normal on barium swallow.

Diagnostic Procedures

- **High-resolution manometry** utilizes pressure sensors along the length of the esophagus allowing for measurement of intraluminal pressure as a continuum along the length of the entire esophagus. This allows for the construction of colored topographic Clouse plots.[30]
- Currently, the Chicago Classification v3.0 provides a hierarchical approach for analyzing HRM recordings. The evaluation is based on ten 5-mL water swallows in patients

without prior esophageal or EGJ surgeries.[31] HRM studies are interpreted in a stepwise fashion as follows:

○ EGJ outflow obstruction. Achalasia manifests with integrated relaxation pressure (IRP) ≥ upper limit of normal and 100% failed swallows or spasm
  ▪ Type 1 achalasia: no contractility
  ▪ Type 2 achalasia: ≥20% panesophageal pressurization
  ▪ Type 3 achalasia: ≥20% spasm (distal latency <4.5 seconds)
○ EGJ outflow obstruction—IRP ≥ upper limit of normal and without features of types 1–3 achalasia.
  ▪ Consider mechanical obstruction or incompletely expressed achalasia.
○ Other major disorders of peristalsis (these are not found in normal health): normal IRP and short distal latency or high distal contractile integral (DCI) or 100% failed peristalsis
  ▪ Diffuse esophageal spasm: ≥20% premature (distal latency <4.5 seconds)
  ▪ Hypercontractile (jackhammer) esophagus: ≥20% DCI >8000 mm Hg/sec/cm
  ▪ Absent contractility: no contraction, achalasia should be considered
○ Minor disorders of peristalsis: normal IRP and ≥50% ineffective swallows (DCI <450 mm Hg/sec/cm)
  ▪ IEM: ≥50% ineffective swallows
  ▪ Fragmented peristalsis: ≥50% fragmented swallows and not ineffective[31]
• **EGD**
  ○ In suspected cases of achalasia, EGD should always be performed to exclude mass lesions as a cause of pseudoachalasia.
  ○ EGD is typically normal in patients with DES, hypercontractile (jackhammer) esophagus, or minor disorders.

TREATMENT

Treatment regimens differ for each class of dysmotility.

Medications

• In achalasia, **endoscopic botulinum toxin injection** of the LES may temporize symptoms and can be used as sole therapy in elderly patients or others where more effective modalities are contraindicated because of comorbidities. Effective therapy requires repeated injection, as efficacy wanes after a median of 9–12 months.[32] Other pharmacologic therapies include calcium channel blockers and nitrates, but these are the least effective treatment options for achalasia.[32]
• Patients with DES and hypercontractile (jackhammer) esophagus can be treated with **nitrates** and **calcium channel blockers** for symptomatic relief. Spastic disorders have a perceptive component to symptomatology, presumably from coexistent visceral hypersensitivity, that may require **neuromodulator therapy** (e.g., low-dose tricyclic antidepressants, particularly for chest pain). Obstructive symptoms (dysphagia, regurgitation) may improve with botulinum toxin injection if abnormal LES relaxation can be demonstrated. **PPI therapy** can also be included in the regimen, if acid reflux is thought to contribute to symptoms.
• The medical treatment of scleroderma should involve aggressive acid control with high-dose PPI.

Nonpharmacologic Therapies

• **Endoscopic pneumatic dilation** of the LES in a graded fashion from 30–40 mm disrupts the LES, and is effective in achalasia patients, often offering immediate relief. Esophageal perforation can occur in 2–5%, requiring emergent surgery in some instances. Predictors of favorable response to dilation include type 2 achalasia, older age, and female sex.[32]

- Endoscopic dilation is typically not useful in DES and nutcracker esophagus.

Surgical Management

- The goal of surgical management in achalasia is disruption of the circular muscle fibers of the LES. The two available approaches are laparoscopic Heller myotomy and peroral endoscopic myotomy (POEM).
- **Surgical myotomy** offers durable efficacy compared with medications and botulinum toxin injection. This procedure is often performed with partial fundoplication, which provides the added benefit of protection against reflux with the fundoplication. Patients with type 2 achalasia respond better than type 1 or 3.[32] Surgical myotomy performs well in young men.
- **POEM** is a newer hybrid surgical/endoscopic procedure that was first performed in 2008. A submucosal tunnel is created in the esophagus proximal to the gastroesophageal junction, and a myotomy of circular muscle layers is distally extended into the cardia. There is now long-term follow-up data showing similar efficacy rates when compared to surgical myotomy. POEM may offer the best option for patients with type 3 achalasia.[32] GERD is the most common postprocedure complication.

MONITORING/FOLLOW-UP

Patients with achalasia have an increased risk of squamous cell esophageal carcinoma (developing in 2–7%) and there is debate whether regular surveillance EGD should be performed.[33]

REFERENCES

1. Kahrilas PJ, Shaheen NJ, Vaezi MF, et al. American Gastroenterological Association medical position statement on the management of gastroesophageal reflux disease. *Gastroenterology*. 2008;135(4):1383–1391.
2. Falk GW. Gastroesophageal reflux disease and Barrett's esophagus. *Endoscopy*. 2001;33(2):109–118.
3. Roman S, Gyawali CP, Savarino E, et al; GERD consensus group. Ambulatory reflux monitoring for diagnosis of gastro-esophageal reflux disease: update of the Porto consensus and recommendations from an international consensus group. *Neurogastroenterol Motil*. 2017;29(10):1–15.
4. Richter JE. The many manifestations of gastroesophageal reflux disease: presentation, evaluation, and treatment. *Gastroenterol Clin North Am*. 2007;36(3):577–599.
5. Patel A, Sayuk GS, Kushnir VM, et al. GERD phenotypes from pH-impedance monitoring predict symptomatic outcome on prospective evaluation. *Neurogastroenterol Motil*. 2016;28(4):513–521.
6. Gyawali CP, Fass R. Management of gastroesophageal reflux disease. *Gastroenterology*. 2018;154(2):302–318.
7. Vaezi MF, Yang YX, Howden CW. Complications of proton pump inhibitor therapy. *Gastroenterology*. 2017;153(1):35–48.
8. Inadomi JM, Jamal R, Murata GH, et al. Step-down management of gastroesophageal reflux disease. *Gastroenterology*. 2001;121(5):1095–1100.
9. Dellon ES, Shaheen NJ. Persistent reflux symptoms in the proton pump inhibitor era: the changing face of gastroesophageal reflux disease. *Gastroenterology*. 2010;139(1):7–13.e3.
10. Leiman DA, Riff BP, Morgan S, et al. Alginate therapy is effective treatment for gastroesophageal reflux disease symptoms: a systematic review and meta-analysis. *Dis Esophagus*. 2017;30(5):1–9.
11. Lundell L, Miettinen P, Myrvold HE, et al. Continued follow-up of a randomized clinical study comparing antireflux surgery and omeprazole in gastroesophageal reflux disease. *J Am Coll Surg*. 2001;192(2):172–181.
12. Madalosso CA, Gurski RR, Callegari-Jacques SM, et al. The impact of gastric bypass on gastroesophageal reflux in morbidly obese patients. *Ann Surg*. 2016;263(1):110–116.

13. Skubleny D, Switzer NJ, Dang J, et al. LINX(R) magnetic esophageal sphincter augmentation versus Nissen fundoplication for gastroesophageal reflux disease: a systematic review and meta-analysis. *Surg Endosc.* 2017;31(8):3078–3084.

14. American Gastroenterological Association; Spechler SJ, Sharma P, Souza RF, et al. American Gastroenterological Association medical position statement on the management of Barrett's esophagus. *Gastroenterology.* 2011;140(3):1084–1091.

15. Heath EI, Limburg PJ, Hawk ET, et al. Adenocarcinoma of the esophagus: risk factors and prevention. *Oncology.* 2000;14(4):507–514.

16. Sikkema M, de Jonge PJ, Steyerberg EW, et al. Risk of esophageal adenocarcinoma and mortality in patients with Barrett's esophagus: a systematic review and meta-analysis. *Clinical Gastroenterol Hepatol.* 2010;8(3):235–244.

17. Brimhall B, Wani S. Current endoscopic approaches for the treatment of Barrett Esophagus. *J Clin Gastroenterol.* 2017;51(1):2–11.

18. Bonacini M, Young T, Laine L. The causes of esophageal symptoms in human immunodeficiency virus infection: a prospective study of 110 patients. *Arch Intern Med.* 1991;151(8):1567–1572.

19. Bonacini M. Medical management of benign oesophageal disease in patients with human immunodeficiency virus infection. *Dig Liver Dis.* 2001;33(3):294–300.

20. Wilcox CM, Monkemuller KE. Diagnosis and management of esophageal disease in the acquired immunodeficiency syndrome. *South Med J.* 1998;91(11):1002–1008.

21. Patel NC, Caicedo RA. Esophageal infections: an update. *Curr Opin Pediatr.* 2015;27(5):642–648.

22. Liacouras CA, Furuta GT, Hirano I, et al. Eosinophilic esophagitis: updated consensus recommendations for children and adults. *J Allergy Clin Immunol.* 2011;128(1):3–20.

23. Noel RJ, Putnam PE, Rothenberg ME. Eosinophilic esophagitis. *N Engl J Med.* 2004;351(9):940–941.

24. Furuta GT, Straumann A. Review article: the pathogenesis and management of eosinophilic oesophagitis. *Aliment Pharmacol Ther.* 2006;24(2):173–182.

25. Akhondi H. Diagnostic approaches and treatment of eosinophilic esophagitis. A review article. *Ann Med Surg (Lond).* 2017;20:69–73.

26. Pregun I, Hritz I, Tulassay Z, et al. Peptic esophageal stricture: medical treatment. *Dig Dis.* 2009;27(1):31–37.

27. Adler DG, Siddiqui AA. Endoscopic management of esophageal strictures. *Gastrointest Endos.* 2017;86(1):35–43.

28. Hoffman RM, Jaffee PE. Plummer-Vinson syndrome. A case report and literature review. *Arch Intern Med.* 1995;155(18):2008–2011.

29. Adler DG, Romero Y. Primary esophageal motility disorders. *Mayo Clin Proc.* 2001;76(2):195–200.

30. Kahrilas PJ, Sifrim D. High-resolution manometry and impedance-pH/manometry: valuable tools in clinical and investigational esophagology. *Gastroenterology.* 2008;135(3):756–769.

31. Kahrilas PJ, Bredenoord AJ, Fox M, et al. The Chicago classification of esophageal motor disorders, v3.0. *Neurogastroenterol Motil.* 2015;27(2):160–174.

32. Patel DA, Lappas BM, Vaezi MF. Achalasia and its subtypes. *Gastroenterol Hepatol (NY).* 2017;13(7):411–421.

33. Streitz JM Jr, Ellis FH Jr, Gibb SP, et al. Achalasia and squamous cell carcinoma of the esophagus: analysis of 241 patients. *Ann Thorac Surg.* 1995;59(6):1604–1609.

14

Gastric Disorders

Jose B. Saenz

Peptic Ulcer Disease

GENERAL PRINCIPLES

- Gastric disorders, especially peptic ulcer disease (PUD), are among the most common illnesses encountered by both internists and gastroenterologists.
- PUD accounts for a significant portion of healthcare expenditures and can lead to potentially life-threatening complications.

Definition

- PUD is characterized by the denudation of mucosa extending into the muscularis propria layer from exposure to gastric acid or other damaging agents.
- Lesions <5 mm in diameter are called *erosions*, whereas lesions >5 mm in diameter are called *ulcers*.
- PUD most commonly occurs in the gastric antrum or duodenal bulb; duodenal ulcers are more common than gastric ulcers in Western countries.

Epidemiology

- PUD is a worldwide problem; the current global annual incidence rate of physician-diagnosed PUD is estimated to be approximately 0.1–0.2%.[1]
- Although the incidence of PUD has fallen since the 1950s with improved hygiene and socioeconomic conditions and decreased *Helicobacter pylori* infection rates, the number of hospital admissions for PUD-related complications does not appear to have decreased.
- The mortality rate of PUD has remained stable over the past two decades and comes mostly from the four major complications of PUD—hemorrhage, perforation, penetration to adjacent organs, and gastric outlet obstruction.
- Duodenal ulcers are slightly more common in men than in women, but gastric ulcers occur with equal frequency in both genders.
- Duodenal ulcers present at a slightly younger age range than gastric ulcers: ages 25–55 years versus ages 40–70 years, respectively. This difference likely derives from the increased use of nonsteroidal anti-inflammatory drugs (NSAIDs), which are associated primarily with gastric ulcers, especially in the elderly population.

Etiology

- Table 14-1 lists etiologies of peptic ulcers. *H. pylori*–associated PUD and NSAID-associated PUD account for >90% of PUDs.
- In patients in whom *H. pylori*, NSAID use, Crohn disease, and Zollinger–Ellison syndrome have been ruled out, no apparent etiology is found in as many as 50% of cases, termed idiopathic PUD. Many of these could still represent partially treated *H. pylori* and NSAID etiologies that have not been determined from routine clinical evaluation and investigation. Other factors include increased acid output and rapid gastric emptying, which have been associated with idiopathic PUD.

TABLE 14-1   ETIOLOGY OF PEPTIC ULCERS

Most Common
Helicobacter pylori–associated
NSAID-associated

Other
Idiopathic
Zollinger–Ellison syndrome
Gastroduodenal Crohn disease
Viral infection
Chemotherapy
Radiation therapy
Vascular insufficiency

NSAID, nonsteroidal anti-inflammatory drug.

- ***Helicobacter pylori*–associated PUD**
  - *H. pylori* is a gram-negative bacillus that lives embedded within the mucus layer overlying gastric epithelium or adherent to gastric epithelial cells, leading to inflammation. *H. pylori* infection is associated with lower socioeconomic status and is typically acquired in childhood.[2]
  - *H. pylori* infection has been traditionally associated with up to 90% of duodenal ulcers and 70–90% of gastric ulcers. The incidence of *H. pylori* infection in PUD is decreasing in the United States. Recent studies have shown that 20–50% of ulcers in the United States are not associated with *H. pylori*, though the proportion of *H. pylori*–negative ulcers elsewhere in the world remains much lower.[3,4]
  - In the case of duodenal ulcers, *H. pylori* is thought to infect the nonacid-secreting gastric antrum or ectopic gastric mucosa in the duodenum, thus stimulating gastrin release and leading to increased acid production from the more proximal acid-secreting corpus mucosa, which is relatively spared from inflammation. This increased gastric acid secretion can result in an increased duodenal acid load and ulceration.[5,6]
  - Conversely, *H. pylori* infection that damages the acid-producing mucosa of the more proximal stomach (i.e., corpus) can lead to hypochlorhydria or achlorhydria and subsequent gastric ulceration.[4]
  - Therefore, gastric ulcers are typically associated with normal or reduced levels of acid secretion, whereas duodenal ulcers are generally characterized by increased levels of acid secretion.[7]
  - Although it does not appear to have a predominant virulence factor, the ability of *H. pylori* to induce gastritis likely stems from a combination of factors.[8]
    - The organism secretes a urease enzyme that breaks down urea in the stomach to produce ammonia, which neutralizes the local acidic gastric environment and thereby protects the bacteria.
    - This urease activity provides the basis for many of the laboratory tests used to evaluate for *H. pylori* infection.
    - *H. pylori* infection is also thought to increase the permeability of the gastric mucus layer to pepsin and acid.
    - Finally, the bacterium produces toxins such as cytotoxin (CagA)[9] and vacuolating cytotoxin A (VacA)[10] that may also contribute to its pathogenicity.
  - *H. pylori* is a risk factor for gastric adenocarcinoma (which develops in 0.1–3% of infected patients)[5,11,12] and gastric mucosa–associated lymphoid tissue (MALT) lymphoma (in <0.01% of infected patients).[13]

- **NSAID-associated PUD**
  - NSAID use has been associated with 30–75% of *H. pylori*–negative ulcers and 15% of *H. pylori*–positive ulcers. It is the secondmost common cause of PUD after *H. pylori* infection.[1]
  - The rate of serious gastrointestinal (GI) complications in patients taking long-term NSAIDs is 7.3 per 1000 patients per year for osteoarthritis and 13 per 1000 patients per year for rheumatoid arthritis.
  - NSAIDs have a direct toxic effect due to their acidic composition and their ability to decrease hydrophobicity of gastric mucus, allowing epithelial injury by acid and pepsin.
  - The predominant mechanism of NSAID-associated PUD is inhibition of endogenous prostaglandin synthesis.[14] Therefore, enteric-coated, parenteral, or rectal NSAIDs present the same risk for ulcers as their oral counterparts. Administration of NSAIDs with food does not decrease ulcer risk.
  - Suppression of prostaglandin synthesis is mediated through inhibition of the cyclooxygenase (COX)-1 enzyme, a "housekeeping" enzyme that maintains integrity of the gastric mucosa where it is constitutively expressed.
  - Inhibition of prostaglandin synthesis decreases mucus production, bicarbonate secretion, mucosal perfusion, epithelial proliferation, and mucosal resistance to injury. These changes impair the integrity of the mucosa, allowing damage by harmful factors such as NSAIDs, pepsin, bile salts, and acid.[15,16]
  - COX-2–selective NSAIDs are less likely to cause GI complications because COX-2 enzyme, which mediates NSAID anti-inflammatory effects, is not expressed in gastric mucosa.[17]
  - NSAID use can cause a spectrum of lesions ranging from superficial erosions to ulcers that bleed or perforate. These affect any area of the stomach, but the gastric antrum is most frequently involved. Endoscopic evidence of mucosal damage has been found in up to two-thirds of patients who use NSAIDs and frank ulceration has been found in 10–25%.
  - Superficial lesions include petechiae and erosions, likely from the direct topical effects of NSAIDs that may occur within hours of NSAID administration. These are typically confined to the mucosa where they do not cause complications.
  - NSAID-associated ulcers can be complicated by hemorrhage and perforation. These complications occur with similar frequency among duodenal and gastric ulcers. Risk of hemorrhage is highest in the early treatment period in first-time users but can occur at any time during the course of treatment.
  - Platelet dysfunction may contribute to the tendency toward hemorrhage, especially with the use of acetylsalicylic acid (ASA).
- **Zollinger–Ellison syndrome**
  - Uncontrolled acid hypersecretion in the setting of gastrin-producing endocrine tumors (gastrinoma) of the pancreas or duodenum, termed Zollinger–Ellison syndrome, accounts for only 0.1% of all peptic ulcers. The syndrome includes multiple peptic ulcers, severe erosive esophagitis, and secretory diarrhea.[18]
  - The increased gastrin levels cause histamine release from enterochromaffin-like cells in the gastric mucosa. The histamine then binds to histamine receptors on parietal cells, causing hypersecretion of hydrochloric acid. Peptic ulcers can develop, as the normal defense mechanisms against acid are overwhelmed by the high gastric acid output.
  - Ulcers typically form in the duodenal bulb but may also be seen in the distal duodenum and jejunum, and multiple ulcers are commonly seen.
  - Diarrhea may also develop because of gastric acid–mediated damage to the small bowel mucosa resulting in net intestinal secretion. The excessive volume of gastric secretion may be contributory.

TABLE 14-2 RISK FACTORS FOR PEPTIC ULCER DISEASE

Infection with *Helicobacter pylori*	First-degree relative with peptic ulcer disease
NSAID use	Emigration from a developing nation
Smoking	African American or Hispanic ethnicity

NSAID, nonsteroidal anti-inflammatory drug.

○ The diagnosis should be suspected in any patient with multiple ulcers in unusual locations or in patients with a family history suggestive of multiple endocrine neoplasia type I.

○ An elevated gastrin level suggests the diagnosis in patients who make gastric acid. This can be assessed by aspirating a small volume of gastric secretions through a nasogastric tube or at endoscopy and testing the pH using litmus paper. A secretin stimulation test or formal fasting gastric acid output analysis helps confirm the diagnosis.

Pathophysiology

- Although the pathophysiology of PUD is not entirely understood, it is believed to arise from an imbalance between gastric mucosal protective factors (provided in part by prostaglandins) and destructive influences that can include *H. pylori,* gastric acid, pepsin, NSAIDs, bile salts, alcohol consumption, and cigarette smoking.[1]

Risk Factors

- Table 14-2 displays a list of known risk factors associated with PUD. The two major risk factors for PUD are *H. pylori* infection and NSAID use.
- Risk factors for the development of NSAID-associated PUD include concomitant corticosteroid use, anticoagulants, and older age (Table 14-3). Corticosteroids alone are not a risk factor for PUD.
- The role of *H. pylori* infection in NSAID-associated PUD remains incompletely defined. It is generally believed, however, that *H. pylori* and NSAIDs may act synergistically to induce PUD.[19]

DIAGNOSIS

In patients who present with symptoms that are suggestive of PUD, the diagnostic approach should attempt both to locate the anatomic abnormality and to explore its cause (often beginning with determining whether *H. pylori* infection is present).

TABLE 14-3 RISK FACTORS FOR NSAID-ASSOCIATED PEPTIC ULCER DISEASE

High NSAID dose	Prior peptic ulcer disease
Concomitant bisphosphonate use	Poor overall health
Concomitant anticoagulant use	Older age
Concomitant corticosteroid use	Female gender

NSAID, nonsteroidal anti-inflammatory drug.

Clinical Presentation

History

- History alone is unreliable in diagnosing PUD. Approximately two-thirds of patients who report dyspepsia have nonulcer or functional dyspepsia, and up to 40% of patients with active PUD have no abdominal pain, or "silent ulcers."
- The classic symptom complex of a patient with a **gastric ulcer** includes pain that occurs 5–15 minutes after oral intake and is relieved with fasting. For this reason, patients with gastric ulcers may learn to avoid food and thus lose weight.
- In contrast, patients with **duodenal ulcer** may have pain that occurs when acid is secreted in the absence of a food buffer and is temporarily relieved with eating but returns 1–2 hours later. However, this temporal relationship between pain and meals can be nonspecific, and the relief afforded by food can also be found in nonulcer dyspepsia.
- Because of the potential for duodenal ulcers to result in right upper quadrant pain, the presentation may mimic that of acute cholecystitis or a biliary colic.
- Perforation of a peptic ulcer may be heralded by an acute change in symptoms and sudden onset of severe diffuse abdominal pain.
- Chronic PUD can lead to scarring and gastric outlet obstruction, when nausea, vomiting, or weight loss may be prominent.
- Patients should be carefully questioned about NSAID and ASA use, including over-the-counter NSAIDs, even if patients have discontinued NSAID use.
- NSAID-associated ulcers are more likely than other forms of peptic ulcers to be painless and present initially with bleeding rather than dyspepsia.

Physical Examination

- In the absence of complicated PUD, the physical examination is not very helpful. Patients may have epigastric tenderness; however, the sensitivity (~65%) and specificity (~30%) of epigastric tenderness on palpation are very limited.[19]
- Patients with perforated peptic ulcers usually exhibit signs of peritonitis.
- Patients with bleeding ulcers may have fecal occult blood, melena, or hematemesis. If patients are hemodynamically compromised, they may be tachycardic or hypotensive.
- Bleeding may be the presenting sign in up to 15% of PUD cases.

Differential Diagnosis

- Table 14-4 lists a differential diagnosis for upper abdominal pain.
- Of note, it is difficult to differentiate functional or nonulcer dyspepsia from PUD on the basis of clinical examination. There are no diagnostic tests for functional dyspepsia, rendering it a diagnosis of exclusion.

TABLE 14-4 DIFFERENTIAL DIAGNOSIS FOR UPPER ABDOMINAL PAIN

Peptic ulcer disease	Functional dyspepsia
Carbohydrate malabsorption	Granulomatous diseases
Biliary pain	Crohn disease
Malignancy (gastric, esophageal, pancreatic)	Hepatoma
Gastroparesis	Medications
Electrolytes (hypercalcemia, hyperkalemia)	Ischemic bowel disease
Chronic abdominal wall pain	Gastroesophageal reflux disease
Parasites (Giardia, Strongyloides)	Systemic (diabetes mellitus, connective tissue diseases)

- Many medications can cause dyspeptic symptoms, including NSAIDs (with or without ulceration), iron, theophylline, and digitalis.
- Granulomatous diseases, including sarcoidosis, eosinophilic granuloma, and Wegener granulomatosis, may also present, albeit rarely, with dyspeptic symptoms.

Diagnostic Testing

Laboratory Testing

- Routine laboratory studies are usually unremarkable. **Complete blood cell count** may show iron-deficiency anemia from chronic fecal occult blood loss or anemia from acute blood loss.
- Patients in whom PUD is established or suspected should be tested for *H. pylori* infection, as this represents the major risk factor for PUD and can represent a contributing factor in ulcers from other causes, such as NSAID use.
  - **Serologic tests for IgG antibodies to *H. pylori***
    - Serology diagnoses *H. pylori* infection rather than the presence of PUD.
    - Because of high sensitivity, serologic tests are more accurate in areas with a high prevalence of *H. pylori*. Specificity is suboptimal in low prevalence areas, hence use is declining in the United States.
    - The most common serologic tests are laboratory-based enzyme-linked immunosorbent assay (ELISA) tests; the accuracy of ELISA testing can extend up to 95%.[20]
    - Less commonly used serology tests are based on immunochromatography and Western blot.
    - Serologic testing is simple and inexpensive, but antibodies to *H. pylori* can remain positive for 1–2 years after eradication of the infection; so it is difficult to evaluate *H. pylori* infection with serology after treatment.
  - **Stool antigen testing** can be more accurate than serology and can detect *H. pylori* only 1 week after discontinuation of proton pump inhibitor (PPI) therapy.
  - **Urease assays** test for the presence of the urease enzyme, which is produced in high amounts by *H. pylori*.
    - These tests include noninvasive urea breath testing as well as biopsy urease tests.
    - They can be used to diagnose active infection and to confirm eradication of infection.
    - False-negative results can occur in the setting of treatment with PPI, histamine 2 (H_2)-receptor blockers, antibiotics, or bismuth-containing medications. Therefore, PPI should be held for at least 7–14 days before testing.
    - In addition, urease breath testing to confirm eradication of *H. pylori* infection should be held until at least 4–6 weeks after completing treatment.
    - The two forms of the urea breath test are the ^{14}C-urea breath test and the ^{13}C-urea breath test.
    - These two breath tests use urea that has been labeled with a radioactive (^{14}C) or nonradioactive (^{13}C) isotope.
    - Labeled urea is given orally to the patient, and in the presence of urease produced by *H. pylori*, the urea is broken down into ammonia and labeled CO_2. After absorption of CO_2 into the circulation, it is expelled into the breath, and $^{13}CO_2$ can be detected by mass spectroscopy and $^{14}CO_2$ by scintillation counting.
    - Radioactive urea breath testing is contraindicated in pregnant women and in children.
    - The theoretical advantage of urea breath testing over biopsy urease tests is a decreased number of false-negative tests deriving from sampling error.[21]
    - Biopsy urease tests may be obtained via endoscopy and are discussed later.
  - **Culture** is not generally performed because it is expensive, time consuming, and difficult. Culture should not be considered unless a patient does not respond to eradication treatment and there is concern about antibiotic resistance.

Histology may be obtained via endoscopy and is discussed later.

Measurement of **serum gastrin levels** and/or **secretin stimulation testing** may be performed if Zollinger–Ellison syndrome is suspected.

Imaging

- Given the advantages of endoscopy, **upper GI radiography** has a limited role in the diagnosis of PUD.
- A radiographic diagnosis of PUD requires demonstration of barium within an ulcer niche, but the sensitivity of barium radiography for detecting PUD depends on the radiologist, and radiography can miss up to half of all duodenal ulcers.[22]

Diagnostic Procedures

- **Upper endoscopy** (esophagogastroduodenoscopy, or EGD) is the most accurate diagnostic test for PUD.
- Decisions regarding EGD for patients with symptoms of PUD should be based on patient symptoms and the risk of gastric cancer. EGD should be performed in patients who have signs or symptoms worrisome for gastric cancer ("alarm symptoms"), including anorexia, dysphagia, epigastric mass, severe vomiting, weight loss, anemia, advanced age, or family history of upper GI cancer.
- Patients with significant dyspepsia, acute GI bleeding, fecal occult blood, or abdominal pain of unclear etiology should also undergo EGD.
- In patients with a high suspicion of PUD, consideration may be given to performing noninvasive testing, such as fecal *H. pylori* antigen testing or urease breath testing without endoscopy, especially if the patient is young and otherwise healthy, as these noninvasive tests are more cost-effective than EGD.
- **Biopsy urease testing** is the best endoscopic method of diagnosing *H. pylori* infection.
  - Biopsy urease tests include the CLOtest, PyloriTek, and Hp-fast.
  - Most of these tests involve a pH-sensitive dye that changes color because of an increase in pH secondary to the production of ammonia from urea.
  - In addition to false-negative results in the setting of prior treatment with PPI, false-negative results can also occur if blood from recent or active bleeding is present.
  - If it is not possible to hold PPI before testing, biopsy samples should be taken from both the antrum and the fundus to increase the likelihood of a positive result.
- **Endoscopic biopsies** are indicated in gastric ulcers because of the risk of malignancy, or in cases of PUD in which urease testing might be falsely negative (i.e., in the setting of PPI use before endoscopy).
- In the case of gastric ulcers, biopsy samples should be obtained from around the ulcer crater and edges to rule out malignancy, but they should also be obtained from other areas of the stomach to test for *H. pylori* infection, which typically presents as a multifocal gastritis.
- Biopsy may be less sensitive in the setting of bleeding ulcers, so other sampling-independent testing, such as serology, should be performed.
- Patients with a gastric ulcer should undergo follow-up EGD at 8–12 weeks to document ulcer healing and exclude malignancy in most instances, as follow-up endoscopy improves survival.[23]
- Duodenal ulcers do not require biopsy or repeat EGD because of the extremely low risk of malignancy.[4,12]

TREATMENT

Medications

- Medications used to treat PUD include antisecretory agents and mucosal protectants such as sucralfate and prostaglandin analogs.

- Duodenal ulcers should be treated with **antisecretory agents** for 4 weeks and gastric ulcers should be treated for 8 weeks. In cases with ulcers >1 cm, complicated PUD, unsuccessful *H. pylori* eradication, or *H. pylori*–negative PUD, it is reasonable to treat with a longer course of antisecretory therapy. Otherwise, maintenance antisecretory therapy after treatment of *H. pylori* infection is not cost-effective and is generally unnecessary.
- Antisecretory agents include H$_2$-receptor antagonists and PPI.
- **H$_2$-receptor antagonists**
  - H$_2$-receptor blockers inhibit acid secretion by blocking the binding of histamine to its receptor on the parietal cell. They inhibit both basal and food-induced acid secretion.
  - The H$_2$-receptor blockers available in the United States include cimetidine, famotidine, nizatidine, and ranitidine.
  - This class of medications is well tolerated, although doses should be adjusted in patients with renal insufficiency. They have largely been replaced by PPIs.
  - In general, when used in the treatment of PUD, H$_2$-receptor blockers are most effective when administered between dinner and bedtime.
- **Proton pump inhibitors**
  - These medications are prodrugs that, when activated by acid, bind to and inhibit the parietal cell H$^+$/K$^+$ adenosine triphosphatase (ATPase).
  - Because they require acid for activation, they are most effectively taken before or with a meal and in the absence of other antisecretory drugs.
  - PPIs pose a theoretical risk of inducing enterochromaffin-like cell hyperplasia and carcinoid tumors, but these medications have been used safely in the United States for the past decade without a notable increase in the incidence of carcinoid tumors.[24]
- **Misoprostol**
  - Misoprostol is a prostaglandin analog.
  - Misoprostol is approved by the U.S. Food and Drug Administration for prophylaxis of NSAID-induced peptic ulcers.
  - Because of its mechanism of action, misoprostol can cause diarrhea or spontaneous abortion.
- **Treatment of *Helicobacter pylori*–associated PUD**
  - Treatment requires both antisecretory and antibiotic therapy, as the **eradication of *H. pylori* infection with antibiotics** significantly lowers the 12-month ulcer recurrence rate from upward of 60% in patients treated with antisecretory therapy alone to <5%.[25]
  - *H. pylori*–associated ulcers may heal spontaneously but frequently recur if the infection is not eradicated.
  - Many regimens have been developed for *H. pylori* eradication, mostly through trial and error, and accepted treatment regimens are listed in Table 14-5.[26] Some regimens are relatively inexpensive but require dosing four times daily, which may decrease compliance.

TABLE 14-5 TREATMENT REGIMENS FOR HELICOBACTER PYLORI ERADICATION

PPI PO BID; amoxicillin, 1000 mg PO BID; clarithromycin, 500 mg PO BID

PPI PO BID; amoxicillin, 1000 mg PO BID; metronidazole (or tinidazole), 500 mg PO BID

PPI PO BID; bismuth subsalicylate, 300 or 525 mg PO QID; metronidazole, 250 or 500 mg PO TID/QID; tetracycline, 500 mg PO QID

PPI, proton pump inhibitor. With the exception of ranitidine bismuth citrate, treatment duration is 14 days.

Effective regimens typically involve more than one antibiotic to maximize the likelihood of eradication and prevent the spread of antimicrobial resistance; monotherapy is inadequate. Amoxicillin and clarithromycin are pH-dependent antibiotics that work more effectively in combination with antisecretory drugs. If this "triple therapy" fails, a salvage course of bismuth-containing "quadruple therapy" can eradicate *H. pylori* infection in an additional three-fourths of patients.

The success rates of these recommended regimens for eradicating *H. pylori* infection appear to have decreased to 70–85% with increasing antibiotic resistance.[25] Treatment failure may be secondary to noncompliance or antibiotic resistance, which occurs most commonly with metronidazole in the United States.

In patients with uncomplicated PUD, confirmation of eradication is not required because recurrence would most likely also be uncomplicated. However, testing for *H. pylori* eradication should be performed in patients with recurrent symptoms, complicated PUD, gastric MALT lymphoma, or early gastric cancer. Because of the high rate of bleeding recurrence in untreated *H. pylori*–positive bleeding ulcers, testing for eradication is critical.

Confirmation of cure can be performed by urea breath testing, but it should be done at least 4–6 weeks after completion of *H. pylori* therapy and 2 weeks after finishing PPI treatment to avoid false-negative results. Serology is less useful to document eradication, as the antibodies to *H. pylori* may remain positive for 1–2 years after successful eradication.

- **Treatment of NSAID-associated PUD**
  - Consideration must be given to **stopping the offending drug**, as continuation of NSAID use delays ulcer healing. However, discontinuing the NSAID is not always practical, and in these cases, GI toxicity may be reduced by decreasing the dose or switching to a less gastrotoxic medication.[27,28] Concomitant corticosteroid, anticoagulant, or bisphosphonate therapy should also be discontinued if possible.
  - Direct treatment of NSAID-induced PUD is **acid suppression with a PPI**.
  - Even with continued NSAID use, acid suppression with PPI therapy results in 85% of NSAID-induced gastric ulcers and >90% of duodenal ulcers healing within 8 weeks, whereas acid suppression with conventional doses of H_2-receptor blockers heals approximately 70% of gastric and duodenal ulcers within 7 weeks. In this manner, PPI therapy is indicated for NSAID-associated PUD and should be continued as long as the patient is being treated with NSAID to reduce the risk of ulcer recurrence.[29]
  - Gastroprotection with either PPI or misoprostol is required during NSAID use in the following: history of a prior ulcer, severe concomitant disease, concomitant warfarin or corticosteroid use, or elderly (>65 years).

Lifestyle/Risk Modification

- Withdrawal of potential contributing agents such as NSAIDs, cigarettes, and excess alcohol is indicated.
- Patients should be instructed to avoid foods that precipitate dyspepsia, although no particular dietary recommendations are necessary.

SPECIAL CONSIDERATIONS

Stress ulcers develop in the stomach and duodenum under situations of severe physiologic stress and intensive care unit (ICU) admission, such as mechanical ventilation, coagulopathy, renal failure, head injuries, burns, and multiple trauma. Pathophysiology involves relative mucosal ischemia and poor mucosal protection from intraluminal acid when splanchnic blood supply is shunted to more important organs during physiologic stress. Erosions and ulcers are demonstrated to form frequently within the first 2–3 days of ICU admission, but complications (bleeding, perforation) are relatively rare in the present day, attributed to better ICU care, attention to hemodynamic stability, and stress ulcer prophylaxis. Patients at risk can be administered intravenous H2-receptor antagonists by infusion; PPIs have also been demonstrated to provide equivalent protection.[30,31] Sucralfate has also been used successfully as a prophylactic agent. If bleeding ensues, management is similar to that of nonvariceal upper GI bleeding from peptic ulcers (Chapter 6).

COMPLICATIONS

- **Hemorrhage**
  - Hemorrhage can occur in approximately 15% of patients with peptic ulcers. See Chapter 6 for further discussion on management of GI bleeding from PUD.
  - NSAID-associated ulcers are overrepresented among hemorrhagic ulcers.
  - Hemorrhage can present as either an acute event with hemodynamic shock or as a slow intermittent blood loss with chronic anemia.
  - If necessary, endoscopic intervention can be utilized to locate the source of bleeding and achieve hemostasis with thermal or laser coagulation, injection sclerotherapy, or mechanical compression with clips.
  - The administration of intravenous PPIs in acute hemorrhage decreases rebleeding rates, the need for blood transfusions, and mortality rates.[32]
- **Perforation** should be suspected in patients with PUD who suddenly develop severe diffuse abdominal pain and other manifestations of peritoneal irritation. Plain abdominal radiography may reveal free air under the diaphragm. Emergent surgery is often indicated for perforation.
- **Obstruction** of the gastric outlet can develop from ulcers in the duodenal bulb and/ or pyloric channel, and patients can present with nausea and vomiting. Management typically involves nasogastric tube placement with measurement of the gastric residual, EGD to facilitate diagnosis (with balloon dilation in patients who do not respond to medical therapy), and intravenous PPI therapy.
- **Penetration** occurs when an ulcer penetrates through the bowel wall without any free perforation or leakage of luminal contents into the peritoneal cavity. Most commonly, ulcers penetrate into the pancreas, gastrohepatic omentum, biliary tract, or liver, but only a small proportion become clinically apparent.

Gastric Adenocarcinoma

GENERAL PRINCIPLES

- In the early 1900s, gastric cancer represented the most common cancer in the United States, but since then, the incidence has decreased dramatically, possibly related to the popularization of refrigeration. Nevertheless, each year >21,000 patients in the United States have a diagnosis of gastric cancer, of whom >11,000 are expected to die.[33]
- As recently as the 1980s, gastric cancer represented the leading cause of cancer deaths worldwide.[34] Of note, *H. pylori* infection appears to be associated with an approximately sixfold increase in the risk of gastric cancer.[35]
- Table 14-6 outlines risk factors for gastric cancer.

DIAGNOSIS

- Many patients with gastric cancer are asymptomatic or present with **nonspecific symptoms** that can include indigestion, epigastric discomfort, anorexia, early satiety, and weight loss. By the time symptoms have been investigated, many gastric cancers are advanced.

TABLE 14-6 RISK FACTORS FOR GASTRIC ADENOCARCINOMA

Helicobacter pylori infection	Prior gastrectomy
Chronic atrophic gastritis	Blood type A
Pernicious anemia	Family history of gastric cancer
Gastric adenoma	Low socioeconomic status

- **Physical examination** may reveal an epigastric mass, ascites, occult blood in stool, or lymphadenopathy.
- An enlarged left supraclavicular lymph node (Virchow node) or periumbilical lymph node (Sister Mary Joseph node) represents a metastatic site.
- **Laboratory evaluation** is of limited use but may demonstrate iron deficiency anemia from chronic blood loss from the cancer.
- **Diagnosis is best made with EGD**, as it allows for direct visualization as well as tissue sampling. Most gastric cancers are exophytic or fungating masses, but some manifest as nonhealing ulcers or with perforation of the gastric wall.
- All gastric ulcers should be aggressively biopsied to exclude malignancy, and repeat EGD should be performed at 8–12 weeks to document healing in any patient with a gastric ulcer.
- Once the diagnosis of gastric adenocarcinoma is established, staging should be performed with endoscopic ultrasonography or abdominal computed tomographic scanning to determine whether surgical resection is an option.

TREATMENT

- **Surgical resection** offers the only chance for cure.
- However, approximately 60% of gastric cancers are deemed unresectable because of local or metastatic spread at the time of diagnosis.
- Depending on location, partial or total gastrectomy may be performed.
- Even with complete resection, 5-year survival rate of patients with advanced/metastatic gastric cancer is <5%.[36]
- **Palliative chemotherapy** can be given to patients who are not surgical candidates, but the median survival is only 6–9 months.[37]

Gastrointestinal Stromal Tumors

GENERAL PRINCIPLES

- Gastrointestinal stromal tumors (GIST) represent 1–2% of all malignant GI tumors. Before the molecular definition of GIST in 1998, these lesions were commonly unrecognized and unreported.
- Despite the increasing recognition of GIST, its true incidence remains unknown, although it has been estimated to be approximately 15 cases per million persons in the United States.
- The median occurrence is in the fifth decade of life, and GIST is found more commonly in women than in men.
- In 1998, the pathophysiology of GIST was discovered to involve mutations in *KIT* signaling pathways leading to tumor proliferation. The definition of GIST has subsequently been narrowed to include a subset of tumors arising from the interstitial cells of Cajal, >90% of which exhibit KIT mutations.
- GIST can be found throughout the GI tract, although 60–70% arise in the stomach.

DIAGNOSIS

- Patients may complain of nonspecific symptoms, such as nausea, vomiting, or early satiety. GIST may also be discovered incidentally on endoscopy or imaging.
- Alternatively, GIST lesions may present after achieving a large size and causing mass effect or obstruction, or with acute upper GI hemorrhage.

TREATMENT

- **Surgical resection** represents the treatment of choice for localized tumors.
- However, if the tumor has metastasized, **chemotherapy** remains an option.
- GIST harbors impressive resistance to traditional cytotoxic chemotherapy agents, but the introduction of the tyrosine kinase inhibitor imatinib mesylate has increased the median survival of patients with advanced GIST from 20–60 months.[38,39]

Gastric Lymphoma

GENERAL PRINCIPLES

- The GI tract represents the predominant site of primary extranodal lymphomas.
- GI lymphomas are most commonly found in the stomach (almost three-fourths of cases) in developed countries. More than 90% of gastric lymphomas are either diffuse large B-cell type or MALT type.
- MALT lymphomas comprise 40% of gastric lymphomas and arise from the transformation of B cells in the marginal zone of the stomach in response to *H. pylori* infection.
- Although *H. pylori* infection is a risk factor, the incidence of MALT in *H. pylori*–infected individuals is between 1 in 30,000 and 1 in 80,000.[40]

DIAGNOSIS

- The most common presenting symptoms are abdominal pain and dyspepsia; B-type symptoms are rare.
- Diagnosis is typically established via EGD with biopsies.

TREATMENT

- Up to three-fourths of patients with low-grade MALT lymphomas experience complete regression after **eradication of *H. pylori* infection**.[25]
- For patients who do not respond to *H. pylori* eradication, radiation, chemotherapy, and surgery represent effective therapeutic options.

REFERENCES

1. Lanas A, Chan FKL. Peptic ulcer disease. *Lancet*. 2017;390(10094):613–624.
2. Sugano K, Tack J, Kuipers EJ, et al. Kyoto global consensus report on Helicobacter pylori gastritis. *Gut*. 2015;64:1353–1367.
3. Andersen LP. Colonization and infection by Helicobacter pylori in humans. *Helicobacter*. 2007;12(Suppl 2):12–15.
4. Graham DY. History of Helicobacter pylori, duodenal ulcer, gastric ulcer and gastric cancer. *World J Gastroenterol*. 2014;20:5191–5204.
5. Ernst PB, Gold BD. The disease spectrum of Helicobacter pylori: the immunopathogenesis of gastroduodenal ulcer and gastric cancer. *Annu Rev Microbiol*. 2000;54:615–640.

6. Malfertheiner P. The intriguing relationship of Helicobacter pylori infection and acid secretion in peptic ulcer disease and gastric cancer. *Dig Dis.* 2011;29:459–464.

7. Saenz JB, Mills JC. Acid and the basis for cellular plasticity and reprogramming in gastric repair and cancer. *Nat Rev Gastroenterol Hepatol.* 2018;15:257–273.

8. Amieva M, Peek RM Jr. Pathobiology of Helicobacter pylori-induced gastric cancer. *Gastroenterology.* 2016;150:64–78.

9. Hatakeyama M. Helicobacter pylori CagA and gastric cancer: a paradigm for hit-and-run carcinogenesis. *Cell Host Microbe.* 2014;15:306–316.

10. Greenfield LK, Jones NL. Modulation of autophagy by Helicobacter pylori and its role in gastric carcinogenesis. *Trends Microbiol.* 2013;21:602–612.

11. Kuipers EJ. Review article: exploring the link between Helicobacter pylori and gastric cancer. *Aliment Pharmacol Ther.* 1999;13(Suppl 1):3–11.

12. Hansson LE, Nyren O, Hsing AW, et al. The risk of stomach cancer in patients with gastric or duodenal ulcer disease. *N Engl J Med.* 1996;335:242–249.

13. Hu Q, Zhang Y, Zhang X, et al. Gastric mucosa-associated lymphoid tissue lymphoma and Helicobacter pylori infection: a review of current diagnosis and management. *Biomark Res.* 2016;4:15.

14. Wallace JL. Prostaglandins, NSAIDs, and gastric mucosal protection: why doesn't the stomach digest itself? *Physiol Rev.* 2008;88:1547–1565.

15. McColl KE. The elegance of the gastric mucosal barrier: designed by nature for nature. *Gut.* 2012;61:787–788.

16. Yandrapu H, Sarosiek J. Protective factors of the gastric and duodenal mucosa: an overview. *Curr Gastroenterol Rep.* 2015;17:24.

17. Huang JQ, Sridhar S, Hunt RH. Role of Helicobacter pylori infection and non-steroidal anti-inflammatory drugs in peptic-ulcer disease: a meta-analysis. *Lancet.* 2002;359:14–22.

18. Komorowski RA, Caya JG. Hyperplastic gastropathy. Clinicopathologic correlation. *Am J Surg Pathol.* 1991;15:577–585.

19. Moayyedi P, Talley NJ, Fennerty MB, et al. Can the clinical history distinguish between organic and functional dyspepsia? *JAMA.* 2006;295:1566–1576.

20. Loy CT, Irwig LM, Katelaris PH, et al. Do commercial serological kits for Helicobacter pylori infection differ in accuracy? A meta-analysis. *Am J Gastroenterol.* 1996;91:1138–1144.

21. Graham DY, Miftahussurur M. Helicobacter pylori urease for diagnosis of Helicobacter pylori infection: a mini review. *J Adv Res.* 2018;13:51–57.

22. Hopper AN, Stephens MR, Lewis WG, et al. Relative value of repeat gastric ulcer surveillance gastroscopy in diagnosing gastric cancer. *Gastric Cancer.* 2006;9:217–222.

23. Leodolter A, Kulig M, Brasch H, et al. A meta-analysis comparing eradication, healing and relapse rates in patients with Helicobacter pylori-associated gastric or duodenal ulcer. *Aliment Pharmacol Ther.* 2001;15:1949–1958.

24. Sheen E, Triadafilopoulos G. Adverse effects of long-term proton pump inhibitor therapy. *Dig Dis Sci.* 2011;56:931–950.

25. Chey WD, Wong BC; Practice Parameters Committee of the American College of Gastroenterology. American College of Gastroenterology guideline on the management of Helicobacter pylori infection. *Am J Gastroenterol.* 2007;102:1808–1825.

26. Fallone CA, Chiba N, van Zanten SV, et al. The Toronto consensus for the treatment of Helicobacter pylori infection in adults. *Gastroenterology.* 2016;151:51–69.e14.

27. Scarpignato C, Pelosini I. Prevention and treatment of non-steroidal anti-inflammatory drug-induced gastro-duodenal damage: rationale for the use of antisecretory compounds. *Ital J Gastroenterol Hepatol.* 1999;31(Suppl 1):S63–S72.

28. Bjarnason I, Scarpignato C, Holmgren E, et al. Mechanisms of damage to the gastrointestinal tract from nonsteroidal anti-inflammatory drugs. *Gastroenterology.* 2018;154:500–514.

29. Scheiman JM, Yeomans ND, Talley NJ, et al. Prevention of ulcers by esomeprazole in at-risk patients using non-selective NSAIDs and COX-2 inhibitors. *Am J Gastroenterol.* 2006;101:701–710.

30. Barbateskovic M, Marker S, Granholm A, et al. Stress ulcer prophylaxis with proton pump inhibitors or histamin-2 receptor antagonists in adult intensive care patients: a systematic review with meta-analysis and trial sequential analysis. *Intensive Care Med.* 2019;45:143–158.

31. Pilkington KB, Wagstaff MJ, Greenwood JE. Prevention of gastrointestinal bleeding due to stress ulceration: a review of current literature. *Anaesth Intensive Care.* 2012;40:253–259.

32. Sachar H, Vaidya K, Laine L. Intermittent vs continuous proton pump inhibitor therapy for high-risk bleeding ulcers: a systematic review and meta-analysis. *JAMA Intern Med.* 2014;174:1755–1762.

33. Ferlay J, Shin HR, Bray F, et al. Estimates of worldwide burden of cancer in 2008: GLOBOCAN 2008. *Int J Cancer*. 2010;127:2893–2917.
34. Plummer M, de Martel C, Vignat J, et al. Global burden of cancers attributable to infections in 2012: a synthetic analysis. *Lancet Glob Health*. 2016;4:e609–e616.
35. The EUROGAST Study Group. An international association between Helicobacter pylori infection and gastric cancer. *Lancet*. 1993;341:1359–1362.
36. Yang D, Hendifar A, Lenz C, et al. Survival of metastatic gastric cancer: significance of age, sex and race/ethnicity. *J Gastrointest Oncol*. 2011;2:77–84.
37. Wohrer SS, Raderer M, Hejna M. Palliative chemotherapy for advanced gastric cancer. *Ann Oncol*. 2004;15:1585–1595.
38. Wang D, Zhang Q, Blanke CD, et al. Phase II trial of neoadjuvant/adjuvant imatinib mesylate for advanced primary and metastatic/recurrent operable gastrointestinal stromal tumors: long-term follow-up results of Radiation Therapy Oncology Group 0132. *Ann Surg Oncol*. 2012;19:1074–1080.
39. Blanke CD, Demetri GD, von Mehren M, et al. Long-term results from a randomized phase II trial of standard- versus higher-dose imatinib mesylate for patients with unresectable or metastatic gastrointestinal stromal tumors expressing KIT. *J Clin Oncol*. 2008;26:620–625.
40. Farinha P, Gascoyne RD. Helicobacter pylori and MALT lymphoma. *Gastroenterology*. 2005;128:1579–1605.

15

Small Bowel Disorders

Martin H. Gregory and Deborah C. Rubin

Introduction

- The small bowel is approximately 600 cm in length, with a functional surface area >600 times that of a hollow tube.
- The following three features unique to the gut enhance the surface area of the small intestine:
  - The plicae circulares, or circular folds, are visible mucosal and submucosal invaginations located predominantly in the duodenum and jejunum.
  - Villi are fingerlike projections, consisting of a layer of epithelial cells overlying the lamina propria, approximately 0.5–1.5 mm long, which protrude into the intestinal lumen and cover the mucosal surface.
  - Microvilli, tubular projections visualized by electron microscopy, are extensions of the apical cell membrane and compose the brush border.
  - These unique mucosal features create an enormous area for digestion, absorption, and secretion.[1]

Malabsorption

GENERAL PRINCIPLES

- Small bowel disorders, pancreatic exocrine insufficiency, and cholestatic liver disease account for most causes of malabsorption.
- Table 15-1 lists the most common causes of malabsorption. Cholestatic liver diseases are discussed in Chapter 20. Pancreatic disorders are discussed in Chapter 23.

Definition

- Malabsorption can be defined as an interruption of normal digestion, absorption, and transport of nutrients and minerals.
- Malnutrition, diarrhea, steatorrhea, electrolyte abnormalities, and weight loss are frequent consequences.
- Clinical manifestations of small bowel disorders often reflect deficiencies of various macro- and micronutrients.

Pathophysiology

- Various disease processes (including celiac disease, Whipple disease, tropical sprue, small bowel bacterial overgrowth, radiation or chemotherapy–induced injury, see subsequent sections) interfere with mucosal luminal digestion, absorption, and nutrient transport.
- The small bowel is primarily responsible for absorbing daily dietary carbohydrates, proteins, fats, electrolytes, and essential nutrients.
- Small bowel disorders can result in selective malabsorption of nutrients depending on the part of the small bowel that is affected. For example, iron, folate, and calcium malabsorption may result from duodenal disease, whereas B12 and bile salt malabsorption

TABLE 15-1 CAUSES OF MALABSORPTION

Small Intestine Disorders	Pancreatic Exocrine Insufficiency
Celiac sprue	Chronic pancreatitis
Ileal resection	Cystic fibrosis
Short bowel syndrome	Pancreatic cancer
Radiation enteritis	Cholestatic liver disease
Small bowel lymphoma	Extrahepatic biliary obstruction
Bacterial overgrowth	Intrahepatic biliary obstruction
Crohn disease	Cirrhosis
Tropical sprue	
Whipple disease	
Acquired immunodeficiency syndrome	
Abetalipoproteinemia	
Diabetes mellitus	
Amyloidosis	
Eosinophilic gastroenteritis	
Protein-losing enteropathy	

occurs with ileal involvement. Fat-soluble vitamins A, D, E, and K deficiencies can occur in proximal small bowel disorders.

DIAGNOSIS

Clinical features and presentation of intestinal malabsorption form the cornerstone of diagnosis and result in effects on numerous organ systems including the gastrointestinal (GI) tract and the hematopoietic, musculoskeletal, endocrine, epidermal, and nervous systems.

Clinical Presentation

- Abdominal pain, cramping, excessive flatus, diarrhea (postprandial or unremitting without prandial exacerbation).
- Weight loss despite appropriate appetite and adequate oral intake.
- Foul-smelling stool with oily character.
- Specific fat-soluble vitamin malabsorption leads to various clinical findings including night blindness (vitamin A), osteopenia/osteoporosis (vitamin D), bleeding diathesis (vitamin K), or neurologic symptoms (vitamin E).
- In addition, amenorrhea, infertility, and impotence may manifest as part of patient history.
- Physical examination findings include glossitis, stomatitis (iron, riboflavin, niacin), tetany (calcium, magnesium, vitamin D), dermatitis (vitamin A, zinc, niacin), peripheral neuropathy (B12, copper, thiamine), and edema (protein-losing enteropathy).

Differential Diagnosis

- Infectious, secretory, and inflammatory causes of diarrhea must be excluded.
- Pancreatic exocrine insufficiency and hepatobiliary disease resulting in intraluminal bile salt deficiency (biliary strictures, cholestatic liver diseases) can result in intraluminal maldigestion and malabsorption.

- Associated malabsorption symptoms must be thoroughly evaluated.
  - For example, alternative causes of weight loss including malignancy, hormonal disorders, and inflammatory/autoimmune disorders should be evaluated.
  - Postprandial abdominal cramping should be evaluated for etiologies such as peptic ulcer disease, cholelithiasis, and pancreatitis.

Diagnostic Testing

Laboratory Testing

- Laboratory test abnormalities include macrocytic (folate, vitamin B12 deficiency) and microcytic (iron deficiency) anemia, elevated INR/prolonged prothrombin time (vitamin K deficiency), and decreased serum calcium (calcium malabsorption or vitamin D deficiency).
- Low serum magnesium and zinc levels, decreased serum albumin, and low cholesterol may also be found. Stool analysis for fat by Sudan red stain or for α_1-antitrypsin for protein-losing enteropathy may be informative.
- **Fecal fat analysis** provides a simple, rapid, inexpensive screening test for malabsorption.[2]
  - Measurement includes fecal fat quantification for 48–72 hours while patient is on a defined intake of fat, typically 100 g/day.
  - Normally, >94% of dietary fat is absorbed; consequently >6 g/day of fecal fat is diagnostic of steatorrhea.
  - Fecal fat analysis does not distinguish among intestinal, hepatobiliary, and pancreatic causes of malabsorption, although the level of steatorrhea associated with pancreatic insufficiency (~50 g) tends to be higher than the level for intestinal disease (~20 g).[3]
- **D-xylose absorption test**
  - This test assesses the absorptive capacity of the small intestine and determines whether a small bowel disorder is present.[2,4]
  - This test is usually performed for further diagnostic purposes once malabsorption is determined.
  - D-xylose is a 5-carbon sugar primarily absorbed passively in the small intestine. Intraluminal digestion is not required and urinary excretion reflects the mucosa's ability to absorb it.
  - This test is performed by administration of 25 g of xylose orally, followed by measurement of urinary excretion, hydrogen breath testing (discussed below), or serum concentration of xylose. A 5-hour urine collection contains at least 5 g of D-xylose.
  - This test can therefore differentiate between pancreatic disorders (D-xylose concentration within normal limits) and true mucosal malabsorptive processes (D-xylose concentration decreased postadministration).[4,5]
- It is important to note that certain bacterial species may metabolize D-xylose causing concurrent bacterial overgrowth–mediated decreased D-xylose levels.
- Low urinary excretion will also occur when delayed gastric emptying, impaired renal function, or ascites is present.
- **Hydrogen breath tests**
  - Hydrogen breath tests are based on the principle that hydrogen is produced by bacterial fermentation of carbohydrates that have escaped absorption in the small intestine. A portion of this hydrogen diffuses into the blood stream and is subsequently exhaled by the lungs and analyzed in breath. Commonly used carbohydrates include lactose, fructose, glucose, and nonabsorbable compounds such as lactulose.[5,6]
  - Hydrogen breath tests can be used to diagnose disaccharidase (lactase) deficiency and lactose intolerance in association with symptoms of abdominal pain, gas, and diarrhea with lactose intake. It is also used for the evaluation of small intestinal bacterial overgrowth (SIBO) (see later).[6]

- Under typical circumstances, only bacterial carbohydrate metabolism is responsible for exhaled hydrogen.
- In disaccharidase deficiency, carbohydrates are not metabolized in the proximal small bowel lumen and travel to the distal small bowel/colon where they are metabolized by colonized bacteria releasing hydrogen.
- Exhaled hydrogen is measured after the patient is given 25–50 g of oral lactose dissolved in water.
- Hydrogen (H_2) levels in end-expiratory breath samples are measured every 15 minutes for up to 3 hours.
- An increase of >20 ppm over basal values for two time points indicates lactose malabsorption. A positive test usually peaks at 2–4 hours.
- False-negative results can occur in setting of colonic flora that do not produce hydrogen, delayed gastric emptying, or prolonged orocecal transit time. False-positive results can occur from oral flora substrate fermentation and hydrogen production. Antibiotic use and fiber intake can also alter the results.
- An early hydrogen peak within 1 hour of ingestion of lactulose may indicate SIBO.
- The lactulose hydrogen breath test suffers from similar false-positive and false-negative results as disaccharidase deficiency workup.
- It is usually performed with an oral load of 10-g lactulose or glucose in a dose of 50–75 g dissolved in water with subsequent hydrogen breath level measurement as above.
- Interpretation of these tests is not uniform; reported sensitivity and specificity of the lactulose hydrogen breath test in detecting SIBO is 52% and 86%, respectively, and for the glucose breath test 63% and 82%, respectively.[6]
- The gold standard remains aspiration of the small bowel contents and subsequent culture. This is not used clinically for diagnosing SIBO.

Imaging

- Imaging for small bowel pathologic processes can be performed with **barium small bowel follow-through** examinations, **single- or double-contrast intubated enteroclysis, computed tomography** (CT) cross-sectional imaging, or magnetic resonance enterography.
- Barium small bowel follow-through and enteroclysis provide fine detail of the mucosal surface.
- **Capsule endoscopy, push endoscopy,** and single- and **double-balloon endoscopy** visualize the mucosal surface of the small bowel. If successfully completed, both capsule endoscopy and double-balloon endoscopy can image the mucosal surface in its entirety.
- Cross-sectional imaging techniques provide good visualization of both superimposed bowel loops and extraluminal findings and complications.
  - **MR enterography (MRE):** Advantages include the lack of ionizing radiation, improved soft tissue contrast, and the ability to provide real-time and functional evaluation.[7]
  - **CT enterography: Advantages include** superior temporal and spatial resolution. Compared with MRE, it is more widely available, and is less expensive.[8]
- Indications for cross-sectional imaging of the small bowel include evaluation of obscure GI bleeding, the presence and activity of Crohn disease, and suspected neoplasia.

Diagnostic Procedures

- **Endoscopic biopsy**
  - Biopsy of the small intestine is extremely useful in patients with suspected malabsorption.
- Specific histologic findings allow diagnosis of the more common causes of malabsorption, such as celiac sprue, as well as more infrequent causes, such as lymphoma and amyloidosis.

Celiac Sprue

GENERAL PRINCIPLES

- Celiac sprue is the most frequently evaluated etiology among the malabsorptive small bowel disorders.
- Sensitive and specific serologies are available and tissue biopsy is usually confirmatory.
- Symptomatic resolution is achieved with avoidance of food products containing gluten.

Definition

Permanent intolerance to the storage proteins or *gluten* found in wheat, rye, and barley results in symptoms of malabsorption including weight loss, abdominal cramping, diarrhea, and excessive flatus.[9]

Epidemiology

Positivity for celiac antibodies is much more common than patients with symptoms. The prevalence of celiac disease in the United States is approximately 1%, similar to Europe.[10]

Pathophysiology

- A consequence of complex adaptive and innate immune responses to dietary gluten, is characterized by chronic inflammation of the proximal intestinal mucosa mediated primarily by T-cell immunologic processes.[9]
- HLA antigen class II DQ molecules DQ2 and DQ8 are necessary but not sufficient for phenotypic expression of the disease.
- Mucosal antigen presenting cells that express HLA DQ2 or HLA DQ8 bind gliadin peptides that are absorbed. Tissue transglutaminase (tTG) deamidates gliadin peptides to allow higher affinity binding to the binding groove of DQ2 or DQ8. The antigen presenting cells then present them to gluten-sensitized CD4+ T cells. These T cells activate B cells to secrete immunoglobulins and activate other CD8+ cells. These release proinflammatory cytokines that mediate damage to the intestinal mucosa.[11]
- Additional innate immune responses are mediated and activated by intraepithelial lymphocytes and act in concert via interleukin-15 produced by enterocytes.
- Since not all people with HLA DQ2 or DQ8 develop celiac disease, other genetic and environmental factors play a role. Some hypothesized factors include the age gluten is introduced and childhood GI infections.

Risk Factors and Associated Conditions

- **High-risk populations** include the following[9]:
  - First-degree relatives of patients with celiac disease (prevalence 10%).
  - Patients with dermatitis herpetiformis (prevalence >90%).
  - Patients with unexplained iron deficiency anemia (prevalence 2–5%).
  - Osteoporosis and bone demineralization (prevalence 1.5–3.0%).
  - Type 1 diabetes mellitus (prevalence 2–5% in adults and 3–8% in children).
  - Patients with liver disease:
    - Elevated transaminase levels of unknown cause (prevalence 1.5–9.0%).
    - Autoimmune hepatitis (prevalence 2.9–6.4%).
    - Primary biliary cirrhosis (prevalence 0–6.0%).
- Genetic disorders (prevalence in patients with Down syndrome ranges from 3–12%).
- Autoimmune thyroid disease (prevalence 1.5–6.7%).
- Reproductive disorders (prevalence in Turner syndrome can range from 2.1–4.1%).
- **Small intestinal lymphoma** is noted to have increasing prevalence with celiac disease. Five-year abstinence from gluten normalizes risk of lymphoma.

DIAGNOSIS

Clinical Presentation

- Intestinal symptoms predominate and include characteristic malabsorption symptoms: weight loss, steatorrhea, fatigue, and abdominal cramps.
- Fatigue can also occur secondary to iron deficiency anemia, which may be the sole manifestation. Osteoporosis may also be the sole manifestation.
- Short stature and failure to thrive may occur in children.
- **Dermatitis herpetiformis**, a pruritic blistering rash on the extensor surfaces, may be seen. Histopathology from the skin lesions, when diagnostic, provides confirmation of celiac sprue.

Diagnostic Criteria

Positive serologic tests coupled with mucosal biopsy suggestive of celiac disease are diagnostic of celiac disease.[9,12]

Differential Diagnosis

In the absence of symptomatic relief with treatment/lifestyle modifications, additional etiologies of malabsorption must be considered:
- Pancreatic exocrine insufficiency
- Hepatobiliary diseases
- Disaccharidase deficiency
- Intestinal lymphoma
- Tropical sprue
- Autoimmune enteropathy
- Common variable immunodeficiency
- Eosinophilic enteritis
- Nonceliac gluten sensitivity. Some patients have symptoms after gluten ingestion without serologic evidence of celiac disease. A subset of these patients have symptoms from foods other than gluten, as many improve with a low fermentable, oligo-, di-, monosaccharides, and polyol (FODMAP) diet.[13]

Diagnostic Testing

Laboratory Testing

- **Serologic testing** with either **tissue transglutaminase (tTG IgA)** or **endomysial (EMA IgA) antibody** is appropriate as an initial screening test in suspected cases of celiac disease.[9] Prevalence of selective IgA deficiency in the celiac disease population is 1.7–3.0%, 10–15 times higher than in the general population. If initial serologic studies are negative and suspicion for celiac disease remains, then measurement of **serum IgA levels** is appropriate. **In patients with IgA deficiency, IgG-deamidated gliadin antibodies or tTG IgG should be measured.**
- All diagnostic testing should be done while patients are eating gluten because all tests, including histology, can normalize with a gluten-free diet. HLA-DQ2/DQ8 testing can be performed on patients who are already on a gluten free diet. A negative result effectively rules out celiac disease.[9]
- **Antigliadin antibody testing** is now rarely performed due to lack of specificity.
- In addition, if small bowel biopsy (see later) and serologic testing remain nondiagnostic, analysis of the **HLA-DQ2/DQ8 alleles** may be helpful to rule out celiac disease.
- Either or both of these alleles are uniformly seen in almost all patients with celiac disease; **absence** of these markers excludes disease, with a negative predictive value close to 100%.
- It is important to evaluate for deficiencies of nutrients that are preferentially absorbed in the proximal small bowel, including iron, folate, and fat-soluble vitamins.

- Elevated transaminases can be seen in celiac disease. Patients with an unexplained elevation in transaminases should be tested for celiac disease.

Diagnostic Procedures
- As noted above, the gold standard for diagnosis, in addition to serologic tests and dietary modification, consists of **duodenal biopsies, including the bulb** confirming the diagnosis.
- Endoscopically, the mucosa can appear scalloped. However, it can look normal and biopsy is required.
- Histologic findings on biopsy include:
  - Atrophy/blunting of the small intestinal villi;
  - Hyperplasia, deepening of crypts; and
  - Infiltration of lamina propria and intraepithelial compartments with chronic inflammatory cells, typically lymphoplasmacytic infiltrate.

TREATMENT

Lifestyle/Risk Modifications
- Successful treatment requires **lifelong adherence to a gluten-free diet**. Wheat, rye, and barley should be removed from the diet.
- This often proves difficult and expensive. Consultation with a dietitian is recommended.
- In addition, it is important to ensure **nutrient deficiency supplementation** (e.g., iron, folate).
- **Screening for concurrent osteoporosis** with bone mineral density scans should also be performed.
- Patients should have repeat serology 6 and 12 months after being on a gluten-free diet and then annually. Persistently positive serology indicates ongoing bowel damage.[12]
- Refractory celiac disease (RCD)
  - Characterized by villous atrophy associated with malabsorptive symptoms in patients who either have not responded to 6 months of therapy with a gluten-free diet, or who have lost response.[10]
  - Enteropathy associated T-cell lymphoma should be considered in this patient population, especially those who were previously well controlled.
  - RCD type 1 has normal intraepithelial lymphocytes and usually responds to strict gluten-free diet adherence and corticosteroids or immunosuppressive agents. RCD type 2 has abnormal intraepithelial lymphocytes and a poorer response to therapy.
- Refractory sprue occurs most often in patients > age 50.
- Alternative etiologies to consider include causes of enteropathy (autoimmune enteropathy, common variable immunodeficiency syndrome, tropical sprue, and eosinophilic gastroenteritis) resulting in hypoalbuminemia and malnutrition.

Small Intestinal Bacterial Overgrowth (SIBO)

GENERAL PRINCIPLES

Several disorders can lead to profound bacterial overgrowth, causing a wide variety of malnutrition symptoms and clinical abnormalities.

Definition
- Classically defined as >10^5 colony-forming units/mL in the proximal small bowel.[6]
- Abnormal, excessive proliferation of bacterial growth within the small bowel intestinal lumen can cause damage to the bowel mucosa, leading to impaired nutrient digestion and absorption. Bacteria can also compete for nutrients contributing to nutrient deficiencies.

Epidemiology

- Prevalence varies widely based on the predisposing condition and definition. Up to 56% of patients with scleroderma have SIBO and have improvement with antibiotics.[14]
- SIBO is an underrecognized etiology of malabsorption in elderly patients. In one series of adults older than 65 years who suffered from malabsorption, SIBO was the most common cause (70.8%).[15]

Etiology

SIBO can be caused by the following:

- **Intestinal stasis:**
  - Motility disorders such as diabetic gastroparesis, hypothyroidism, postsurgical ileus, medication-induced (i.e., opiates), and rheumatologic/infiltrative conditions (i.e., scleroderma, amyloidosis);
  - Structural lesions such as strictures in the setting of Crohn disease, radiation enteritis, postsurgical adhesions, and malignancy;
- **Fistulas, abnormal connections between small and large intestines**, such as those seen in Crohn disease or postsurgically in bypass patients who have blind bowel loops;
- **Reduced gastric acid secretion** and consequent decreased acid barrier to ingested bacteria. This can sometimes be seen in the setting of excessive acid suppression, postvagotomy, impaired gastric acid secretion postgastrectomy, or pernicious anemia;
- **Immunodeficiency syndromes.**

Pathophysiology

- Direct bacterial overgrowth–mediated toxin production can damage bowel lumen epithelium, impairing digestion and absorption.
- Bacteria can deconjugate bile salts, leading to more proximal small bowel bile salt reabsorption and impairment of fat-soluble nutrient absorption.
- Bacteria can coat the bowel wall, metabolize certain nutrients (i.e., vitamin B12), and reduce availability.
- The role of SIBO in irritable bowel syndrome (IBS) is controversial,[15] but rifaximin, commonly used for SIBO, is approved in the United States for diarrhea-predominant IBS.

DIAGNOSIS

Clinical Presentation

- Presentation can be similar to other malabsorptive states, with findings of abdominal distention, cramping, excessive flatus, significant vitamin and carbohydrate malnutrition, and weight loss.
- Patients often have medical histories predisposing them to states of impaired intestinal motility, immunodeficiency, or reduced gastric acid secretion.

Differential Diagnosis

- Includes alternative etiologies of malabsorption including hepatobiliary diseases, autoimmune-mediated processes, such as celiac disease, refractory sprue, intestinal lymphoma, and infections such as tropical sprue or Whipple disease.

Diagnostic Testing

Laboratory Testing

- Typical malabsorptive vitamin (vitamins A, D, E, K, and B12) and electrolyte/micronutrient (iron and calcium) deficiencies are noted.
- Bacteria can make folic acid, leading to elevated serum folate levels, which in combination with low B12 is suggestive of SIBO.

- Additional findings include macrocytic or microcytic anemia, elevated prothrombin time and INR leading to bleeding diathesis.

Diagnostic Procedures

- Gold standard for diagnosis remains microbiologic culture of >10^5 colony-forming units/mL small bowel aspirate.[15]
- Because of the time-consuming, expensive, and invasive nature of small bowel aspirate culture, hydrogen breath tests using glucose or lactulose are often used. Anaerobic fermentation of carbohydrates by colonic bacteria that have colonized the small intestine leads to absorption of hydrogen into the bloodstream. Some of the hydrogen is exhaled and its concentration can be measured. An elevated concentration of hydrogen is suggestive of SIBO.
- Given the difficulty with these tests, some clinicians treat empirically for SIBO in patients with symptoms and predisposing conditions.

TREATMENT

- Focus is twofold:
  - Eradication of the abnormal proliferating intraluminal bacteria.
  - Reversal of predisposing risk factors that precipitate SIBO if possible.

Medications

- **Antibiotics** are typically used to treat enteric gut flora.
- **Rifaximin** is commonly used to treat SIBO. Other agents include **quinolones, amoxicillin/clavulanic acid, doxycycline or metronidazole**. Repeat courses of antibiotics are often required, particularly if the predisposing factors cannot be corrected.
- **Agents to augment altered intestinal motility** (e.g., metoclopramide, erythromycin) have been tried but long-term use can be associated with significant adverse effects.
- In the setting of systemic disorders associated with altered intestinal motility, attention should be focused on **treating the underlying disease etiology** (i.e., diabetes control, thyroid supplementation in setting of hypothyroidism, immunosuppressive agents in scleroderma, etc.).

Surgical Management

- Reversal of structural abnormalities that can predispose intestinal stasis should be considered. Correction of postsurgical blind loops may prevent recurrence of bacterial overgrowth in those bowel segments.
- Elimination of postsurgical or inflammatory disease–mediated adhesions or strictures either endoscopically or surgically.

Short Bowel Syndrome (SBS)

GENERAL PRINCIPLES

Definition

- Resection of large segments of small bowel (usually resulting in <200 cm of small intestine remaining) can culminate in symptoms and clinical presentation ranging from mild nutritional deficiencies to debilitating diarrhea and malnutrition.
- Functional SBS may result from extensive small bowel mucosal disease.[16]

Etiology

- In infants, congenital SBS can occur as a consequence of intestinal atresia and other congenital intestinal anomalies.[1,17]
- SBS in adults is an acquired condition resulting from multiple resections for refractory complications from Crohn disease, or from catastrophic vascular events, volvulus, trauma, intestinal adhesions, complications of gastric bypass surgery such as internal herniation, or intestinal tumors.

Pathophysiology

- Resection of small intestine can reduce the surface area for nutrient absorption.
- If the resected segment length is not significant, patients remain asymptomatic and do not suffer from consequences of SBS.
- Postsurgically, the length of remaining small bowel and continuity with the colon determines disease severity.[17]
- Nutritional risk remains greatest for those with intestinal failure, defined as inability to maintain proper hydration or protein energy, electrolyte or micronutrient balances on an oral diet.[16,18,19]
- Anatomic definitions of intestinal failure include[16,19]:
    - Jejunoileal anastomosis, with <35 cm of jejunum but presence of IC valve and colon;
    - Jejunocolic or ileocolic anastomosis, with <60 cm of residual small bowel and no ileocecal valve;
    - End jejunostomy, with <115 cm of residual small bowel and resection of the ileocolic valve.
- Intestinal adaptive response to resection involves an increase in absorptive surface area that results from crypt cell hyperplasia and increase in villus height.[17]
- Ileal resection cannot be compensated by jejunal hypertrophy, and a resultant loss in vitamin B12, bile salts, and fat-soluble vitamin resorption occurs.
- Consequently, nutrient malabsorption depends on location and extent of small bowel resection.
- Altered intestinal motility often develops postsurgically (e.g., ileocecal valve resection) predisposing to bacterial colonization and resulting in SIBO.
- Postresection, there are alterations in the release of distal ileal and colonic hormones (glucagon-like peptide-2, neurotensin) stimulated by fat or bile salts.
- Rapid gastric emptying may be precipitated from this process causing significant volume losses.
- In the setting of ileal compromise, further diarrhea can be precipitated by bile acid–mediated irritation of the bowel lumen.

DIAGNOSIS

Clinical Presentation

Symptoms in patients having had recent surgical resection vary from malabsorption, weight loss, and increased frequency of bowel movements, especially postprandially, to significant malnutrition, profuse diarrhea, and dehydration.

Diagnostic Testing

Diagnosis in these patients is relatively simple and requires a history of prior surgical intervention, routinely for the above etiologies.

- Malabsorption (carbohydrate, vitamin, nutrient deficiencies) can be significant in these patients.
- In addition, significant electrolyte abnormalities, renal insufficiency, and varying degrees of acid/base disturbances result from the profound diarrhea and dehydration that occur in SBS.

TREATMENT

- Teduglutide is an SBS-specific therapy that increases gut mucosal growth.[16,20] It is a recombinant analog of glucagon-like peptide-2, a hormone secreted by intestinal enteroendocrine L cells, that has trophic effects on the intestinal mucosa and reduces PN requirements overall by 20%. It is indicated for treatment of patients who are either TPN or IV fluid dependent.
- Treatment is otherwise primarily supportive.[17,18] Principles of management include the following:
  - **Appropriate hydration and volume resuscitation.**
  - **Encouragement of hyperphagia, adequate nutrition and supplementation with micronutrients and vitamins.**
  - Often, **supplemental enteral feeding** (via nasogastric/orogastric tubes) is required on a short-term basis before possible transition to **total parenteral nutrition**.
  - To ensure adequate time for absorption, agents such as **diphenoxylate–atropine** or **loperamide** can be used to slow intestinal motility.
  - If the suspicion of concurrent SIBO is high, **antibiotics** such as quinolones, metronidazole, or rifaximin can be used.
  - For possible bile acid–mediated diarrhea, **bile acid–binding agents** such as cholestyramine may provide additional relief in patients with a residual colon.
  - Growth hormone (somatropin) is FDA approved for SBS, but multiple side effects from chronic use including type 2 diabetes mellitus, musculoskeletal pain, carpal tunnel syndrome, and edema among others have precluded its long-term use.[16,21]

Small Bowel Neoplasms

GENERAL PRINCIPLES

- The small bowel comprises 75% of the length of the entire GI tract and 90% of the mucosal surface. However, <2% of GI malignancies originate in the small bowel.
- Age-adjusted incidence of small bowel malignancies is 2.3 per 100,000.[22]

Classification

- **Benign tumors** consist of the following:
  - Leiomyomas are the most frequent symptomatic benign tumors of the small bowel. These occur most commonly in the sixth or seventh decade of life.
  - Other benign tumors include adenomas, lipomas, and hamartomas.
- Several **malignant tumors** can occur in the small bowel.
  - Adenocarcinomas are the most common primary malignant tumors of the small bowel, accounting for 30–50% of malignant tumors.[23] Annual incidence is 3.9 cases per million, with a slight male predominance, most commonly presenting in the sixth or seventh decade.
  - Carcinoids account for 25–30% of malignant tumors.
  - Lymphomas account for 15–20% of malignant tumors.
- **Gastrointestinal stromal tumor (GIST)** are tumors of mesenchymal cell origin that can be found throughout the GI tract.

Risk Factors

- Certain hereditary conditions predispose individuals to small intestinal tumors.
  - **Peutz–Jeghers syndrome** is characterized by hamartomatous polyps primarily in the jejunum and ileum. They can develop adenomas and carcinomas throughout the GI tract.

- **Familial adenomatous polyposis** (FAP) can be associated with small bowel adenomas, which can progress to adenocarcinoma. One of the most common extracolonic malignancy in FAP patients is periampullary duodenal cancer. Duodenal cancer is a leading cause of death in FAP patients who have undergone colectomy.[24]
- **Lynch syndrome/Hereditary nonpolyposis colorectal cancer** is associated with an increased risk of small bowel malignancy, but screening is not currently recommended.
- **Celiac sprue** can be complicated by enteropathy-associated T-cell lymphoma, a particularly aggressive lymphoma. It should be suspected in a previously well patient with Celiac disease who decompensates despite adherence to a gluten-free diet.
- **Crohn disease.** There is a 20- to 40-fold increase in risk of small bowel adenocarcinoma with Crohn disease compared with the general population.[25]

DIAGNOSIS

Clinical Presentation

- Small bowel tumors can cause intermittent abdominal pain, anemia, bleeding (either overt or occult, manifesting in the setting of chronic anemia), or structural abnormalities resulting in obstruction. Presentation can be insidious and nonspecific. In one large series, mean time to diagnosis was 7 months.
- **Symptomatic presentation is more likely to be seen with malignant tumors**, whereas benign tumors are often discovered incidentally, often at surgery for small bowel obstruction.
- **Leiomyomas** are highly vascular tumors that can present with bleeding (65%), often from the duodenum, or with obstruction or intussusception (25%).
- **Adenomas and adenocarcinomas**, specifically those located in the duodenum with periampullary involvement, can present with signs of obstructive jaundice when the distal common bile duct is involved. Typically, manifestations are nonspecific and occur late in the disease course.
- **Lymphoma** often presents with abdominal pain, weight loss, occult or overt GI bleeding, abdominal mass, perforation, or obstruction.
- **Carcinoid tumors** often present similar to other small bowel tumors. Features of the carcinoid syndrome (episodic flushing, diarrhea, hypotension, bronchospasm, and carcinoid heart disease) can be seen if carcinoid tumors metastasize.
- **GISTs** can be found incidentally on endoscopy performed for other reasons. Large tumors can cause abdominal pain or intussusception and if ulcerated can cause GI bleeding.

Differential Diagnosis

- Small bowel tumors are often appreciated incidentally in the setting of unremitting abdominal pain, unexplained anemia, lower GI bleeding, and small bowel obstruction.
- Alternative etiologies for all these presenting symptoms must be considered prior to endoscopic or invasive diagnostic testing. This can include inflammatory strictures, adhesions as a cause for small bowel obstruction, and other common causes for GI bleeding (see Chapters 6 and 7).

Diagnostic Testing

Laboratory Testing

- Patients can present with laboratory abnormalities consistent with malabsorption from luminal obstruction and consequent impaired nutrient absorption.
- Unexplained anemia can be seen if occult bleeding is a chronic manifestation.

- Urinary 5-HIAA and serum chromogranin A are often elevated in patients with carcinoid tumors.
- Patients with an ampullary adenoma should undergo colonoscopy for colonic adenomas. If colorectal adenomas are present or if other extracolonic features of FAP are present, patient should be referred for genetic counseling and testing for FAP or MUTYH mutations.[24]
- Patients with small bowel adenocarcinoma and colorectal cancer should have their tumors tested for microsatellite instability due to the possibility of Lynch syndrome.[26]
- Patients with two or more hamartomatous polyps characteristic of Peutz–Jeghers syndrome should undergo genetic testing for STK11 mutations.[24]
- Individuals with juvenile polyps in the small bowel should undergo genetic testing for SMAD4 and BMPR1A mutations to identify the juvenile polyposis syndrome.[24]

Imaging
- Luminal irregularities consistent with intestinal tumors can be seen in barium contrast studies, specifically with small bowel follow-through series, contrast enteroclysis, or CT/MRE.
- For patients suspected of having a carcinoid tumor but negative cross-sectional imaging, functional imaging with indium[111] pentetreotide or galium[68] DOTATATE can be used to localize the tumor.[27]

Diagnostic Procedures
- **Endoscopic diagnosis with histopathologic confirmation** remains the ideal confirmatory test prior to surgical resection, when possible.
- **Leiomyomas** are most frequently found in the jejunum, followed by the ileum and the duodenum. Endoscopically, they appear as single, firm, grayish-white, well-defined masses with central umbilication and ulceration, often covered with normal epithelium.
- **Adenomas** can be found anywhere in the small bowel, but most commonly in the duodenum.
- Large size or findings of prominent villus component or atypia increase the risk for malignancy.
- **Adenocarcinomas** are most often found in the proximal small bowel, with the duodenum, and more specifically, the periampullary region being the most common location.
- **Lymphomas** can be diagnosed with endoscopic visualization and biopsy, but may require exploratory laparotomy for tissue diagnosis.

TREATMENT

- In general, resection (endoscopic or surgical) is indicated whenever possible for all tumors without metastases, or in patients presenting with obstruction, perforation, or severe bleeding.
- Radiation or chemotherapy is used to treat in tumors that have metastasized.

Surgical/Endoscopic Management

- Adenomas should be removed or ablated as first-line treatment endoscopically if possible.
- Duodenal polyps are often amenable to endoscopic resection. Endoscopic resection of periampullary tumors may be feasible, but larger tumors, those with significant growth into the pancreatic or common bile duct, or those in association with advanced polyposis may require pancreaticoduodenectomy.
- Surgery is the only curative therapy for adenocarcinomas. Unfortunately, many patients have unresectable disease upon presentation.
- Pancreaticoduodenectomy (Whipple procedure) is often required for tumors of the first or second part of the duodenum. Distal duodenal, ileal, and jejunal tumors can be removed with segmental resection.
- Localized carcinoid tumors and GISTs should be resected. Endoscopic resection is sometimes feasible.

Other Therapies

- In the setting of metastatic disease or incomplete surgical resection of small bowel adenocarcinoma, chemotherapy can provide a survival benefit, but prognosis remains dismal.
- Lymphomas are often treated with a combination of surgery, chemotherapy, and/or radiation therapy since they frequently present with advanced disease.
- Somatostatin analogs may help control symptoms in patients with metastatic carcinoid tumors.
- The tyrosine kinase inhibitor imatinib is used in patients with invasive GISTs.

MONITORING/FOLLOW-UP

- When incidental adenomas are found on endoscopy, they should be resected. Endoscopic surveillance is recommended to ensure complete ablation and to monitor for recurrence.
- More aggressive surveillance is indicated in the setting of adenocarcinoma or lymphoma after curative management.
- Patients with FAP should begin screening at age 25–30 with a side viewing endoscope for periampullary duodenal cancer.[24]
- Though they are at increased risk, screening for small bowel cancers in patients with Lynch syndrome is not recommended.[26]
- Patients with Peutz–Jeghers syndrome should undergo screening with video capsule endoscopy every 3 years beginning at age 8.[24]

OUTCOME/PROGNOSIS

- Small bowel adenocarcinoma prognosis remains dismal despite aggressive management, with an overall 5-year survival rate as low as 30%.
- Prognosis for adenomas, however, is excellent for those who lack malignant change or in which malignancy is confined to superficial layers on biopsy.
- Surgical resection is the only curative therapy for carcinoid tumors. Prognosis in patients with metastatic disease varies, but some tumors are slow growing and managed expectantly until the disease progresses.[27]
- Prognosis for lymphoma varies by subtype, stage, and performance status. For example, patients with enteropathy-associated T-cell lymphoma often die within months of diagnosis. Others, such as follicular lymphoma, are slow-growing and often managed expectantly.[28]

REFERENCES

1. Rubin DC, Shaker A. Small intestine: anatomy and structural anomalies. In: Yamada Y, Alpers DH, Kaplowitz N, et al., eds. *Textbook of Gastroenterology*. 6th ed. Philadelphia, PA: Lippincott Williams & Wilkins; 2016:73–92.
2. Thomas PD, Forbes A, Green J, et al. Guidelines for the investigation of chronic diarrhea, 2nd edition. *Gut*. 2003;52(Suppl 5):1–15.
3. Bai JC, Andrush A, Matelo G, et al. Fecal fat concentration in the differential diagnosis of steatorrhea. *Am J Gastroenterol*. 1989;84(1):27–30.
4. Craig RM, Atkinson AJ Jr. D-xylose testing: a review. *Gastroenterology*. 1989;97(1):246–247.
5. Nikaki K, Gupte GL. Assessment of intestinal malabsorption. *Best Pract Res Clin Gastroenterol*. 2016;30(2):225–235.
6. Grace E, Shaw C, Whelan K, et al. Small intestinal bacterial overgrowth—prevalence, clinical features, current and developing diagnostic tests, and treatment. *Aliment Pharmacol Ther*. 2013; 38(7):674–688.

7. Fidler J. MR imaging of the small bowel. *Radiol Clin N Am*. 2007;45(2):317–331.

8. Macari M, Megibow A, Balthazar E. A pattern approach to the abnormal small bowel: observations at MDCT and CT enterography. *AJR Am J Roentgenol*. 2007;188(5):1344–1355.

9. Rubio-Tapia A, Hill ID, Kelly CP, et al. ACG clinical guidelines: diagnosis and management of celiac disease. *Am J Gastroenterol*. 2013;108(5):656–676.

10. Rubio-Tapia A, Ludvigsson JF, Bratner TL, et al. The prevalence of celiac disease in the United States. *Am J Gastroenterol*. 2012;107(10):1538–1544.

11. Shannahan S, Leffler DA. Diagnosis and updates in celiac disease. *Gastrointest Endosc Clin N Am*. 2017;27(1):79–92.

12. Husby S, Murray JA, David A, et al. AGA clinical practice update on diagnosis and monitoring of celiac disease-changing utility of serology and histologic measures: expert review. *Gastroenterology*. 2019;156(4):885–889.

13. Biesiekierski JR, Peters SL, Newnham ED, et al. No effects of gluten in patients with self-reported non-celiac gluten sensitivity after dietary reduction of fermentable, poorly absorbed, short-chain carbohydrates. *Gastroenterology*. 2013;145(2):320-8.e1–320-8.e3.

14. Pittman N, Rawn SM, Wang M, et al. Treatment of small intestinal bacterial overgrowth in systemic sclerosis: a systematic review. *Rheumatology*. 2018;57(10):1802–1811.

15. Quigley EM. Small intestinal bacterial overgrowth: what it is and what it is not. *Curr Opin Gastroenterol*. 2014;30(2):141–146.

16. Jeppesen PB. Gut hormones in the treatment of short bowel syndrome and intestinal failure. *Curr Opin Endocrinol Diabetes Obes*. 2015;22(1):14–20.

17. Buchman AL, Scolapio J, Fryer J. AGA technical review on short bowel syndrome and intestinal transplantation. *Gastroenterology*. 2003;124(4):1111–1134.

18. Boutte HJ, Rubin DC. Short bowel syndrome. In: Bardan E, Shaker R, eds. *Gastrointestinal Motility Disorders*. Heidelberg, Germany: Springer; 2018:343–351.

19. Carbonnel F, Cosnes J, Chevret S, et al. The role of anatomic factors in nutritional autonomy after extensive small bowel resection. *JPEN J Parenter Enteral Nutr*. 1996;20(4):275–280.

20. Schwartz LK, O'Keefe SJD, Fujioka K. Long-term teduglutide for the treatment of patients with intestinal failure associated with short bowel syndrome. *Clin Transl Gastroenterol*. 2016;7:e142.

21. Scolapio JS. Short bowel syndrome: recent clinical outcomes with growth hormone. *Gastroenterology*. 2006;130(2 Suppl 1):S122–S126.

22. Noone AM, Howlader N, Krapcho M, et al., eds. *SEER Cancer Statistics Review, 1975–2015*. Bethesda, MD: National Cancer Institute; 2018. Available at https://seer.cancer.gov/statfacts/html/smint.html. Based on November 2017 SEER data submission, posted to the SEER web site, April 2018.

23. Delaunoit T, Neczyporenko F, Limburg PJ, et al. Pathogenesis and risk factors of small bowel adenocarcinoma: a colorectal cancer sibling? *Am J Gastroenterol*. 2005;100(3):703–710.

24. Syngal S, Brand RE, Church JM, et al. ACG clinical guideline: genetic testing and management of hereditary gastrointestinal cancer syndromes. *Am J Gastroenterol*. 2015;110(2):223–262.

25. Beaugerie L, Sokol H, Seksik P. Noncolorectal malignancies in inflammatory bowel disease: more than meets the eye. *Dig Dis*. 2009;27(3):375–381.

26. Giardiello FM, Allen JI, Axilbund JE, et al. Guidelines on genetic evaluation and management of lynch syndrome: a consensus statement by the US Multi-Society Task Force on Colorectal Cancer. *Am J Gastroenterol*. 2014;109(8):1159–1179.

27. Raphael MJ, Chan DL, Law C, et al. Principles of diagnosis and management of neuroendocrine tumours. *CMAJ*. 2017;189(10):E398–E404.

28. Lightner AL, Shannon S, Gibbons MM, et al. Primary gastrointestinal non-Hodgkin's lymphoma of the small and large intestines: a systematic review. *J Gastrointest Surg*. 2016;20(4):827–839.

Colon Neoplasms

Ricardo Badillo, Rama Suresh,
and Dayna S. Early

16

GENERAL PRINCIPLES

Background

- Though rates of colorectal cancer (CRC) incidence and cancer-related deaths have progressively declined in the past few decades due to advances in early detection and treatment, there is an estimate over 135,000 new cases and over 50,000 deaths attributed to CRC in the United States each year; and CRC remains the second leading cause of cancer death in the United States.[1,2]
- Prognosis is closely linked to stage at diagnosis. The 5-year survival rate for localized cancers is >90%, whereas the 5-year survival rate for those with invasive cancer is <10%.
- Nearly all CRC develops from colorectal adenomas; a progression that occurs over 5–15 years.
- Screening colonoscopy and polypectomy have been shown to reduce mortality from CRC.[3] The high survival rate of patients with localized CRC and the ability to detect and resect precursor polyps make screening a vital tool in the treatment and prevention of CRC.

Epidemiology

- The prevalence of adenomatous polyps in asymptomatic patients varies from 23–41%.
- The lifetime incidence of CRC is roughly 5% for average risk individuals, with 90% of cases occurring after age 50 years.
- Different ethnic populations carry varying risks for developing colorectal adenomas and cancer. CRC incident rates are higher in non-Hispanic blacks and lowest in Asian and Pacific Islander Americans. Elderly African American males have a higher risk for interval CRC than Caucasian counterparts.[2]
- There are also disparities related to gender and geographical distribution. Men have a reported 30% higher CRC incidence rate than women.[2] In the last several decades, there has been a geographical shift in CRC death rates with more deaths in the South and Midwest United States.[2]
- Developing countries have lower rates of CRC than North America, Australia, and Europe. This may be due to diets high in red meat and fat and low in fruits, vegetables, and fiber in developed countries.
- These disparities suggest that lifestyle and environmental influences are additional risk factors in the development of CRC.
- Distribution of polyps is fairly uniform throughout the colon. In patients older than 60 years and in women, adenomas tend to be more common in the proximal colon. In recent years, the incidence of proximal (ascending colon and cecal) CRC has increased.

Etiology

- Adenomatous polyps are believed to develop in a stepwise fashion as a result of a series of genetic mutations and arise in colonic crypts.[4]
- Histologically, tubular adenomas are the most common type of adenomatous polyp, representing 80–86% of all adenomatous polyps. These lesions tend to be small and

exhibit only mild dysplasia, seen microscopically as a complex network of branching adenomatous glands.

- Villous adenomas tend to have a higher degree of dysplasia, with adenomatous glands extending through to the center of the polyps, thereby appearing grossly as fingerlike projections.
- Villous (papillary) and tubulovillous adenomas are three times more likely to become malignant than tubular adenomas.
- Traditional serrated adenomas and sessile serrated adenomas share some histologic features with hyperplastic polyps. These lesions, however, are associated with CRC risk similar to classic adenomas. Sessile serrated adenomas are more common in the proximal colon, and traditional serrated adenomas are more common in the rectosigmoid colon.
- Overall, only a small percentage of colon adenomas develop into carcinomas.

Pathophysiology

- With the exception of CRC that develops in patients with inflammatory bowel disease, CRC develops from colorectal adenomas.
- Several studies including the National Polyp Study found that removal of adenomas resulted in a significantly lower incidence of CRC.[3] In confirmed colon cancers, residual adenomatous tissue can be found within cancerous tissue. Additionally, surgically resected CRC may contain adjacent adenomatous polyps in one-third of cases.
- The progression from adenoma to carcinoma occurs as a result of a series of DNA mutations. However, the exact sequence of mutations necessary for malignant progression is unclear.
  - Among the earliest mutations is inactivation of the adenomatous polyposis coli (APC) gene.[5]
  - Later changes include mutations of the KRAS proto-oncogene, DNA hypomethylation, 18q inactivation, and p53 (tumor suppressor gene) inactivation.[5]
  - The accumulation of abnormalities results in a stepwise progression over an average of 10 years from normal mucosa to adenoma to carcinoma.
  - Detection of these mutations from sloughed cells in stool samples is the basis of a new screening test for early CRC detection (fecal DNA test).

Risk Factors

- Several factors predict the risk of developing colorectal adenomas and cancer.
- Older age is the most important risk factor and is associated not only with a higher prevalence of polyps but also with multiple polyps, severe dysplasia, and larger adenoma size.
- Non-Hispanic African Americans have a higher risk of developing colon cancer than other races.[6]
- Personal history of CRC or adenomatous polyps is associated with increased risk.
- Inflammatory bowel disease, such as ulcerative colitis and Crohn disease involving the colon, can increase the risk of developing colon cancer. Elevated risk is associated with younger age at disease onset, involvement of the entire colon, and more severe disease.
- Several genetic syndromes, most notably familial adenomatous polyposis and hereditary nonpolyposis CRC (Lynch syndrome), substantially increase the risk of developing colon cancer (see Table 16-1).
- Family history of colon cancer:
  - The overall colon cancer risk in those with multiple first-degree relatives or a single first-degree relative with a diagnosis before age 45 years is three to four times higher than the general population.
  - In patients with a single first-degree relative with CRC or adenoma diagnosed before age 60 years, risk of developing CRC is twice that of the general population.

TABLE 16-1 GENETIC SYNDROMES ASSOCIATED WITH COLORECTAL CANCER

	Genetic Mutation	Phenotype	Risk for CRC	Age to Begin Screening	Type of Screening	Other Cancers
Hereditary nonpolyposis colorectal cancer	Autosomal dominant, DNA mismatch repair genes	CRC without polyposis	75%	25 or 10 yrs younger than earliest case in family	Colonoscopy every 1–2 yrs (most CRC are right sided)	GYN, GU, UGI tract
FAP	Germline mutation of APC gene	Hundreds to thousands of adenomatous polyps	100%	10–12 yrs, perform colectomy when polyps found	Flexible sigmoidoscopy	Duodenal (especially ampullary) and gastric
• Gardner syndrome	Same as FAP	Same as FAP	Same as FAP	Same as FAP	Same as FAP	Desmoid tumors, osteomas, CHRPE, thyroid, adrenal, hepatobiliary tumors
• Attenuated FAP	Same as FAP	Much fewer number of adenomas	Same as FAP, slightly older	Same as FAP	Same as FAP	Same as FAP
Peutz–Jeghers syndrome	Autosomal dominant, STK11 mutation	Mucocutaneous pigmentation Hamartomatous polyps, small bowel, and CRC	Up to 66%	Age 8 yrs for UGI and CRC Age 25 yrs for pancreatic cancer	EGD, colonoscopy, and video capsule endoscopy every 3 yrs if polyps found Endoscopic ultrasonography every 1–2 yrs	Genital, breast, pancreas
Familial juvenile polyposis	Autosomal dominant, SMAD4 mutation	≥10 hamartomatous/"juvenile" polyps	Up to 20%	Mid-teens	FOBT every 1–2 yrs or colonoscopy every 3–5 yrs Small bowel examination every 1–2 yrs	Possible association with hereditary hemorrhagic telangiectasia

CHRPE, congenital hypertrophy of the retinal pigment epithelium; EGD, esophagogastroduodenoscopy; FAP, familial adenomatous polyposis; FOBT, fecal occult blood testing; GU, genitourinary; GYN, gynecologic; STK11, serene/threonine kinase 11; UGI, upper gastrointestinal.

- Tobacco and alcohol use may increase the risk of developing colorectal polyps and CRC.[7]
- Other medical conditions, including diabetes mellitus, high BMI, acromegaly, uretero-colic anastomoses, and pelvic radiation, have also been associated with an increased risk of developing CRC.[7]

Prevention

- For screening purposes, individuals are stratified into average or high risk.[8]
    - Average risk individuals are those with no family or personal history of CRC or adenoma and no history of ulcerative colitis.
    - High-risk populations include those with prior CRC or adenoma, family history of CRC, family history of adenoma before age 60, and long-standing ulcerative colitis.[9]
    - Current recommendations do not take into account gender, dietary, or environmental risks modifiers.
- Screening for CRC should begin at age 50 years for average risk individuals. New recommendations indicate screening African Americans starting at age 45.[10]
- Individuals deemed to be at high risk due to family history should be screened starting at age 40, or 10 years earlier than the age of the youngest CRC diagnosis in the family, whichever is earlier.
- CRC screening is unique in that national organizations provide a "menu" of screening options from which to choose, and they generally do not endorse one screening test over another.
    - Options for screening include fecal immunochemical testing (FIT), fecal occult blood testing (FOBT), flexible sigmoidoscopy (FS), CT colonography, colonoscopy, and stool DNA testing.
    - These tests used alone and in combination reduce CRC incidence and mortality.
- Multiple studies have shown extremely low population screening rates, generally <50%. Extensive public education of the community has modestly increased screening rates over the past few years.

Fecal Occult Blood Testing (FOBT) and Fecal Immunochemical Testing (FIT)

- FOBT is a guaiac-based test that detects pseudoperoxidase activity of heme in stool. FIT is an immunochemical test that detects human globin. FOBT and FIT are relatively sensitive, but nonspecific, and are associated with minimal initial cost.[11]
- When used as a screening test, FOBT or FIT should be performed yearly.
    - Two samples from each of three consecutive stool samples should be evaluated during FOBT. A single sample is not recommended.
    - A restricted diet and avoidance of red meat for 3 days before testing are recommended.
    - Two samples from two consecutive stools should be used for FIT. No dietary restrictions are necessary for FIT testing.
    - There is no need to rehydrate the slide because this increases the false-positive rate.
- Abnormal FIT and FOBT should be further evaluated with colonoscopy. There is insufficient evidence to recommend noninvasive methods such as FIT or fecal DNA for surveillance after adenomatous polyps have been found.[10,12]

Flexible Sigmoidoscopy

- FS is very low risk and of moderate cost, but it only examines approximately one-fourth of the colon.
- Sigmoidoscopy should be offered every 5 years when used as a screening test. At least partial bowel prep is required.

- Case-controlled studies have shown a reduced mortality rate for CRC in individuals who undergo FS; however, there is no reduction in CRC risk in the uninspected proximal colon.[13]
- Patients having FS should have a diagnostic colonoscopy if an adenoma is identified because distal adenomas (within reach of FS) are associated with high rates of more proximal adenomas.
- Up to one-half of individuals with a proximal adenoma have no distal adenoma, raising concern about the use of FS as a screening modality.

Colonoscopy

- Colonoscopy is the most sensitive and specific test, but it involves the greatest cost and carries a small risk of complications.[14]
- Colonoscopy as a screening method should be offered every 10 years for average risk individuals. Full bowel prep is required prior to the procedure.
- It is the "preferred" screening test according to the American College of Gastroenterology and the US Multi-Society Task Force (USMSTF).
- Colonoscopy with polypectomy has been shown to reduce the incidence and mortality of CRC.[15]
- Colonoscopy allows examination of the entire colon, despite higher risks and cost. It also allows for biopsy and polypectomy if indicated.
- Detection rates of adenomas appear to be directly related to longer times for scope withdrawal, and adequate bowel cleansing.[16]

Computed Tomography Colonography (CTC)

- Screening for average risk individuals using CTC is recommended every 5 years.
- CTC requires oral contrast as well as bowel preparation. A small-caliber, flexible rectal catheter is used for colonic distension, generally with CO_2.
- The colonic preparation does allow for same-day colonoscopy if colon polyps are found.
  - Patients with large polyps (>10 mm) or multiple moderate size polyps (>6 mm) are referred for colonoscopy.
  - Colonoscopy is recommended for patients with one to two polyps between 6 and 9 mm, although some advocate enrolling those patients in a CTC surveillance program every 1–2 years. This program is associated with cumulative radiation exposure which carries risk.
  - Polyps <5 mm are not reported, which raises concerns about CTC, since small polyps can harbor advanced histology (although rare).
- Many factors limit CTC use for screening, including lower sensitivity of detecting small polyps, cost-effectiveness, bowel preparation, risks of cumulative radiation exposure, and questions regarding management of the small polyps seen on CTC.[17]
- Additionally, the issue of extracolonic findings on CTC adds to the complexity and cost of the procedure.

Fecal DNA Testing

- Fecal DNA testing detects the presence of DNA alterations that are shed from colorectal adenomas and CRC (see Chapter 25).
- Studies have shown fecal DNA testing to be more sensitive than guaiac tests for cancer and advanced neoplasms with comparable specificity.[18]
- Unlike FOBT and FIT, in order to perform a fecal DNA test, a full bowel movement sample must be collected from the patients and shipped with an ice pack.
- Currently, screening with fecal DNA testing is performed every 5 years for average-risk individuals, but no standardized interval has been established.
- Hypermethylation of genes associated with CRC has led to investigation of new assays, which would detect aberrant methylation in stool as a marker for cancer.[19]

DIAGNOSIS

Clinical Presentation

History

- Most patients with colonic polyps are asymptomatic but may occasionally present with occult or overt bleeding from the gastrointestinal tract. Villous adenomas >3 cm can cause a secretory diarrhea, which can lead to volume depletion and electrolyte abnormalities.
- Many adenocarcinomas are asymptomatic but may occasionally present with multiple symptoms, including abdominal pain (44%), change in bowel habit (43%), hematochezia or melena (40%), weakness (20%), anemia without other gastrointestinal symptoms (11%), or weight loss (6%).[20,21]
  - Right-sided cancers may grow and become large before producing symptoms because of the larger luminal caliber of the cecum and ascending colon. Iron deficiency anemia is often the only manifestation of right-sided cancer.
  - Tumors in the left side of the colon may present with symptoms of partial or complete obstruction, including abdominal distention, bloating, and constipation.
  - Rectal or sigmoid cancers often cause hematochezia, constipation, or thinning of the stools. Tenesmus, melena, or weight loss may also be symptoms.
- An infection with *Streptococcus bovis* or *Clostridium septicum* also warrants evaluation of the colon because 10–25% of these individuals have CRC.[22]
- Consequently, new-onset hematochezia, anemia, or change in bowel habits, especially in older patients, mandates colonoscopic evaluation.

Physical Examination

- Examination of patients should focus on confirming information obtained in the history.
  - An abdomen examination should be performed to evaluate for abdominal pain, distension, mass, and bowel sounds.
  - Signs of iron deficiency anemia would present typically as pale conjunctiva, skin, or nail beds.
- Roughly 20% of patients have distant metastatic disease at presentation, with the most common sites being regional lymph nodes, liver, lungs, and peritoneum.[23] Thus, right-sided abdominal pain, hepatomegaly, abdominal distension, supraclavicular adenopathy, or periumbilical nodules could signify advanced disease.

Differential Diagnosis

- Not all colorectal polyps have malignant potential, but visual inspection cannot predict polyp histology; accordingly, all visualized polyps should be removed and evaluated by surgical pathology.
- Hyperplastic polyps consist of hyperplastic mucosal proliferation. Small hyperplastic polyps are considered to have no malignant potential.
  - Approximately one-third of colon polyps are hyperplastic.
  - A subset of large hyperplastic polyps may be premalignant and are felt to progress to carcinoma through the pathway of serrated adenomas.
- Juvenile polyps (also known as hamartomas) are tumors of the mucosa; in contrast, hyperplastic and adenomatous polyps result from epithelial proliferation.
- Other polypoid lesions in the colon can include lymphoma, carcinoid, Kaposi sarcoma, or metastatic disease.
- Symptoms of CRC are nonspecific and other colonic diseases, including diverticulosis and inflammatory bowel disease, can present with similar symptoms of abdominal pain, hematochezia, and change in bowel habits.

Diagnostic Testing

- **Diagnostic colonoscopy** is the test of choice for identifying CRC and adenomas.
- Barium enema and CTC can suggest CRC or adenoma, but only colonoscopy allows for tissue sampling of tumors and removal of adenomatous polyps.

TREATMENT

- Most polyps found with FS or colonoscopy can be resected completely. The specific technique used is based on the size, location, and gross appearance of the polyp.
- Current guidelines for treatment of adenomatous polyps include complete resection by colonoscopy or surgery.[3]
- Polyps that contain intramucosal cancer can be considered resected for cure by polypectomy if the entire polyp is resected with a negative margin.
- **Staging:**
  - Once CRC is diagnosed, further workup, including a chest radiograph, CT of the abdomen and pelvis, complete blood cell count, chemistry panel, and carcinoembryonic antigen level, is required to determine the extent of local and distant extent of the disease.
    - Magnetic resonance imaging of the liver can also be used to identify hepatic metastatic lesions.
    - Endoscopic ultrasound is a technique to evaluate the depth of invasion and nodal status in rectal cancer.
  - Staging of cancers is done using the TNM (tumor, node, metastasis) universal system (Table 16-2), which was recently updated.

Surgical Management

- For patients diagnosed with CRC, the treatment of choice is surgical resection.
  - The goal of surgery is removal of the affected segment of bowel as well as surrounding lymph nodes. The extent of resection is determined by the distribution of blood vessels and lymphatic drainage.
  - For patients with rectal cancer, the surgical approach depends on the location, size, and extent of involvement.
  - Proximal rectal cancer can be resected with low anterior resection, while distal and locally advanced rectal cancers are treated with neoadjuvant chemoradiotherapy, followed by low anterior resection.
  - Abdominoperineal resection is rarely performed in the current era.
- In patients with CRC, synchronous polyps can occur in 20–40% of cases and synchronous cancers in 3–5%; thus, preoperative colonoscopy is recommended in patients before undergoing resection.
  - The USMSTF recommends patients undergo high-quality perioperative clearing with colonoscopy or within 3–6 months interval after surgery if there is an obstructive lesion that prevents preoperative colonoscopy.[12]
  - If the tumor is obstructing and cannot be traversed by the colonoscope, barium enema or CTC may be performed to evaluate the proximal colon.
- Patients with obstructing metastatic cancers can have palliative resection or endoscopic stenting as a bridge to surgery, to prevent complete obstruction.

Chemotherapy

- Adjuvant chemotherapy after surgical resection typically consists of 5-fluorouracil, leucovorin plus oxaliplatin, or capecitabine plus oxaliplatin.[24,25] Treatment has been shown to have a survival benefit and increases the probability of remaining tumor free in patients with Stage III CRC.

TABLE 16-2 TUMOR, NODE, METASTASIS (TNM) STAGING SYSTEM FOR COLORECTAL CANCER

Stage	Criteria	Estimated 5-yr Survival (%)
0	Tis, N0, M0	N/A
I	T1–2, N0, M0	93
IIA	T3, N0, M0	85
IIB	T4a, N0, M0	72
IIC	T4b, N0, M0	
IIIA	T1–2, N1/N1c, M0	83
	T1, N2a, M0	
IIIB	T3–4a, N1/N1c, M0	64
	T2–3, N2a, M0	
	T1–2, N2b, M0	
IIIC	T4a, N2a, M0	44
	T3–4a, N2b, M0	
	T4b, N1–2, M0	
IVA	T(any), N(any), M1a	5–7
IVB	T(any), N(any), M1b	

TX, primary tumor cannot be assessed; T0, no evidence of primary tumor; Tis, carcinoma in situ; T1, tumor invades submucosa; T2, tumor invades muscularis propria; T3, tumor invades through the muscularis propria into pericolorectal tissues; T4a, tumor penetrates to the surface of the visceral peritoneum; T4b, tumor directly invades or is adherent to other organs or structures.

NX, regional lymph nodes cannot be assessed; N0, no metastases in regional lymph nodes; N1, metastases in one to three regional lymph nodes (N1a, metastasis in one regional lymph node; N1b, metastasis in two to three regional lymph nodes; N1c, tumor deposit(s) in the subserosa, mesentery, or nonperitonealized pericolic or perirectal tissues without regional nodal metastasis); N2, metastases in four or more regional lymph nodes (N2a, metastasis in four to six regional lymph nodes; N2b, metastasis in seven or more regional lymph nodes).

MX, presence or absence of distant metastases cannot be determined; M0, no distant metastases detected; M1, distant metastases detected (M1a, metastasis confined to one organ or site [e.g., liver, lung, ovary, nonregional node]; M1b, metastases in more than one organ per site or the peritoneum).

- American Society of Clinical Oncology (ASCO) panel supports adjuvant chemotherapy for Stage II CRC with high-risk factors for recurrence (based on indirect evidence from Stage III colon cancer data)[26]: poorly differentiated histology (exclusive of those cancers that are microsatellite instability high [MSI-H]), lymphatic/vascular invasion, bowel obstruction, <12 lymph nodes examined, perineural invasion, localized perforation, and close, indeterminate, or positive margins.[27] Among patients with Stage II and III CRC, tumors that have DNA mismatch repair (MMR) deficiency or MSI-H are associated with longer survival than MMR-proficient tumors despite being poorly differentiated in many patients.[27]
- Prospective studies show prolonged survival and enhanced quality of life for patients with metastatic disease who receive chemotherapy.
  - Irinotecan and oxaliplatin are used in combination with fluoropyrimidines.[28]
  - Targeted therapies like anti-VEGF monoclonal antibodies (bevacizumab, aflibercept, ramucirumab) and anti-EGFR monoclonal antibodies (cetuximab, panitumumab) have shown to improve survival when used in combination with chemotherapy.[29–32]

Tumor mutational status of RAS or BRAF V600E plays a role in efficacy of anti-EGFR antibodies: these mutations do not respond to anti-EGFR antibodies.[33-35]

Regorafenib is an inhibitor of angiogenic tyrosine kinases. It is FDA approved for the treatment of patients with metastatic CRC previously treated with fluoropyrimidine combination therapy.[36]

Trifluridine–tipiracil (TAS-102) is an oral cytotoxic agent that inhibits trifluridine metabolism and has antiangiogenic properties as well. TAS-102 was associated with a significant prolongation in median overall survival in the RECOURSE study, irrespective of prior regorafenib use.[37]

Immunotherapy is being investigated in treatment of metastatic CRC. FDA recently approved pembrolizumab (anti PD-1 antibody) for the treatment of unresectable or metastatic CRC that is MSI-H or MMR.[38]

- Preoperative adjuvant chemotherapy and conventional radiotherapy are commonly used for rectal adenocarcinomas. For T3–T4 lesions, compared to postoperative therapy, preoperative therapy is associated with decreased relapse rates, increased rates of sphincter-sparing resections, and comparable overall survival rates. Study results are less definitive with T1 and T2 lesions. Treatment choice remains an area of study, but fluoropyrimidine-based therapy is frequently used.[39]

Lifestyle/Risk Modifications

- Intense interest surrounds the issue of prevention and risk reduction with lifestyle modification and supplementation.
- Calcium and aspirin have been demonstrated to reduce colorectal neoplasia risk in randomized controlled trials.[40]
- Hormone replacement therapy and estrogen, statins, nonsteroidal anti-inflammatory drugs, magnesium, vitamin B6, folic acid, and physical activity have all been thought to be protective against CRC, but data are inconclusive.[40]
- Folic acid was evaluated in a randomized, double-blind, placebo-controlled trial for secondary prevention of adenoma with negative results. The timing of folate administration appears to be important, because folate may act as a preventive agent if given before preneoplastic lesions arise, but it may increase tumor development if given after a preneoplastic lesion exists.[41]
- Diets high in meat fat are thought to increase risk of CRC.

SURVEILLANCE

- Surveillance intervals after polypectomy should be based on the number, size, and histology of polyps. Surveillance intervals should be modified if subsequent adenomas or cancers are found, if a family history of CRC is present, or if a hereditary cancer syndrome is suspected.
- Table 16-3 lists the surveillance recommendations for patients with colorectal adenomas.[42]
- Screening intervals for individuals at high risk because of family history is generally every 5 years, unless an inherited syndrome is suspected or confirmed.[10]
- For large polyps removed via piecemeal resection, a shortened interval colonoscopy (< 1 year) may be considered if there is uncertainty regarding complete resection.
- Individuals with small distal hyperplastic polyps are not at increased risk for development of CRC, and colonoscopy every 10 years is sufficient. The exceptions are individuals felt to have hyperplastic polyposis syndrome, wherein many or large hyperplastic polyps are present. These individuals should be screened similarly to individuals with adenomas.
- Surveillance after resection of CRC is generally at 1 year after surgery or perioperative colonoscopy, followed by 3 years, and then every 5 years if no subsequent adenomas or tumors are found.

TABLE 16-3 COLONOSCOPIC SURVEILLANCE FOR COLORECTAL POLYPS

	Risk	Repeat Colonoscopy
One or two adenomas, <1 cm, low-grade dysplasia	Low	5–10 yrs
Three or more adenomas, or any adenoma ≥1 cm, or any adenoma with villous architecture, high-grade dysplasia, or both	Moderate	3 yrs
Malignant polyps, large sessile adenomas, multiple adenoma	High	Complete removal is mandatory and then revert to 3-yr surveillance Consider genetic counseling when hereditary syndrome suspected
Hyperplastic polyps (unless hyperplastic polyposis syndrome and then treated as moderate risk)	None	10 yrs

- Due to higher rates of local recurrence compared to CRC, the interval length of surveillance for minimally invasive resection of rectal cancer without neoadjuvant chemoradiation should be shortened to every 3–6 months for the first 2–3 years after surgery.[10,12]
- Genetic counseling is recommended for any individual in whom a hereditary cancer syndrome is suspected. Features of hereditary cancer syndromes are outlined in the Special Considerations section.
- Poor quality colonoscopies in which detection of lesions >5 mm may be missed should be considered for a repeat colonoscopy within 1 year.

PROGNOSIS

- At diagnosis of CRC, symptomatic patients have a worse prognosis than asymptomatic patients, with a 5-year survival rate of 49% versus 71%, respectively.[43]
- CRC survival is excellent for those with limited stage disease at the time of diagnosis (Table 16-2).[44]
- The development in the past decade of new chemotherapeutic agents has led to a significant increase in treatment options for CRC and improved survival.
- Survival of patients with advanced CRC has increased from a median survival of 10–12 months with fluoropyrimidines only to >20 months with combination therapy (fluoropyrimidine, irinotecan, and oxaliplatin or cytotoxic chemotherapy with targeted therapy, or immunotherapy).[38,45-51]

SPECIAL CONSIDERATIONS

- **Hereditary syndromes with CRC risk:** A number of hereditary syndromes are associated with increased CRC risk and are summarized in Table 16-1. These syndromes are addressed in more detail in Chapter 25. Management of patients with these syndromes should be multidisciplinary, including genetic counselors, gastroenterologists, and colorectal surgeons.[52]

- **Inflammatory bowel disease:**
  - Surveillance colonoscopy is effective in reducing the mortality from CRC for patients with Crohn colitis or ulcerative colitis.
  - Risk of dysplasia is associated with duration, extent, and activity of disease; current recommendations are to perform surveillance colonoscopy every 1–3 years on patients with pancolitis for >8 years or left-sided colitis for >15 years. Patients should have random biopsies taken every 10 cm throughout the entire colon. Chromoendoscopy should be considered to identify areas for targeted biopsies.
  - Patients with ulcerative colitis may have inflammatory polyps as well as adenomas.
    - Sporadic adenomas that are not associated with active inflammation can be managed similarly to polyps in patients without ulcerative colitis.
    - Adenomas or flat lesions with dysplasia found in the setting of active inflammation should be managed by proctocolectomy.
    - The finding of high-grade dysplasia mandates colectomy, whereas low-grade dysplasia is more controversial, with many experts also recommending colectomy.

REFERENCES

1. Jemal A, Siegel R, Xu J, et al. Cancer statistics, 2010. *CA Cancer J Clin*. 2010;60(5):277–300.
2. Siegel RL, Miller KD, Fedewa SA, et al. Colorectal cancer statistics, 2017. *CA Cancer J Clin*. 2017;67(3):177–193.
3. Winawer SJ, Zauber AG, Ho MN, et al. Prevention of colorectal cancer by colonoscopic polypectomy. The National Polyp Study Workgroup. *N Engl J Med*. 1993;329(27):1977–1981.
4. Correa P. Epidemiology of polyps and cancer. *Major Probl Pathol*. 1978;10:126–152.
5. Vogelstein B, Fearon ER, Hamilton SR, et al. Genetic alterations during colorectal-tumor development. *N Engl J Med*. 1988;319(9):525–532.
6. Bach PB, Pham HH, Schrag D, et al. Primary care physicians who treat blacks and whites. *N Engl J Med*. 2004;351(6):575–584.
7. Bailie L, Loughrey MB, Coleman HG. Lifestyle risk factors for serrated colorectal polyps: a systematic review and meta-analysis. *Gastroenterology*. 2017;152(1):92–104.
8. Winawer SJ, Fletcher RH, Miller L, et al. Colorectal cancer screening: clinical guidelines and rationale. *Gastroenterology*. 1997;112(2):594–642.
9. Burt RW. Impact of family history on screening and surveillance. *Gastrointest Endosc*. 1999;49 (3 Pt 2):S41–S44.
10. Rex DK, Boland CR, Dominitz JA, et al. Colorectal cancer screening: recommendations for physicians and patients from the U.S. Multi-Society Task Force on Colorectal Cancer. *Gastroenterology*. 2017;153(1):307–323.
11. Lieberman D. Colorectal cancer screening in primary care. *Gastroenterology*. 2007;132(7):2591–2594.
12. Kahi CJ, Boland CR, Dominitz JA, et al. Colonoscopy surveillance after colorectal cancer resection: recommendations from the US Multi-Society Task Force on Colorectal Cancer. *Gastroenterology*. 2016;150(3):758–768.e711.
13. Selby JV, Friedman GD, Quesenberry CP Jr, et al. A case-control study of screening sigmoidoscopy and mortality from colorectal cancer. *N Engl J Med*. 1992;326:653–657.
14. Lieberman DA, Weiss DG, Bond JH, et al. Use of colonoscopy to screen asymptomatic adults for colorectal cancer. Veterans Affairs Cooperative Study Group 380. *N Engl J Med*. 2000;34(3): 162–168.
15. Zauber AG, Winawer SJ, O'Brien MJ, et al. Colonoscopic polypectomy and long-term prevention of colorectal-cancer deaths. *N Engl J Med*. 2012;366(8):687–696.
16. Barclay RL, Vicari JJ, Doughty AS, et al. Colonoscopic withdrawal times and adenoma detection during screening colonoscopy. *N Engl J Med*. 2006;355(24):2533–2541.
17. Kim DH, Pickhardt PJ, Hoff G, et al. Computed tomographic colonography for colorectal screening. *Endoscopy*. 2007;39(6):545–549.

18. Imperiale TF, Ransohoff DF, Itzkowitz SH, et al. Fecal DNA versus fecal occult blood for colorectal-cancer screening in an average-risk population. *N Engl J Med.* 2004;351(26):2704–2714.

19. Nagasaka T, Tanaka N, Cullings HM, et al. Analysis of fecal DNA methylation to detect gastrointestinal neoplasia. *J Natl Cancer Inst.* 2009;101(18):1244–1258.

20. Speights VO, Johnson MW, Stoltenberg PH, et al. Colorectal cancer: current trends in initial clinical manifestations. *South Med J.* 1991;84(5):575–578.

21. Steinberg SM, Barkin JS, Kaplan RS, et al. Prognostic indicators of colon tumors. The Gastrointestinal Tumor Study Group experience. *Cancer.* 1986;57(9):1866–1870.

22. Panwalker AP. Unusual infections associated with colorectal cancer. *Rev Infect Dis.* 1988;10(2): 347–364.

23. Jemal A, Siegel R, Ward E, et al. Cancer statistics, 2009. *CA Cancer J Clin.* 2009;59(4):225–249.

24. André T, Boni C, Navarro M, et al. Improved overall survival with oxaliplatin, fluorouracil, and leucovorin as adjuvant treatment in stage II or III colon cancer in the MOSAIC trial. *J Clin Oncol.* 2009;27(19):3109–3116.

25. Schmoll HJ, Tabernero J, Maroun J, et al. Capecitabine plus oxaliplatin compared with fluorouracil/folinic acid as adjuvant therapy for stage III colon cancer: final results of the NO16968 randomized controlled phase III trial. *J Clin Oncol.* 2015;33(32):3733–3740.

26. Benson AB, Schrag D, Somerfield MR, et al. American Society of Clinical Oncology recommendations on adjuvant chemotherapy for stage II colon cancer. *J Clin Oncol.* 2004;22(16): 3408–3419.

27. Lanza G, Gafà R, Santini A, et al. Immunohistochemical test for MLH1 and MSH2 expression predicts clinical outcome in stage II and III colorectal cancer patients. *J Clin Oncol.* 2006; 24(15):2359–2367.

28. Van Cutsem E, Cervantes A, Adam R, et al. ESMO consensus guidelines for the management of patients with metastatic colorectal cancer. *Ann Oncol.* 2016;27(8):1386–1422.

29. Hurwitz HI, Tebbutt NC, Kabbinavar F, et al. Efficacy and safety of bevacizumab in metastatic colorectal cancer: pooled analysis from seven randomized controlled trials. *Oncologist.* 2013; 18(9):1004–1012.

30. Van Cutsem E, Tabernero J, Lakomy R, et al. Addition of aflibercept to fluorouracil, leucovorin, and irinotecan improves survival in a phase III randomized trial in patients with metastatic colorectal cancer previously treated with an oxaliplatin-based regimen. *J Clin Oncol.* 2012; 30(28):3499–3506.

31. Tabernero J, Yoshino T, Cohn AL, et al. Ramucirumab versus placebo in combination with second-line FOLFIRI in patients with metastatic colorectal carcinoma that progressed during or after first-line therapy with bevacizumab, oxaliplatin, and a fluoropyrimidine (RAISE): a randomised, double-blind, multicentre, phase 3 study. *Lancet Oncol.* 2015;16(5):499–508.

32. Van Cutsem E, Köhne CH, Láng I, et al. Cetuximab plus irinotecan, fluorouracil, and leucovorin as first-line treatment for metastatic colorectal cancer: updated analysis of overall survival according to tumor KRAS and BRAF mutation status. *J Clin Oncol.* 2011;29(15):2011–2019.

33. Allegra CJ, Rumble RB, Hamilton SR, et al. Extended RAS gene mutation testing in metastatic colorectal carcinoma to predict response to anti-epidermal growth factor receptor monoclonal antibody therapy: American Society of Clinical Oncology provisional clinical opinion update 2015. *J Clin Oncol.* 2016;34(2):179–185.

34. Pietrantonio F, Petrelli F, Coinu A, et al. Predictive role of BRAF mutations in patients with advanced colorectal cancer receiving cetuximab and panitumumab: a meta-analysis. *Eur J Cancer.* 2015;51(5):587–594.

35. Rowland A, Dias MM, Wiese MD, et al. Meta-analysis of BRAF mutation as a predictive biomarker of benefit from anti-EGFR monoclonal antibody therapy for RAS wild-type metastatic colorectal cancer. *Br J Cancer.* 2015;112(12):1888–1894.

36. Grothey A, Van Cutsem E, Sobrero A, et al. Regorafenib monotherapy for previously treated metastatic colorectal cancer (CORRECT): an international, multicentre, randomised, placebo-controlled, phase 3 trial. *Lancet.* 2013;381(9863):303–312.

37. Mayer RJ, Van Cutsem E, Falcone A, et al. Randomized trial of TAS-102 for refractory metastatic colorectal cancer. *N Engl J Med.* 2015;372(20):1909–1919.

38. Le DT, Uram JN, Wang H, et al. PD-1 blockade in tumors with mismatch-repair deficiency. *N Engl J Med.* 2015;372(26):2509–2520.

39. Sauer R, Liersch T, Merkel S, et al. Preoperative versus postoperative chemoradiotherapy for locally advanced rectal cancer: results of the German CAO/ARO/AIO-94 randomized phase III trial after a median follow-up of 11 years. *J Clin Oncol.* 2012;30(16):1926–1933.

40. Burt RW, Winawer SJ, Bond JH, et al. *Preventing Colorectal Cancer: A Clinician's Guide. American Gastroenterological Association Monograph.* Washington, DC: The American Gastroenterological Association; 2004.

41. Cole BF, Baron JA, Sandler RS, et al. Folic acid for the prevention of colorectal adenomas: a randomized clinical trial. *JAMA.* 2007;297(21):2351–2359.

42. Winawer S, Fletcher R, Rex D, et al. Colorectal cancer screening and surveillance: clinical guidelines and rationale—Update based on new evidence. *Gastroenterology.* 2003;124(2):544–560.

43. Beahrs OH, Sanfelippo PM. Factors in prognosis of colon and rectal cancer. *Cancer.* 1971;28(1):213–218.

44. O'Connell JB, Maggard MA, Ko CY. Colon cancer survival rates with the new American Joint Committee on Cancer sixth edition staging. *J Natl Cancer Inst.* 2004;96(19):1420–1425.

45. Douillard JY, Cunningham D, Roth AD, et al. Irinotecan combined with fluorouracil compared with fluorouracil alone as first-line treatment for metastatic colorectal cancer: a multicentre randomized trial. *Lancet.* 2000;355:1041–1047.

46. Hochster HS, Hart LL, Ramanathan RK, et al. Safety and efficacy of oxaliplatin and fluoropyrimidine regimens with or without bevacizumab as first-line treatment of metastatic colorectal cancer: results of the TREE Study. *J Clin Oncol.* 2008;26:3523–3529.

47. Van Cutsem E, Köhne CH, Láng I, et al. Cetuximab plus irinotecan, fluorouracil, and leucovorin as first-line treatment for metastatic colorectal cancer: updated analysis of overall survival according to tumor KRAS and BRAF mutation status. *J Clin Oncol.* 2011;29:2011–2019.

48. Douillard JY, Siena S, Cassidy J, et al. Final results from PRIME: randomized phase III study of panitumumab with FOLFOX4 for first-line treatment of metastatic colorectal cancer. *Ann Oncol.* 2014;25:1346–1355.

49. Kopetz S, Grothey A, Yaeger R, et al. Encorafenib, binimetinib, and cetuximab in BRAF V600E-mutated colorectal cancer. *N Engl J Med.* 2019;381:1632–1643.

50. Overman MJ, McDermott R, Leach JL, et al. Nivolumab in patients with metastatic DNA mismatch repair-deficient or microsatellite instability-high colorectal cancer (CheckMate 142): an open-label, multicentre, phase 2 study. *Lancet Oncol.* 2017;18:1182–1191.

51. Overman MJ, Lonardi S, Wong KYM, et al. Durable clinical benefit with nivolumab plus ipilimumab in DNA mismatch repair-deficient/microsatellite instability-high metastatic colorectal cancer. *J Clin Oncol.* 2018;36:773–779.

52. Rhodes M, Bradburn DM. Overview of screening and management of familial adenomatous polyposis. *Gut.* 1992;33(1):125–131.

Inflammatory Bowel Disease

Kelly C. Cushing and Matthew A. Ciorba

17

GENERAL PRINCIPLES

- In 1932, Burrill Crohn, Leon Ginzburg, and Gordon Oppenheimer first described inflammatory bowel disease (IBD) as an idiopathic disorder, which they designated *terminal ileitis*. Later descriptions included *regional enteritis* and granulomatous colitis before the eventual eponym of *Crohn disease* was adopted.
- Chronic ulcerative colitis has been recognized as a clinical entity distinct from infectious enteritis since the late 1800s.
- Understanding of IBD genetics and molecular pathophysiology are rapidly evolving and will continue to be translated into targeted and patient-centered clinical management strategies over the next decade.

Definition

- IBD is a spectrum of chronic intestinal inflammation of uncertain etiology.
- **Crohn disease** (CD) and **ulcerative colitis** (UC) comprise the two main clinical entities and are often discussed together for ease of comparison and contrast. It is possible that CD and UC constitute a continuum of disease and manifest as varying clinical phenotypes. **Microscopic colitis (MC)** is also included under the umbrella of IBD.

Epidemiology

- IBD is more common in well-developed areas and is particularly prevalent in Caucasian Northern Europeans and North Americans. However, incidence of IBD is rapidly increasing in less well-developed countries.
- There are currently an estimated 1.6–3.1 million cases of adult IBD in the United States.[1,2]
- Prevalence was initially reported highest in the Jewish population, particularly in Ashkenazi Jews, but there is clearly now a presence of IBD across culture and race.
- IBD can present any time from infancy to old age. However, incidence peaks between the ages 15 and 30 years, with a second minor peak between ages of 50 and 80 years. There is no gender specificity.

Etiology

- The precise etiology of IBD has not yet been defined. Genetic, autoimmune, and environmental factors are implicated in disease development and progression.
- A leading hypothesis indicates that IBD is the result of an overly aggressive immune response to a subset of commensal enteric bacteria in a genetically susceptible host exposed to an environmental trigger(s).

Pathophysiology

- Although most affected patients have no family history of IBD, first-degree relatives are five times more likely to develop the disease. Twin studies show higher concordance rates of IBD, greater in CD than in UC. Both UC and CD can occur in the same family, an observation now supported by the identification of susceptibility genes associated with both conditions.

- **Molecular characteristics of IBD**[3-6]
  - Multicenter and multinational genome-wide association studies (GWAS) have identified 200 genetic loci associated with IBD risk. Despite low relative risk for polymorphisms in most of these genes, important pathways in disease development are linked to these polymorphisms, including **autophagy** and **defects in handling of host–microbe interactions** by the innate and adaptive immunoregulation. Epithelial barrier function is also highly represented.
  - The initial events in IBD development are linked to **aberrancies of innate immunity**, whereas the chronic state has an **overactive adaptive immune response** to commensal luminal microbiota.
  - CD is associated with elevated levels of tumor necrosis factor (TNF)-α, interferon γ, IL-1β, and the cytokines of the IL23–TH17 pathway. Elevated levels of TNF-α, IL-17, and cytokines of the Th2 cells are found in UC. Several of these cytokines and pathways are targets for new or investigational therapeutics.
  - The gene encoding NOD2 (an intracellular sensor of bacterial peptidoglycan important in innate immunity) is associated with CD. NOD2 polymorphisms are more common in Europeans than in African Americans or Asians. NOD2 polymorphism carrier status is linked to ileal and fibrostenosing disease phenotype. In heterozygous individuals, the risk of CD is increased up to fourfold, whereas individuals with two allelic variants have an 11- to 27-fold increase of relative risk.
  - Autophagy is a process by which cells degrade and control or clear intracellular pathogens and organelles. Genes directly (ATG16L1 and IRGM) or indirectly (NOD2) involved in autophagy are associated with CD.
- Colitis is a nonspecific manifestation that can result from alterations in many genes involved in the mucosal barrier epithelium or mucosal immune system, backing up the polygenic hypothesis.
- Several lines of evidence support the importance of **gene–environment interactions** in disease development and activity. Bacteria, viruses, and fungi have been implicated as important luminal factors. Genetically susceptible mice raised in sterile conditions do not develop IBD. Antibiotics have therapeutic efficacy in some forms of IBD. In CD, surgical diversion attenuates inflammation in the gastrointestinal (GI) tract distal to the ostomy.
- So far, it is estimated that only 20% of genetic variability associated with IBD susceptibility has been identified. Multiple genes have been associated with both CD and UC, supporting the overlap between them. This novel information can lead to new directly targeted therapies for IBD.

Pathologic Features

- **Crohn disease**
  - CD can affect any portion of the luminal GI tract, from mouth to anus.
  - CD is characterized by chronic, progressive, potentially **transmural inflammation** with mucosal damage and fissuring that can lead to fibrosis, strictures, fistulae, and obstruction. Early disease is characterized by inflammatory activity, whereas fibrosis and stricturing are more common with long-standing disease.
  - There is a sharp demarcation, both macro- and microscopically, between diseased and adjacent unaffected bowel with asymmetric and discontinuous inflammatory changes.
  - Noncaseating granulomas can be seen on histopathology.

TABLE 17-1 MONTREAL CLASSIFICATION OF INFLAMMATORY BOWEL DISEASE

Crohn Disease			Ulcerative Colitis
Age at Diagnosis	Location	Behavior	Extent of Disease
A1: <16 yr	L1: ileal	B1: nonstricturing, nonpenetrating	E1: ulcerative proctitis, distal to rectosigmoid junction
A2: 17–40 yr	L2: colonic	B2: stricturing (fibrostenotic)	E2: left sided: distal to splenic flexure
A3: >40 yr	L3: ileocolonic	B3: penetrating (fistulizing)	E3: extensive: extending proximal to splenic flexure
	L4: upper GI disease	p: perianal disease	

L4 can be added to L1, L2, or L3 as needed.
p (perianal disease) can be added to any behavior.

- Roughly 80% of patients have small bowel involvement, a third with exclusively ileitis (usually with terminal ileum involvement), and one-half with ileocolitis. Approximately 20% of patients have disease limited to the colon, and about one-half of these patients have rectal sparing.
- About 7% of patients have predominant oral or gastroduodenal involvement, and even fewer patients (5%) have esophageal or proximal small bowel involvement. This can be concurrent with the ileocolonic involvement. These patients are typically younger at disease onset. About a third of patients have perianal disease, including fistula and fissures.
- Extraintestinal manifestations are common, often related to inflammatory disease activity, and are more frequent with colonic involvement.
- The Montreal classification of CD uses age at diagnosis, location, and behavior to characterize the disease. This is particularly useful for CD due to its variable phenotypes. See Table 17-1.[7]
- **Ulcerative colitis**
  - UC is a chronic, relapsing, ulceroinflammatory disease limited to the colon extending proximally from the rectum.
  - UC is a systemic disorder with frequent extraintestinal manifestations, including hepatic involvement as primary sclerosing cholangitis (PSC).
  - Lesions affect predominantly the mucosa and submucosa in a circumferential and uninterrupted distribution.
  - Well-formed granulomas and fistulae are absent in UC. Islands of regenerating mucosa protrude into the lumen to create pseudopolyps.
  - The extent of disease is the basis for the Montreal classification of UC. See Table 17-1.[7]

Risk Factors

- Patients who have **first-degree relatives with IBD** have an increased risk of having IBD themselves (see *Pathophysiology*).
- **Smoking**

Current smokers' risk of developing UC is lower, about 40% that of nonsmokers. Former smokers, however, have a 1.7 times increased risk for UC over lifetime nonsmokers.

Smoking is associated with a twofold increased risk of CD and increases rates of disease flares. Current smoking is associated with resistance to medical therapy in CD.

- **Concomitant infections** (*Clostridium difficile*, Cytomegalovirus, etc.) and their treatment (antibiotics) can exacerbate IBD.
- **Nonsteroidal anti-inflammatory drugs** (NSAIDs) are often cited as worsening IBD, but the data are conflicting. Short courses of cyclo-oxygenase-2 inhibitors (e.g., celecoxib) may be safer than nonselective NSAID in patients with UC in remission.
- Appendectomy before age 20 for appendicitis or lymphadenitis may protect against developing UC but not CD.
- Stress and psychopathology do not increase the onset of IBD, but stress may increase exacerbations of IBD possibly via activation of the enteric nervous system and elaboration of proinflammatory cytokines.
- Controversy remains as to whether oral contraceptive or isotretinoin (Accutane) use puts individuals at increased risk of IBD.

DIAGNOSIS

Clinical Presentation

- **Crohn disease**
  - Clinical manifestations of CD are more variable than those of UC because of the transmural nature and the variability of disease locations. CD may present with GI symptoms, extraintestinal symptoms, or both.
  - Ileal and colonic CD can present with chronic diarrhea, abdominal pain, weight loss, fatigue, and fever, with or without rectal bleeding (bleeding is less common than in UC). CD patients do not uniformly have diarrhea (Table 17-2).
  - Coexistent irritable bowel syndrome (IBS) can contribute to symptoms of pain and diarrhea highlighting the importance of using objective measures when determining disease activity.
  - Signs can include cachexia, abdominal tenderness or mass (most commonly in the right lower quadrant), perianal fissures, fistulas, or abscess.
  - Gastric and duodenal CD is commonly asymptomatic, but may present with nausea and vomiting, epigastric pain, or gastric outlet obstruction.
  - Oral and esophageal CD can present as oral ulcers, gum pain, dysphagia, and odynophagia.
  - A proposed **severity classification** is as follows[8]:
    - **Mild–moderate disease:** Patients are able to tolerate oral intake without signs of systemic toxicity.
    - **Moderate–severe disease:** Patients have failed therapy for mild–moderate disease, or have abdominal pain, nausea, vomiting, fevers, dehydration, anemia, or weight loss of >10%.
    - **Severe–fulminant disease:** Persistent symptoms after corticosteroid therapy, or the presence of high fevers, obstruction, cachexia, surgical abdomen, or abscess formation.
    - **Remission:** Asymptomatic patients who have no evidence of disease after medical or surgical intervention.
- **Ulcerative colitis**
  - Patients with UC can have varying symptoms and signs dictated by anatomic extent and disease severity (Table 17-2).

TABLE 17-2 COMPARISON BETWEEN CROHN DISEASE AND ULCERATIVE COLITIS

	Crohn Disease	Ulcerative Colitis
Disease location	Anywhere in GI tract; terminal ileum most common	Colon only; begins in rectum
Clinical presentation	Abdominal pain or mass (right lower quadrant), diarrhea, weight loss, vomiting, perianal disease	Rectal bleeding, diarrhea, passage of mucus, crampy pain, increased bowel movement frequency/urgency
Endoscopy	Rectal sparing, skip lesions, aphthous ulcers, cobblestoning, linear ulceration	Rectal involvement, continuous, friability, loss of vascularity
Radiology	Small bowel and terminal ileal disease, segmental, strictures, fistulae	Colon disease, loss of haustra, continuous ulceration, no fistulae
Histology	Transmural disease, aphthous ulcers, noncaseating granulomas	Abnormal crypt architecture, superficial inflammation
HLA antigen association	HLA-A2, HLA-DR1, HLA-DQw5	HLA-DR2
IBD genes	NOD-2, ATG16L1; IL23R	IL23R
Cigarette smoking	Increases risk development, recurrence rates and complicates treatment	Current smoking decreases risk
Appendectomy	No effect	Decreases risk (if prior to onset)
Antibiotics	Some response in colonic disease	No response
p-ANCA/ASCA	ASCA associated	p-ANCA associated
PSC	~3% develop	~5% develop PSC

ASCA, anti-*Saccharomyces cerevisiae* antibodies; HLA, human leukocyte antigen; IBD, inflammatory bowel disease; p-ANCA, perinuclear antineutrophil cytoplasmic antibodies; PSC, primary sclerosing cholangitis.

- **Rectal bleeding** is much more common in UC than in CD. UC can involve mucus passage, urgency, diarrhea, or fever.
- **Tenesmus** (the constant feeling of the need to empty the bowel with false alarms), **pain, and cramping** are common.
- The Montreal classification of symptoms severity is helpful for determining UC management[7]:
  - **Clinical remission:** asymptomatic

- **Mild disease:** ≤ fewer than 4 loose stools a day (may be bloody) and no signs of systemic toxicity, normal erythrocyte sedimentation rate (ESR)
- **Moderate UC:** >4 stools per day and minimal signs of systemic toxicity
- **Severe UC:** ≥6 loose stools per day, with blood, pulse rate of >90 beats per minute, higher temperatures of ≥37.5°F, hemoglobin <10.5 g/dL, ESR ≥ 30 mm/hour
- **Fulminant colitis** was previously used to describe >10 stools a day, continuous bleeding, and tenderness or distension and dilation on imaging but is along the continuum with severe colitis.
- **Toxic megacolon** can develop with severe systemic manifestations in addition to fulminant colitis. Potential precipitants include opiates, electrolyte abnormalities, antimotility agents, and intercurrent infectious colitis. The colon can be dilated up to 5–6 cm with a precipitous decrease in bowel movement frequency; rarely, the colon may not be dilated. Complications include sepsis, hemorrhage, and perforation.
- **Extraintestinal manifestations**
  - Extraintestinal complications are frequent in both CD and UC.[9] These involve almost any organ system and contribute considerably to patient morbidity (Table 17-3).
  - Extraintestinal manifestations may parallel or be independent of intestinal disease activity. These are typically associated with UC or colonic CD.
  - The presence of one manifestation increases the likelihood of having others. Extraintestinal manifestations represent autoimmune-related processes, with antibodies against antigens shared among the colon and four common locations (skin, joints, eyes, and liver).
  - **Ankylosing spondylitis and sacroiliitis** are more common in CD than in UC. Other joint manifestations include pauciarticular, asymmetric, peripheral arthritis of the larger joints, and a polyarticular, symmetric arthritis of the small joints.
  - **Osteoporosis** is common and is multifactorial in origin. Steroid use, low intake or absorption of dietary calcium and vitamin D, low body weight, and relative hypogonadism have all been implicated.
  - **Primary sclerosing cholangitis** (PSC) is seen in about 5% of patients with UC, more commonly than in CD. Conversely, most patients with PSC have IBD.

TABLE 17-3	EXTRAINTESTINAL MANIFESTATIONS OF INFLAMMATORY BOWEL DISEASE
Manifestation	**Parallels Intestinal Disease Activity**
Erythema nodosum	Yes
Pyoderma gangrenosum	Yes
Peripheral arthropathy	Yes
Episcleritis or scleritis	Yes
Anterior uveitis	No
Spondyloarthropathy (ankylosing spondylitis, sacroiliitis)	No
Osteoporosis (often steroid induced)	No
Primary sclerosing cholangitis (usually ulcerative colitis)	No
Nephrolithiasis (usually Crohn disease)	No
Cholelithiasis (after ileal resection)	No

○ Rates of both **venous and arterial thromboembolism** are increased in IBD. IBD-associated hypercoagulable state can occur both dependent and independent of disease activity.

○ **Nephrolithiasis** with oxalate stones can be related to ileal CD. Fat malabsorption in CD leads to increased absorption of free dietary oxalate, which then binds to available calcium ions to form kidney stones. Calcium supplementation has therapeutic benefit in this scenario.

○ Generally, manifestations that parallel disease activity are managed by intensification of intestinal IBD therapy, whereas the other conditions are treated symptomatically.

History

A careful history should be obtained to include the following:
- Epidemiology and risk factors such as smoking and family history
- Disease onset and duration and severity of current symptoms
- Presence or absence of constitutional symptoms
- Extraintestinal manifestations
- Symptoms of infections, risk factors for superimposed infections
- Quality of life and impairment of daily activities
- Prior clinical course including medication and surgical history

Physical Examination

A full physical examination should be performed.
- **Vital signs** should be reviewed along with weight trends.
- A careful **abdominal examination** is essential. The abdomen should be auscultated for high-pitched or absent bowel sounds. The abdomen may be tender in both CD and UC. Right lower quadrant tenderness and fullness is classic in CD involving the terminal ileum. A palpable mass is also more common in CD than in UC. UC patients may have fullness or tenderness localizing to disease activity, typically in the left lower quadrant. Peritoneal signs are concerning for an intestinal perforation.
- A **perianal examination** should be performed for evaluating skin tags, anal fissures, and fistulae or abscesses that would suggest CD rather than UC. Although a digital rectal examination is not requisite in most patients, gross or occult blood on the examining finger may indicate active disease.
- **Skin, joint, and eye examinations** should also be performed to evaluate for the presence of extraintestinal manifestations or skin malignancy complicating therapy (Table 17-3).

Differential Diagnosis

- The differential diagnosis of IBD is extensive (Table 17-4) and includes infectious as well as noninfectious causes. Chronic symptoms of 3 months or longer are suggestive of IBD.
- At initial presentation and during exacerbations, it is important to rule out infectious disease. *Salmonella, Shigella, Campylobacter, Aeromonas, Escherichia coli* 0157:H7, *C. difficile, Cytomegalovirus,* and sexually transmitted diseases can all cause bloody diarrhea.
- Findings suggestive of CD include rectal sparing; small bowel involvement; absence of gross bleeding; presence of perianal disease; and the presence of skip lesions, granulomas, or fistula (Table 17-3).
- In about 10–15% of patients with colonic IBD, the distinction between CD and UC cannot be made, and these are termed **inflammatory bowel disease, type unclassified (IBDU)**. **Indeterminate colitis** is reserved for whom pathologic diagnosis cannot be made even after colectomy and full examination of the colon. In the future, combined genetic and serologic markers may assist in distinguishing CD and UC.

TABLE 17-4	DIFFERENTIAL DIAGNOSIS OF INFLAMMATORY BOWEL DISEASE	
Infectious Etiologies		
Bacterial	**Mycobacterial**	**Viral**
Salmonella	Tuberculosis	Cytomegalovirus
Shigella	Mycobacterium avium	Herpes simplex
Toxigenic Escherichia coli	Parasitic	HIV
Campylobacter	Amebiasis	Fungal
Yersinia	Isospora	Histoplasmosis
Clostridium difficile	Trichuris trichiura	Candida
Gonorrhea	Hookworm	Aspergillus
Chlamydia trachomatis	Strongyloides	
Noninfectious Etiologies		
Inflammatory	**Neoplastic**	**Drugs and Chemicals**
Appendicitis	Lymphoma	NSAID
Diverticulitis	Metastatic carcinoma	Phospho-soda
Diversion colitis	Carcinoma of the ileum	Cathartic colon
Collagenous/Lymphocytic colitis	Carcinoid	Gold
	Familial polyposis	Oral contraceptives
Ischemic colitis		Cocaine
Radiation colitis/enteritis		Chemotherapy
Eosinophilic gastroenteritis		
Neutropenic colitis		
Behçet syndrome		
Graft-versus-host disease		

HIV, human immunodeficiency virus; NSAID, nonsteroidal anti-inflammatory drug.

Diagnostic Testing

The diagnosis of IBD is made with a combination of clinical, laboratory, radiographic, endoscopic, and pathologic findings.

Laboratory Testing

- Laboratory tests can help support, but not confirm, the diagnosis in clinical presentations consistent with IBD.
- Evaluation should include a **complete blood cell** count to assess for anemia and leukocytosis. A **complete metabolic panel** evaluates for electrolyte and metabolic abnormalities related to IBD.

- Elevated levels of **C-reactive protein are nonspecific** but are observed in active IBD. This is generally higher in CD than in UC.
- **Stool studies** (*C. difficile,* culture, ova, and parasites) should be sent to evaluate for superimposed infections that may mimic IBD. Some clinicians use fecal calprotectin or lactoferrin to distinguish inflammatory from noninflammatory diarrhea.
- **Autoantibodies** have been detected in IBD patients. The two most commonly used antibody tests are **antineutrophil cytoplasmic antibodies (p-ANCA)**, which is more common in UC, and **anti-*Saccharomyces cerevisiae* antibodies (ASCA)**, which along with **anti-OmpC antibody and antibody against CBir1 flagellin**, are more common in CD. Combination serologic testing is available commercially and is used by some physicians to distinguish between CD and UC.

Imaging

- A **plain abdominal radiograph** is helpful in the acute setting to evaluate for toxic megacolon or bowel obstruction.
- **Small bowel follow-through** x-ray series can provide evaluation of the small bowel in CD. Typical features are luminal narrowing with "string" sign, nodularity and ulceration, a "cobblestone" appearance, and fistulae or abscess formation.
- **Air-contrast barium enema** may be used to confirm the anatomic pattern and extent of disease in UC and Crohn colitis. Barium studies may be normal despite endoscopically evident mild disease. Barium enema must be avoided in severely ill patients because of the risk of precipitating ileus with toxic megacolon.
- **Computed tomography** and **magnetic resonance enterography** are useful in evaluating specific complications (e.g., abscesses, strictures, and fistulas). Magnetic resonance enterography has the advantage of avoiding radiation exposure and for this reason has become an imaging modality of choice at many institutions for nonemergent evaluations.

Diagnostic Procedures

- **Colonoscopy with ileoscopy and biopsy** can usually differentiate CD, UC, and disorders that mimic IBD. Colonoscopy assesses disease location, extent, and severity to confirm IBD diagnosis, obtains tissue for histologic evaluation, and assesses response to therapy.
- Endoscopic features common to both CD and UC include pseudopolyps (UC > CD), loss of haustral folds, fibrotic strictures, and linear superficial scars.
- In CD, specific endoscopic features include discrete aphthous ulcers, "cobblestoning" (formed by deep linear ulcers), discontinuous "skip" lesions, rectal sparing, and involvement of the terminal ileum.
- In UC, endoscopy shows contiguous and circumferential involvement, beginning at the anal verge and extending proximally to a transition to normal mucosa. Erythema, loss of the fine vascular pattern, mucosal granularity, friability, and edema are seen.
- On histopathology, aphthoid ulcers, focal crypt abscesses, and chronic transmural inflammatory infiltrates can be seen only in CD. **Noncaseating granulomas** are pathognomonic for CD but are captured on biopsy in <50% of patients.
- Continuous, diffuse inflammatory infiltrate confined to the mucosa and submucosa, cryptitis, and crypt abscesses are common in UC.
- Complete colonoscopy is typically not performed in patients with severe colitis or toxic megacolon because of the increased risk of perforation. Flexible sigmoidoscopy is often performed in these circumstances to rule out a complicating superinfection with *C. difficile* or Cytomegalovirus.
- **Capsule endoscopy** can be useful in diagnosing CD of the small bowel when diseased areas cannot be reached by endoscopy, but risk of intestinal obstruction exists if the capsule lodges in a tight stricture. The use of a **"patency capsule"** prior to the capsule

endoscopy may help avert this complication; many centers obtain a barium small bowel follow-through series prior to a capsule study. Balloon-assisted enteroscopy is another increasingly used option.

TREATMENT

Medications

- Medical therapy for both CD and UC includes induction and maintenance phases of therapy.[10–13]
- Choice of treatment modality takes disease location or extent, severity, complications, and extraintestinal manifestations into consideration.
- Initiation of longer-term immunosuppressant or immunomodulator therapy requires ruling out any superimposed infections. Steroids may be initiated in acute flares while studies are pending.
- *5-Aminosalicylic acid compounds*
  - 5-Aminosalicylic acid (5-ASA) drugs are used for induction and maintenance of remission in mild to moderate IBD. In CD, they may have modest efficacy in delaying postoperative recurrence or treating colonic disease.
  - Available formulations in the United States are **mesalamine** (Pentasa, Asacol, Asacol HD, Apriso, Lialda), **sulfasalazine**, and **balsalazide** (Colazal), as well as **rectal mesalamine** (Canasa, Rowasa). These formulations differ in the mechanism of release of 5-ASA (Table 17-5).
  - Therapeutic effects of sulfasalazine are derived primarily from the 5-ASA moiety, whereas side effects are mostly caused by its sulfa moiety. Nausea, vomiting, malaise, anorexia, and headache are dose related, whereas hypersensitivity reactions (rash, fever, hemolytic anemia, agranulocytosis, hepatitis, pancreatitis, and worsening of colitis) are idiosyncratic. Non-sulfa 5-ASA derivatives are better tolerated than sulfasalazine and can be escalated to higher doses of 5-ASA.
  - In patients with colonic disease and associated peripheral arthropathy, sulfasalazine has benefit as a disease-modifying antirheumatic drug.
  - Other potential side effects of all 5-ASA drugs are diarrhea and abdominal pain. 5-ASA drugs should be used with caution in patients with salicylate or sulfa allergy. Some mesalamines have carrier products (phthalates) which may be associated with abnormalities of the reproductive system in male offspring.
  - There are reports of nephrotoxicity from interstitial nephritis with 5-ASA compounds. This is more frequent in the first year of therapy but can occur at any time. Serum creatinine level is usually measured before and monitored during treatment.
  - Topical rectal therapies are useful in induction and maintenance for ulcerative proctitis. These agents provide added benefit to orally administered 5-ASA preparations in the treatment of more extensive colitis.
  - Once remission is achieved, lower doses of sulfasalazine (2 g daily) or mesalamine (1.5–2.4 g daily) may maintain remission in UC or potentially reduce postoperative relapse rates in CD.
  - Maintenance 5-ASA treatment may reduce risk of developing colorectal cancer (CRC).
- *Antibiotics*: Although a specific causative microorganism has not been identified in IBD, antibiotics have a role in disease therapy.
  - **Antibiotic use in Crohn disease:**
    - **Metronidazole** (10 or 20 mg/kg/day) **with or without ciprofloxacin** (500 mg PO BID) has use in the treatment of mild to moderately active mucosal inflammation in luminal CD.

TABLE 17-5 AMINOSALYCYLIC ACID THERAPIES

5-ASA Compound	Indication	Dosage
Diffusion dependent[a]		
Mesalamine controlled release (Pentasa)	Proximal disease Severe diarrhea (release not affected by rapid transit) Strictures Pouchitis Postoperative anastomosis	Pentasa = 2.4–4.8 g
pH dependent[b]		
Mesalamine delayed release (Asacol) MMX (multimatrix) mesalamine (Lialda) Mesalamine delayed and extended release (Apriso)	Ileocolonic disease	Asacol = 2.4–4.8 g daily in divided doses. Asacol as 400 mg tablets; Asacol HD as 800-mg tablets Lialda = 1.2-g tablet (once-daily dosing as 2–4 tablets for a 2.4–4.8 g daily dose) Apriso = 1.5 g (0.375 g capsules, 4 capsules once daily)
Colonic bacteria dependent		
Sulfasalazine (Azulfidine)	Colonic disease (bacteria required to cleave azo-bond)	Sulfasalazine = 2–6 g daily in divided doses, usually TID
Balsalazide (Colazal)	Universal and distal UC	Balsalazide = 6.75–13.5 g
Diazo compound with 5-ASA bonded to the sulfonamide sulfapyridine (sulfasalazine) or inert carrier (balsalazide)	Colonic CD Arthropathy	
Directly acting (topical)		
Mesalamine suppositories (Canasa) Mesalamine enema (Rowasa)	Left-sided colitis and proctitis	Canasa = 500 mg Rowasa = 4 g

[a]Timed release begins in the upper small intestine, continues through the colon.
[b]Released at pH 6–7 in terminal ileum/colon. Of note 2.4 g mesalamine = 6 g sulfasalazine = 6.75 g balsalazide.
CD, Crohn disease; UC, ulcerative colitis.

- Metronidazole, ciprofloxacin, tetracycline, or combinations thereof are often used for extended periods in CD patients who have fistulas, abscesses, or perianal disease.
- Antibiotics are indicated for bacterial overgrowth, seen with small bowel strictures or after ileocolic resection.
- **Patients taking long-term metronidazole need to be monitored closely for peripheral neuropathy**, which can be irreversible. Ciprofloxacin use has been associated with tendon inflammation and/or rupture, especially in patients using concurrent steroids, age >60 years, or organ transplant recipients.
- **Antibiotic use in ulcerative colitis:** In fulminant colitis, antibiotics reduce the risk of bacterial translocation. Otherwise, antibiotics do not have a role in the management of UC.
- *Corticosteroids*
  - In UC and CD:
    - Corticosteroids have long been **used to induce remission** in moderate to severe IBD, and to treat patients who have active disease despite other simpler therapies (e.g., 5-ASA).
    - Steroids are **ineffective in *maintaining* remission or *preventing* relapse**, and their use should be limited, given their numerous side effects.
    - Superimposed infections, such as Cytomegalovirus or *C. difficile,* and complications, including toxic megacolon or perforation, should be considered in patients starting or taking steroids. Cultures should be sent at time of starting a steroid therapy.
    - Both **oral prednisone** (40–60 mg daily) and **intravenous methylprednisolone** (40–60 mg daily) induce remission in patients with active disease compared with placebo. Doses are typically tapered (about 5 mg/wk) when a clinical response has been achieved. Tapers should be slow (over 2–3 months), as rapid tapers lead to return of symptoms.
    - As >50% of patients treated acutely with steroids become steroid dependent or refractory, a maintenance strategy (such as an immunomodulator or a biologic agent) needs to be considered when initiating steroids.
  - In ileal colonic Crohn disease: **Budesonide** (up to 9 mg daily) is a controlled-release corticosteroid with high local potency and lower systemic activity due to high first-pass hepatic metabolism. It is an alternative to prednisone in patients with distal small bowel disease and may reduce systemic side effects.
  - In left sided ulcerative colitis or rectal Crohn disease:
    - **Budesonide MMX** (Uceris) has a pH-dependent release allowing for activation of drug in the terminal ileum followed by targeted release throughout the length of the colon. It is beneficial in patients with predominantly colonic disease, such as ulcerative colitis.
    - **Steroid enemas** (e.g., Cortenema) **or foams** (e.g., Cortifoam, Proctofoam, or Budesonide foam) can be used to treat rectal disease and **may be used as an alternative to oral/systemic steroid therapy to treat rectal disease.**
    - If tapering leads to a return of symptoms despite 5-ASA treatment, an immunomodulator or biologic should be considered.
- *Immunomodulator therapy*
  - Oral **azathioprine** (AZA; 2.5–3 mg/kg/day) and its metabolite **6-mercaptopurine** (6-MP; 1.5–2 mg/kg/day) are used to achieve maintenance of steroid-free remission in CD and UC, especially with recurrent disease flares as steroid-sparing agents.
  - In CD, these agents have a role in fistulous CD and perianal disease and in preventing postoperative relapses.
  - Onset of action is generally delayed for as long as 8–12 weeks, and full therapeutic effect can take 3–6 months of continued use. Time to efficacy can be shortened by starting at full-weight–based dose rather than using a titration approach.

Side effects of thiopurines

- Bone marrow suppression (including agranulocytosis), pancreatitis, allergic reactions, hepatitis, and life-threatening infections have been reported, but are usually reversible on discontinuation of therapy. Allergic symptoms, such as joint aches, fevers, nausea, and malaise, typically occur within the first 1–2 weeks of use; pancreatitis occurs around week 3 and leukopenia by week 4.
- Susceptibility to early, severe leukopenia can be predicted before initiation by measuring **thiopurine S-methyltransferase (TPMT)** enzyme activity. TPMT is responsible for drug metabolism. However, TPMT testing does not substitute for monitoring blood counts. 6-MP and AZA should be avoided in patients with very low TPMT activity, and the starting dose should be lowered with intermediate activity. See Chapter 25 for further discussion.
- **Blood counts should be followed every 7–10 days the first 4 weeks and after dose increases.** Once the goal dose has been reached, a complete blood cell count should be checked every 3 months. If the leukocyte count falls below 3000 cells/μL, the dose should be lowered or held.
- An increased risk of lymphoma is reported with azathioprine or 6-MP, but the overall absolute risk still remains quite low. The risk of hepatosplenic T-cell lymphoma is modestly elevated when used concurrently with anti-TNF agents.
- Although controversial, expert opinion suggest that since the risk of harm to a developing fetus is low and active disease is associated with poor fetal outcomes, that the risks and benefits of discontinuing therapy during pregnancy should be carefully considered in a pregnant female on azathioprine.

Monitoring response to therapy

- 6-Thioguanine nucleotide (6-TGN), the active metabolite of 6-MP, can be checked to assess for adequate therapeutic levels of the medications. Low 6-TGN levels can indicate underdosing, high metabolism, or nonadherence. Adequate levels of 6-TGN without a clinical response may indicate the need to change to other therapies.[14]
- The second metabolite that is measured is 6-MMP, which is inactive. Patients who preferentially produce large amounts of 6-MMP can be given allopurinol to shift the metabolism toward increased production of 6-TGN. The addition of allopurinol is accompanied by a decrease in the dose of the immunomodulator to 25% of the original dose due to drug–drug interactions. If this technique is used, close monitoring of blood counts is obligatory.

CD-specific immunomodulators. Subcutaneous or intramuscular **methotrexate** (25 mg weekly) is more effective than placebo in inducing remission in patients with severe CD, with trials showing an effective dose for maintenance of remission at 15 mg weekly. Current evidence is less robust in support of methotrexate for UC.

UC-specific immunomodulators

- **Intravenous cyclosporine** (2–4 mg/kg/day) has been shown effective in fulminant UC, but side effects include grand mal seizures, opportunistic infection, and bowel perforation. Use of cyclosporine as a rescue agent is becoming less common given alternative options and potential organ toxicities. If planning to use, prescribers should be familiar with its use pattern and toxicities. Cyclosporine probably has little role in most cases of CD.
- Oral small molecule **Janus kinase (JAK) inhibition** with tofacitinib (Xeljanz) is currently an approved therapy for UC. Induction dosing is at 5 or 10 mg BID with planned tapering to the lowest effective dose at 8 weeks. Side effects are dose dependent for tofacitinib and include changes in lipid profiles, cytopenias, liver function abnormalities, infectious complications (herpes zoster in particular), and rare thromboembolic events. Prophylactic vaccination against zoster and laboratory monitoring are recommended. Promising trials of other JAK inhibitors will likely extend this therapeutic class to CD.

- **Biologic (antibody-based) therapy**
  - TNF-α is an important cytokine in the pathogenesis of both CD and UC. Three **monoclonal antibodies against TNF** are used in CD (infliximab, adalimumab, and certolizumab) and UC therapy (infliximab, adalimumab, and golimumab) (Table 17-6).[15-24]
  - Targeted blockade of lymphocyte migration to the gut is an additional therapeutic mechanism of action. One monoclonal antibody against $\alpha_4\beta_7$ integrin is approved for the therapy of CD and UC: vedolizumab (Table 17-6).[25,26]
  - IL-12 and -23 are important mediators of T-cell differentiation and have been implicated in the pathogenesis of CD. One monoclonal antibody targeting a shared p40 subunit is approved for the therapy of CD and UC: ustekinumab (Table 17-6).[27]
  - Please see Table 17-6 for information on natalizumab, a humanized monoclonal antibody α_4 subunit of the integrin molecule.[28]
  - **Considerations with biologic therapy**
    - Randomized trials of biologic-naive patients with CD and UC suggest benefit to combination therapy with infliximab and AZA as compared with infliximab or AZA alone (SONIC and UC-SUCCESS). The extrapolation of this concept to other biologics is less well established.[29]
    - Clinical experience with infliximab and adalimumab demonstrates that increases in dosing or dose frequency are sometimes required to maintain therapeutic effect. Assessment of drug concentration and antidrug antibody levels can help guide therapeutic management in IBD in primary nonresponders or those who lose response. Low trough levels with high antidrug antibodies suggest need for an alternative biologic agent.[30]
  - **Important side effects**
    - **Acute infusion reactions** and **delayed-type hypersensitivity** reactions are more common with repeat infusions of infliximab, especially after a prolonged interval since the previous infusion (over 12 weeks). Development of human antidrug antibodies occur in 10–15% of cases and are associated with decreased efficacy.
    - **Reactivation of latent tuberculosis** can occur; therefore, a purified protein-derivative skin or blood-based test must be performed and confirmed negative before therapy. Congestive heart failure and drug-induced lupus have also been reported. In endemic areas, other fungal infections (histoplasmosis) should be considered if symptoms arise during therapy. Other mild and self-limited side effects include headache, upper respiratory infection, and nausea.
    - Side effects of subcutaneously administered biologic agents include **injection site reactions** or **pain**. Other side effects, including risk for infections and lymphoma, are similar in all anti–TNF-α biologic categories.
    - Natalizumab, though effective in CD, has been associated with **progressive multifocal leukoencephalopathy (PML)** and is now rarely used. No cases of PML have been reported with use of vedolizumab, a gut-specific antileukocyte trafficking therapy.
  - There are multiple novel biologics currently being developed for CD. These new therapies utilize unique targets based on modern understanding of CD genetics and pathogenesis.
- **Antidiarrheal agents**
  - Antidiarrheal agents, such as **loperamide** (Imodium), **codeine,** or **tincture of opium** may decrease the frequency and volume of diarrhea.
  - These agents should be withheld if intestinal infection or severely active disease is suspected because of the risk of toxic megacolon.

Surgical Management
- **Crohn disease**
  - Surgical management is often necessary for certain complications, including intractable hemorrhage, perforation, persistent obstruction from stricturing disease, abscess,

TABLE 17-6 BIOLOGIC THERAPY IN INFLAMMATORY BOWEL DISEASE

Name (Trade Name)	Target	Route	Dosing	Indications	Representative Trials
Infliximab (Remicade)	TNF-α (chimeric monoclonal Ab)	IV infusion	5–10 mg/kg body weight over 2 hrs at weeks 0, 2, and 6 and then every 8 wks for maintenance	CD (luminal and fistulizing), UC	CD: ACCENT 1[15] UC: ACT 1 and ACT 2[16]
Adalimumab (Humira)	TNF-α (human Ab)	Subcutaneous	160 mg → 80 mg → 40 mg (weeks 0, 2 and then every 2 wks)	CD (luminal), UC	CD: CLASSIC I[17] and CHARM[18] UC: ULTRA 1[19] and 2[20]
Certolizumab (Cimzia)	TNF-α (PEGylated Fab' fragment of humanized Ab)	Subcutaneous	400 mg at weeks 0, 2, and 4 and then every 4 wks	CD (luminal)	Induction: PRECISE 1[21] Maintenance: PRECISE 2[22]
Golimumab (Simponi)	TNFα (human Ab)	Subcutaneous	200 mg at week 0, 100 mg at week 2, then 100 mg every 4 wks	UC	Induction: PURSUIT-SC[23] Maintenance: PURSUIT-M[24]
Vedolizumab (Entyvio)	α4β7-Integrin (humanized monoclonal Ab; selective to the gut)	IV infusion	300 mg at 0, 2, and 6 weeks then every 8 wks	CD (luminal), UC	UC: GEMINI 1[25] CD: GEMINI 2[26]
Ustekinumab (Stelara)	IL-12/23 (human monoclonal Ab)	One IV infusion then subcutaneous thereafter	Weight-based IV infusion (260 mg up to 55 kg, 390 mg 55–85 kg, and 520 mg if >85 kg) then 90 mg SQ every 8 wks	CD (luminal), UC	Induction: UNITI 1 and 2 Maintenance: IM Uniti[27]
Natalizumab (Tysabri)	α4-Integrin (selective adhesion molecule humanized IgG4 monoclonal Ab)	IV infusion	300 mg every 4 wks	CD (luminal)	ENCORE[28]

Ab, antibody; CD, Crohn disease; IV, intravenous; UC, ulcerative colitis.

or disease activity intractable to medical therapy. Abscesses often require drainage under radiographic guidance or with surgery.

Surgical resection is **not curative** in CD, with clinical recurrence rates of 10–15% annually. Postoperative management with immunomodulators, metronidazole, or mesalamine may lower recurrence rates. Infliximab has been associated with reduced rates of postoperative endoscopic recurrence, but not clinical recurrence.[31,32]

Smoking increases recurrence rates.

Suppurative perianal disease is often treated surgically with the placement of **a noncutting seton (silastic band)**.

Therapeutic options for strictures include strictureplasty, endoscopic balloon dilation, and local injection of steroids or biologic glues. All strictures should be biopsied to exclude malignancy.

- **Ulcerative colitis**
  - Medically refractory disease activity is the most common reason for surgery in UC. Less commonly, total colectomy is required for acutely ill patients with megacolon or systemic toxicity not responding to medical therapy within 48 hours.
  - **Proctocolectomy is curative** in UC. The mortality of colectomy is low even in severe cases. Advances in surgical technique allow for the creation of an ileal pouch–anal anastomosis, and a permanent ileostomy is typically not required.[33]
  - **Pouchitis**, or inflammation of the surgically created ileal reservoir, is the most common complication of this surgery and occurs at least in a mild form in approximately 50% of the population. Symptoms include increased stool frequency, urgency, hematochezia, abdominal pain, and fever, but the diagnosis is made endoscopically and histologically. First-line therapy is typically with **antibiotics** (metronidazole or ciprofloxacin); **probiotics** (such as VSL#3) may be useful for prevention. Recurrent or refractory pouchitis may represent misdiagnosed CD, which is typically confirmed when significant inflammation is identified proximal to the pouch. Pouch excision is required in 5% of patients.
  - **Cuffitis** is inflammation of the short section of retained rectal mucosa. It is treated with topical steroids or 5-ASA suppositories.

Lifestyle/Risk Modification

- No dietary factors have been shown to either cause or cure IBD. On an individual basis, certain foods may trigger symptomatic exacerbations and may need avoidance.
- In stricturing disease, a **low-residue diet** (avoidance of pulps, peels, and whole leaf vegetables) is recommended to avoid obstruction.
- Maintenance of adequate nutrition is essential in the care of CD patients. Approximately, 75% of CD patients admitted to the hospital are malnourished.
- **Nutritional deficiencies** are typically related to decreased oral intake, malabsorption, and blood loss. Vitamin and nutrient supplementation may be needed after small bowel resection or in the setting of extensive bowel involvement. For example, patients with ileitis may need vitamin B12 supplementation.
- Common deficiencies in CD include vitamins B12, A, and D, calcium, potassium, iron, and zinc. In UC, common deficiencies are folate, vitamin D, and iron, and less commonly vitamin B12. Levels should be measured. Repletion and prophylactic supplementation may be beneficial.
- To meet nutritional needs, **enteral feeding** is generally preferable to parenteral (total parenteral nutrition [TPN]). TPN is efficacious in refractory CD when used in conjunction with bowel rest and medical therapy. In these instances, discontinuation of TPN may be associated with high relapse rates.
- Some **probiotics** have shown efficacy in maintenance of remission in UC (VSL#3, *E. coli* Nissle). They also have a role in the treatment of pouchitis (VSL#3). Despite patient enthusiasm, the evidence for probiotics in CD is poor.

SPECIAL CONSIDERATIONS

- **Pregnancy in IBD**
  - Pregnancy has been associated with both improvement and worsening of disease activity.[34]
  - High disease activity is associated with poor fetal outcomes, mainly preterm delivery. Thus, achieving remission prior to conception is optimal.
  - Medical therapy of IBD in pregnancy should be addressed by gastroenterologists and obstetricians experienced with such care. The risk to benefit ratio for biologic or immunomodulator therapy should be considered.
  - Increased rates of congenital anomalies or preterm birth have not been demonstrated in pregnant women exposed to anti-TNF therapy.[35]
  - Anti-TNF drug levels have been detected in infants up to 1 year.[36] A careful risk–benefit analysis should be conducted before exposing infants to a live vaccination in the first year of life. If necessary, an infant drug level may be helpful in further risk stratification.
  - Systemic steroids should be avoided in the first trimester but may be the therapy of choice in the third trimester. Methotrexate is a known teratogen.
- **Microscopic colitis (MC)**
  - MC consists of a group of diseases characterized by chronic, watery, nonbloody diarrhea, with largely normal endoscopic findings. MC is less common than CD and UC.
  - The two main types of MC are **collagenous colitis** and **lymphocytic colitis**, although mixed forms and variants have also been described. On histology, a thickened subepithelial collagenous band is seen with collagenous colitis. Lymphocytic colitis is marked by a subepithelial lymphocytic infiltrate.
  - Etiology is unknown, and it is doubtful that a single pathogenetic mechanism exists.
  - Collagenous colitis has a female-to-male predominance of 9 to 15:1, whereas lymphocytic colitis has equal incidence in both genders. Onset typically occurs after age 50.
  - Collagenous colitis may be caused by abnormal collagen metabolism, particularly reduced matrix degradation rather than enhanced synthesis. Vascular endothelial growth factor may play a role in this collagen balance. Celiac disease, bacterial toxins, NSAIDs, selective serotonin reuptake inhibitors, and other drugs have been linked to the development of MC.
  - The **clinical presentation** of collagenous and lymphocytic colitis consists of progressively increasing watery diarrhea that is often refractory to over-the-counter antidiarrheal medications. Associated symptoms can include nausea, abdominal pain, and fecal urgency. Many patients have a diagnosis of a diarrhea predominant IBS until colonic pathology is examined, stressing the importance of colonoscopy and random biopsies of normal appearing mucosa.
  - Although the disease course is generally benign, relapsing and remitting symptoms can be debilitating. Patients should be reassured that MC is not associated with increased mortality or an increased risk of developing CRC. NSAIDs or other drugs associated with MC should be discontinued if possible. Patients should be tested for celiac disease.
  - **Antidiarrheal agents,** such as loperamide and Lomotil, can be first tried. Most cases referred to a gastroenterologist lead to a trial of **budesonide** (9 mg daily for a month, followed by a taper over next 2 months). Bismuth subsalicylate, cholestyramine, and mesalamine products are effective in some patients. In refractory cases, immunomodulators, systemic corticosteroids, and even biologic-based therapy have been tried.

REFERRAL

With advances in newer biologic therapies as well as improved understanding of existing medications, treatment of moderate or severe IBD is best orchestrated by physicians with significant experience in IBD management or in specialized centers focusing on IBD.

MONITORING/FOLLOW-UP

- **Response to therapy**
  - In addition to symptomatic improvement, mucosal healing is an important endpoint, as it can indicate better long-term outcomes, including decreased rates of hospitalization and surgical resections. Routine endoscopy with biopsies is recommended.
- **Osteoporosis**
  - Osteoporosis is a source of significant morbidity, impaired quality of life, and costs in IBD.
  - IBD itself only modestly lowers bone mineral density but increases the risk of fractures by 40% over the general population.
  - Bone densitometry (DEXA) scan is indicated in all postmenopausal women and those with exposure to corticosteroids.
  - Other useful tests include an alkaline phosphatase, calcium level (corrected for serum albumin), creatinine, testosterone level (males), and 25-OH-vitamin D level.
  - All patients should be educated about the importance of regular weight-bearing exercise and avoiding smoking and excessive alcohol intake.
  - Adequate intake of vitamin D (800 IU daily) and calcium (1000 to 1500 mg daily) is recommended.
  - Bisphosphonates are used in patients at highest risk for fractures.
- **Malignancy**
  - Patients with UC and colonic CD are at increased risk for **colorectal cancer** (CRC) compared with the general population (see also Chapter 16). The level of risk is related to the duration, severity, and colonic extent of inflammation. Risks are higher with a family history of CRC. Because CRC is generally preceded by dysplasia, surveillance is recommended to detect and intervene when dysplasia is found.[37]
  - In patients with UC and pancolitis, CRC risk seems to increase after 8–10 years of symptoms. The cumulative incidence of CRC in UC is reported to be as high as 5–10% after 20 years and 12–20% after 30 years of disease, although recent studies report lower incidences.
  - For left-sided colitis, CRC risk may increase after 15–20 years. Distal colitis and proctosigmoiditis probably do not increase the risk of CRC. Patients with UC with PSC have an even higher increased risk for developing CRC.
  - Surveillance colonoscopy is recommended beginning after 8 years of pancolitis and after 15 years of left-sided colitis and then repeated every 1–3 years thereafter. No screening is recommended for ulcerative proctitis.
  - Surveillance colonoscopy with chromoendoscopy, the application of a dye (such as methylene blue or indigo carmine) to enhance mucosal surface abnormalities, is recommended to improve dysplasia detection.[38] Random biopsy protocols also remain in use.
  - Patients with an ileal pouch should undergo flexible sigmoidoscopy with biopsies every other year.
  - Colectomy is generally recommended for carcinoma, high-grade dysplasia, and multifocal low-grade dysplasia.

In CD, patients with long-standing colitis or age >30 years at diagnosis are at greatest risk. Recommended surveillance strategies are similar to those for UC.

- **Other health maintenance issues**[39]
  - IBD patients on immunomodulators and biologic therapy should be up-to-date in **vaccinations against preventable illnesses**. Considerations include hepatitis A/B, yearly *influenza, pneumococcus, meningococcus,* tetanus. After immunosuppressive therapy has begun, live-attenuated vaccines (e.g., varicella) should be avoided.
  - Pap smears should also be performed regularly, as there is an increased risk of abnormal pap smears with thiopurine therapy. Vaccination against malignancy-associated human papillomavirus (Gardasil) should be offered.

OUTCOME/PROGNOSIS

- Both CD and UC are chronic diseases with intermittent exacerbations of mild to severe symptoms alternating with periods of varying levels of remission.
- About 10–20% of patients with CD will experience a very prolonged remission after initial presentation. Conversely, predictors of a severe course include age <40 years, presence of perianal disease, smoking, initial requirement of corticosteroids, and perforating disease. CD can be associated with a modest decrease in overall life expectancy.
- The course of UC depends on extent of disease. Proctitis and distal colitis usually have a more benign course, resolving spontaneously in about 20% of cases.
- In UC, increased relapse rates are seen in younger patients (ages 20–30 years), older patients (>70 years), women, those with more than five prior relapses, and those with basal plasmacytosis on rectal biopsy. Approximately 30% undergo colectomy after 15–25 years of disease. Overall mortality is only slightly increased compared with the general population.

REFERENCES

1. Shivashankar R, Tremaine WJ, Harmsen WS, et al. Incidence and prevalence of Crohn's Disease and ulcerative colitis in Olmsted County, Minnesota from 1970 through 2010. *Clin Gastroenterol Hepatol.* 2017;15:857–863.
2. Dahlhamer JM, Zammitti EP, Ward BW, et al. Prevalence of inflammatory bowel disease among adults aged ≥18 years—United States, 2015. MMWR *Morb Mortal Wkly Rep.* 2015;65:1166–1169.
3. Abraham C, Cho JH. Inflammatory bowel disease. *N Engl J Med.* 2009;361:2066–2078.
4. Xavier RJ, Podolsky DK. Unravelling the pathogenesis of inflammatory bowel disease. *Nature.* 2007;448:427–434.
5. Uniken Venema WT, Voskuil MD, Dijkstra G, et al. The genetic background of inflammatory bowel disease: from correlation to causality. *J Pathol.* 2017;241:146–158.
6. Abraham C, Medzhitov R. Interactions between the host innate immune system and microbes in inflammatory bowel disease. *Gastroenterology.* 2011;140:1729–1737.
7. Satsangi J, Silverberg MS, Vermeire S, et al. The Montreal classification of inflammatory bowel disease: controversies, consensus, and implications. *Gut.* 2006;55:749–753.
8. Lichtenstein GR, Hanauer SB, Sandborn WJ. Management of Crohn's disease in adults. *Am J Gastroenterol.* 2009;104:465–483; quiz 464, 484.
9. Rothfuss KS, Stange EF, Herrlinger KR. Extraintestinal manifestations and complications in inflammatory bowel diseases. *World J Gastroenterol.* 2006;12:4819–4831.
10. Terdiman JP, Gruss CB, Heidelbaugh JJ, et al. American Gastroenterological Association Institute guideline on the use of thiopurines, methotrexate, and anti-TNF-alpha biologic drugs for the induction and maintenance of remission in inflammatory Crohn's disease. *Gastroenterology.* 2013;145:1459–1463.
11. Kornbluth A, Sachar DB. Ulcerative colitis practice guidelines in adults: American College Of Gastroenterology, Practice Parameters Committee. *Am J Gastroenterol.* 2010;105:501–523; quiz 524.
12. Danese S, Fiocchi C. Ulcerative colitis. *N Engl J Med.* 2011;365:1713–1725.
13. Danese S, Vuitton L, Peyrin-Biroulet L. Biologic agents for IBD: practical insights. *Nat Rev Gastroenterol Hepatol.* 2015;12:537–545.

14. Ha C, Dassopoulos T. Thiopurine therapy in inflammatory bowel disease. *Expert Rev Gastroenterol Hepatol.* 2010;4:575–588.
15. Hanauer SB, Feagan BG, Lichtenstein GR, et al. Maintenance infliximab for Crohn's disease: the ACCENT I randomised trial. *Lancet.* 2002;359:1541–1549.
16. Rutgeerts P, Sandborn WJ, Feagan BG, et al. Infliximab for induction and maintenance therapy for ulcerative colitis. *N Engl J Med.* 2005;353:2462–2476.
17. Hanauer SB, Sandborn WJ, Rutgeerts P, et al. Human anti-tumor necrosis factor monoclonal antibody (adalimumab) in Crohn's disease: the CLASSIC-I trial. *Gastroenterology.* 2006;130:323–333; quiz 591.
18. Colombel JF, Sandborn WJ, Rutgeerts P, et al. Adalimumab for maintenance of clinical response and remission in patients with Crohn's disease: the CHARM trial. *Gastroenterology.* 2007;132:52–65.
19. Reinisch W, Sandborn WJ, Hommes DW, et al. Adalimumab for induction of clinical remission in moderately to severely active ulcerative colitis: results of a randomised controlled trial. *Gut.* 2011;60:780–787.
20. Sandborn WJ, van Assche G, Reinisch W, et al. Adalimumab induces and maintains clinical remission in patients with moderate-to-severe ulcerative colitis. *Gastroenterology.* 2012;142:257–265.e1-3.
21. Sandborn WJ, Feagan BG, Stoinov S, et al. Certolizumab pegol for the treatment of Crohn's disease. *N Engl J Med.* 2007;357:228–238.
22. Schreiber S, Khaliq-Kareemi M, Lawrance IC, et al. Maintenance therapy with certolizumab pegol for Crohn's disease. *N Engl J Med.* 2007;357:239–250.
23. Sandborn WJ, Feagan BG, Marano C, et al. Subcutaneous golimumab induces clinical response and remission in patients with moderate-to-severe ulcerative colitis. *Gastroenterology.* 2014;146:85–95; quiz e14-5.
24. Sandborn WJ, Feagan BG, Marano C, et al. Subcutaneous golimumab maintains clinical response in patients with moderate-to-severe ulcerative colitis. *Gastroenterology.* 2014;146:96–109.e1.
25. Feagan BG, Rutgeerts P, Sands BE, et al. Vedolizumab as induction and maintenance therapy for ulcerative colitis. *N Engl J Med.* 2013;369:699–710.
26. Sandborn WJ, Feagan BG, Rutgeerts P, et al. Vedolizumab as induction and maintenance therapy for Crohn's disease. *N Engl J Med.* 2013;369:711–721.
27. Feagan BG, Sandborn WJ, Gasink C, et al. Ustekinumab as induction and maintenance therapy for Crohn's disease. *N Engl J Med.* 2016;375:1946–1960.
28. Targan SR, Feagan BG, Fedorak RN, et al. Natalizumab for the treatment of active Crohn's disease: results of the ENCORE Trial. *Gastroenterology.* 2007;132:1672–1683.
29. Dulai PS, Siegel CA, Colombel JF, et al. Systematic review: monotherapy with antitumour necrosis factor alpha agents versus combination therapy with an immunosuppressive for IBD. *Gut.* 2014;63:1843–1853.
30. Melmed GY, Irving PM, Jones J, et al. Appropriateness of testing for anti-tumor necrosis factor agent and antibody concentrations, and interpretation of results. *Clin Gastroenterol Hepatol.* 2016;14:1302–1309.
31. Lu KC, Hunt SR. Surgical management of Crohn's disease. *Surg Clin North Am.* 2013;93:167–185.
32. Regueiro M, Feagan BG, Zou B, et al. Infliximab reduces endoscopic, but not clinical, recurrence of Crohn's disease after ileocolonic resection. *Gastroenterology.* 2016;150:1568–1578.
33. McLaughlin SD, Clark SK, Tekkis PP, et al. Review article: restorative proctocolectomy, indications, management of complications and follow-up—a guide for gastroenterologists. *Aliment Pharmacol Ther.* 2008;27:895–909.
34. Mahadevan U, McConnell RA, Chambers CD. Drug safety and risk of adverse outcomes for pregnant patients with inflammatory bowel disease. *Gastroenterology.* 2017;152:451–462.e2.
35. Nguyen GC, Seow CH, Maxwell C, et al. The Toronto consensus statements for the management of inflammatory bowel disease in pregnancy. *Gastroenterology.* 2016;150:734–757.e1.
36. Julsgaard M, Christensen LA, Gibson PR, et al. Concentrations of adalimumab and infliximab in mothers and newborns, and effects on infection. *Gastroenterology.* 2016;151:110–119.
37. Velayos F, Kathpalia P, Finlayson E. Changing paradigms in detection of dysplasia and management of patients with inflammatory bowel disease: is colectomy still necessary? *Gastroenterology.* 2017;152:440–450.e1.
38. Laine L, Kaltenbach T, Barkun A, et al. SCENIC international consensus statement on surveillance and management of dysplasia in inflammatory bowel disease. *Gastrointest Endosc.* 2015;81:489–501.e26.
39. Moscandrew M, Mahadevan U, Kane S. General health maintenance in IBD. *Inflamm Bowel Dis.* 2009;15:1399–1409.

18

Irritable Bowel Syndrome

Ted Walker and Gregory S. Sayuk

GENERAL PRINCIPLES

Background and Definition

- Functional gastrointestinal disorders (FGIDs) are disorders of gut–brain interaction.
- The hallmark feature of FGIDs is visceral hypersensitivity, manifested as abdominal discomfort or pain.
- Motility disturbances, altered mucosal and immune function, shifts in gut microbiota, disordered central nervous system processing, and psychosocial disturbances all have purported pathophysiologic relevance in some patients.
- Importantly, by definition, FGIDs lack identifiable structural abnormalities on diagnostic evaluations.
- FGID symptoms can arise from any portion of the GI tract (esophagus to anus), and frequently multiple FGIDs may be identified in the same individual.
- These functional syndromes, as defined by the Rome criteria,[1] are listed in Table 18-1.
- The prototypical and most common functional GI disorder is irritable bowel syndrome (IBS), which is characterized by abdominal pain associated with defecation or a change in bowel habit and features of disordered defecation (constipation and/or diarrhea).
- IBS and other FGIDs impose substantial burdens on patient well-being and, in turn, result in frequent visits to both primary care physicians and gastroenterologists.

Classification

- Several historical diagnostic criteria for IBS exist, with the Rome IV criteria (Table 18-2) representing the most recent criteria.[2] These criteria were devised primarily as a tool for devising clinical studies rather than for routine clinical application.
- When implemented in clinical practice, these criteria have a high positive predictive value (>95%).
- Although not requisite for an IBS diagnosis, several supportive symptoms (Table 18-3) help to solidify the diagnosis and further characterize the disorder into IBS with constipation (IBS-C), IBS with diarrhea (IBS-D), mixed IBS (IBS-M), or unsubtyped IBS.

Epidemiology

- IBS is frequently seen in both primary care and specialty care settings and is one of the most common diagnoses seen by gastroenterologists.[3]
  - Estimates place the prevalence of IBS anywhere from 1–20% worldwide.
  - Systematic reviews suggest 5–10% of individuals in North America are affected with IBS.[4]
  - Population surveys of adults have shown IBS to be more prevalent in women than in men, with a ratio of 2 to 3:1.
  - Symptom onset tends to occur before the fifth decade, but it can occur at any age.
  - When considering a new diagnosis of IBS in older individuals, exclusion of other mimicking conditions (celiac disease, inflammatory bowel disease, small intestinal bacterial overgrowth [SIBO]) is essential.

TABLE 18-1 ROME IV DESIGNATIONS OF FUNCTIONAL GASTROINTESTINAL DISORDERS

Esophageal Disorders

Functional chest pain
Functional heartburn
Reflux hypersensitivity
Globus
Functional dysphagia

Gastroduodenal Disorders

Functional dyspepsia
Belching disorders
Nausea and vomiting disorders
Rumination syndrome

Bowel Disorders

Irritable bowel syndrome
Functional constipation
Functional diarrhea
Functional abdominal bloating/distension
Unspecified functional bowel disorder
Opioid-induced constipation

Centrally Mediated Disorders of Gastrointestinal Pain

Centrally mediated abdominal pain syndrome (CAPS)
Narcotic bowel syndrome (NBS)/Opioid-induced GI hyperalgesia

Gallbladder and SO Disorders

Functional gallbladder disorder
Functional biliary sphincter of Oddi disorder
Functional pancreatic sphincter of Oddi disorder

Anorectal Disorders

Fecal incontinence
Functional anorectal pain
Functional defecation disorders

TABLE 18-2 THE ROME IV IRRITABLE BOWEL SYNDROME CRITERIA

Recurrent abdominal pain, on average, at least 1 day/wk in the last 3 months associated with two or more of the following:

1. Related to defecation
2. Associated with a change in frequency of stools
3. Associated with a change in form (appearance) of stool

From Mearin F, Lacy BE, Chang L, et al. Bowel disorders. *Gastroenterology*. 2016;160: 1393–1407.

TABLE 18-3	SUPPORTIVE SYMPTOMS OF IRRITABLE BOWEL SYNDROME

Abnormal stool frequency (*abnormal* defined as more than three bowel movements per day or fewer than three bowel movements per week)
Abnormal stool form (lumpy/hard or loose/watery stool)
Abnormal stool passage (straining, urgency, or feeling of incomplete evacuation)
Passage of mucus
Bloating or feeling of abdominal distention

- Up to 75% of affected individuals do not seek medical care.
    - Still, the cost of IBS to society is considerable, accounting for over 3.6 million physician visits and $1.6 billion in direct medical costs each year.
    - Indirect costs in the form of work absenteeism may exceed $20 billion per annum.
- The burden on the patient is also considerable with health-related quality-of-life scores similar to patients with diabetes and worse than patients with chronic kidney disease and gastroesophageal reflux disease.[5]

Pathophysiology

- No single pathophysiologic abnormality has been found that adequately explains the manifestations of IBS in all cases.
- Multiple factors, including abnormalities of intestinal motility, visceral hypersensitivity, GI tract inflammatory processes, the microbiome, disturbances along the brain–gut axis, and psychological factors, all have been examined as potentially causative in IBS.
- A portion of patients with IBS will exhibit exaggerated motility, and enhanced sensory responses to stressors, meals, and balloon inflation in the GI tract.
    - These motility responses, however, are neither uniformly identifiable in patients with IBS nor consistently detectable in the same individual.
    - Nonetheless, accelerated transit times collectively are associated with diarrhea-predominant IBS while slowed transit times in constipation-predominant IBS.
- IBS may result from sensitization of afferent neural pathways from the gut such that normal intestinal stimuli induce pain. In experimental settings, IBS patients have a lower pain threshold to balloon distention of the colon than healthy volunteers, while retaining normal sensitivity to somatic stimuli.
- Intestinal inflammation has also been hypothesized as playing a role in the development of IBS, particularly as it relates to persistent neuroimmune interactions following infectious gastroenteritis ("postinfectious IBS").
- Approximately one-third of patients with IBS report symptom onset after an episode of acute gastroenteritis.
- Seven percent to 30% of patients presenting with an acute enteric infection go on to develop IBS-like symptoms.
- Psychological distress (particularly somatization) seems to be an important cofactor in determining who develops persistent functional symptoms following an enteric infection.
- The role of SIBO in the development of IBS has been a focus of recent investigations.[6] The evidence for the role of SIBO in IBS remains incompletely understood and likely is relevant to only a subset of IBS patients.[7]
- The CNS (and its interpretation of peripheral enteric nerve signals) is receiving increasing attention in investigational settings because of the potential mechanistic significance in IBS.

- Differential responses of brain activation to both noxious rectal stimulation and antici-pated rectal discomfort can be appreciated in patients with IBS.
  - These connections are both the focus of intense research and the potential target for novel therapies.
  - Psychological factors (anxiety, depression, somatization) are important in their poten-tial to further modulate this afferent pain network.[8]
- Convincing evidence exists for genetic basis for IBS.
  - IBS clusters in families and early-life influences are important.[9]
  - No single genetic defect reliably accounts for all IBS cases.
  - Genetic polymorphisms predict endophenotypes and gene–gene interactions and environmental influences are likely key to genetic predisposition.[10]

DIAGNOSIS

Clinical Presentation

- IBS is a symptom-based diagnosis founded on a reporting of abdominal pain and alter-ation in stool pattern.
- IBS diagnosis requires an element of chronicity (per Rome criteria, 1 day per week over the preceding 3 months).
- The diagnosis of IBS should be made after organic causes have been considered, so a careful search for alarm symptoms should be conducted. Important alarm symptoms include weight loss of ≥10 lb (≥4.5 kg), recurrent fever, persistent diarrhea, hematoche-zia, age >50 years, and family history of GI malignancy, inflammatory bowel disease, or celiac sprue.
- A brief history of rapidly progressive symptoms suggests organic disease. The presence of any such "red flag" features warrants an early, entailed investigation before establishing a diagnosis of IBS.
- The physical examination should be focused to exclude organic disease.
  - Diffuse abdominal tenderness is commonly present because of the heightened visceral sensitivity noted in this population. Peritoneal signs should be absent.
  - Physical examination alarm signs include the presence of ascites, jaundice, organo-megaly, abdominal mass, adenopathy, or heme-positive stool.

Diagnostic Testing

- **Laboratory and invasive testing should be kept to a minimum**, because extensive or repetitive investigations may be costly and promote illness behavior.
- Initial laboratory testing should include a complete blood cell count, C-reactive protein, and fecal occult blood test when appropriate.
- These tests, along with a complete metabolic profile, stool culture, and *Clostridium difficile* toxin assay can be ordered in the proper setting, but likely are low yield for most IBS patients.
- **Testing for celiac sprue (serum tissue transglutaminase IgA + quantitative IgA or deamidated gliadin IgG) should be considered in all IBS patients** (particularly in IBS-D and IBS-M).
- Sensitivity and specificity of glucose and lactose breath tests are inadequate to evaluate for SIBO, and these are not recommended for use in IBS patients.[4]
- Small bowel aspirates and culture are cumbersome and expensive; these tests also are reserved for research settings.
- For IBS-D type a few additional testing strategies can be considered.
  - Measurement of fecal calprotectin can discriminate between IBS and IBD with good accuracy.[11]

- A meta-analysis showed more than 1 in 4 persons has evidence of bile acid diarrhea and a therapeutic trial of a bile acid sequestrant can be used as a diagnostic approach.[12]
- Recent research has focused on developing novel biomarkers to aid in diagnosis.
  - Biomarkers that have shown promising results include antibodies to a bacterial toxin produced by *Campylobacter jejuni* (cytolethal distending toxin, CdtB) and vinculin.
  - These antibodies can distinguish IBS from non-IBS controls with good specificity (92% for *C. jejuni* and 84% for vinculin) but low sensitivity (44% for CdtB and 33% for vinculin).[13] Testing in "real-world" setting is still needed.
- Endoscopy (esophagogastroduodenoscopy and colonoscopy) may be unnecessary, especially in young patients with classic features of IBS and without any alarm symptoms.
  - Colonoscopy should be considered in all patients older than 50 years (also important part of routine colon cancer screening).[4]
  - In this setting, colonoscopy offers the following advantages:
    - Rule out inflammation or tumors (especially in patients older than 50 years).
    - Identify melanosis coli indicative of laxative abuse.

TREATMENT

- The approach to therapy in IBS is multifaceted and should be tailored to the patient, given the individual's constellation and severity of symptoms.[14]
- **Two key factors that determine therapy** are as follows:
  - Dominant symptoms (diarrhea, constipation, pain, other)
  - Symptom severity (intensity, bother, effects on quality of life)
- Current management approaches include gut-targeted peripherally acting agents, centrally acting agents, and psychological–behavioral therapy.
- Cases with mild or intermittent symptoms can be managed with symptomatic treatment using peripherally acting agents administered on an as-needed basis.
- Patients with moderate symptoms (as designated by intermittent interference with daily activities) may benefit from regular use of peripheral agents as an initial approach, with the option of introducing centrally acting agents if this approach incompletely resolves symptoms.
- Patients with severe symptoms (regular interference with daily activities and concurrent affective, personality, and psychosomatic disorders) benefit from combinations of peripherally and centrally acting agents, but may also need contemporary pharmaceutical agents and cognitive behavioral therapy (CBT) to manage their overlapping affective, personality, and psychosomatic disorders.
- Although medical therapy is available and new drugs are currently in development, IBS is a lifelong condition with exacerbations and remissions, and medications should be minimized to the extent possible.
- Clearly, **narcotics have no role in the management of IBS**. Narcotic bowel syndrome may result with paradoxical worsening of abdominal pain.
- Given the lack of identifiable biomarkers, trials of medications are frequently part of the IBS diagnostic process.
- These trials should be pursued for at least 4 weeks before moving on to different strategies.
- If failure to respond to a single agent in a drug class is experienced, response to a different drug in the same class may still be observed.
- It is important to recognize the substantial (up to 50%) placebo response rates present in this patient population.
- **Patient education and reassurance** while establishing a therapeutic relationship are cornerstones in the management of this condition.

TABLE 18-4	GENERAL APPROACH TO IRRITABLE BOWEL SYNDROME AND THE FUNCTIONAL BOWEL DISORDERS

Assess for typical symptoms and the absence of "red flag" alarm symptoms
Minimize invasive testing, targeted to exclude other disorders as appropriate
Avoid repetitive testing unless necessary
Determine patient expectations and goals
Education and reassurance with emphasis on benign nature of condition
Dietary modifications and fiber supplementation are first-line therapy
Medications for more persistent or difficult cases
Behavioral or psychological interventions for refractory and motivated patients with IBS

- The strength of the physician's relationship with the patient correlates to higher rates of patient satisfaction and fewer return visits.
- Table 18-4 summarizes general management principles for patients with IBS or other functional bowel disorders.

Peripherally Acting Agents

- **Therapies for constipation-predominant IBS** (IBS-C)
  - Increasing the amount of **dietary fiber** is a simple, inexpensive option in mild IBS-C and can be instituted as an early approach.
  - A systematic review and meta-analysis of seven trials showed that soluble fiber was beneficial in management of IBS.[4,15]
  - Natural fiber sources (e.g., psyllium) or synthetic fibers (e.g., methylcellulose) are available.
- In patients who complain of bloating or gas, fiber supplementation can be associated with an increase in those symptoms and slow titration and exclusion of flatulogenic foods should be encouraged.
- Use of a **low-fermentable oligosaccharides, disaccharides, monosaccharides, and polyols (FODMAP)** diet has come into favor, with randomized, controlled trial evidence demonstrating improvement in IBS symptom scores, bloating, and pain with the low-FODMAP diet.[16]
- **Osmotic laxatives** such as milk of magnesia, sorbitol, lactulose, or polyethylene glycol may also be considered for patients with IBS-C. Currently, there are no randomized controlled trial data to support their use.[4]
- These agents are generally safe for long-term use and are preferable to stimulant laxatives.
- Nonabsorbable carbohydrates such as lactulose and sorbitol can be fermented by gut bacteria, inducing bloating symptoms; hence, they are best avoided.
- **Lubiprostone** (Amitiza) is a chloride channel activator indicated in the treatment of IBS-C in women at a dose of 8 μg twice daily.
  - Lubiprostone has shown benefit in reducing global IBS symptom scores.[4]
  - Side effects include nausea, diarrhea, and headache.
- **Linaclotide** (Linzess) is a guanylate cyclase-C agonist that upregulates secretion of anions including chloride, followed by sodium and fluid into the bowel lumen. It has been approved for IBS-C at a dose of 290 μg daily.
  - It has been shown to improve bowel movement frequency and IBS pain.[17,18]
  - Main side effect is diarrhea experienced by up to 20% treated with this higher dose. The diarrhea diminishes with continued use, and may be improved by administering medication with meals.
  - Linaclotide is not absorbed and thus has negligible concern for drug interactions.

- **Plecanatide** (Trulance) is another guanylate cyclase-C agonist which has been approved for chronic idiopathic constipation and IBS-C at 3 mg a day dosing.
- The 5-HT$_4$ agonist **prucalopride** has been used in Europe and Canada (Resotran) for several years for IBS-C, and now is available in the United States (Motegrity) as well.
- **Tegaserod** (Zelnorm) is another 5-HT$_4$ agonist first available in the United States in 2002 for IBS-C treatment. It was later withdrawn from the market over concerns for cardiovascular (CV) events. However, it is once again FDA approved, with an indication in women with IBS-C and low CV risk.
- **Therapies for diarrhea-predominant IBS** (IBS-D)
  - The antidiarrheal **loperamide** (2–4 mg up to four times daily) is effective as a short-term agent to control diarrhea; it is not intended for long-term use, and is minimally effective at addressing pain symptoms.
  - On the basis of its mechanism of action, **diphenoxylate** 2.5 mg **with atropine** 0.025 mg (Lomotil, up to QID) may also be used.[4]
  - Suspension forms of these medications are available for patients who need dose titrations.
  - **Cholestyramine** (Questran), **colestipol** (Colestid), and **colesevelam** (WelChol) can be considered as an adjunct, or for early use when diarrheal symptoms exacerbated by cholecystectomy. May be more effective when bile acid malabsorption can be established (SeHCAT scanning; abnormal in 1–10% of patients with IBS-D in research settings); serum markers C4 and FGF-19 identify IBS patients with bile acid malabsorption, and are gaining use in clinical settings.
  - **Alosetron** (Lotronex), a selective 5-HT$_3$ receptor antagonist, was approved for treatment of women with IBS-D.
    - Alosetron was voluntarily withdrawn from the market in 2000 because of a possible relationship with acute ischemic colitis and severe constipation induced by this medication (1.1 and 0.66 cases per 1000 patient-years, respectively).
    - It was reapproved by the U.S. Food and Drug Administration in 2002 for chronic, severe IBS-D that has failed to respond to conventional therapy; currently, its use requires prescriber registration.
  - **Eluxadoline** (Viberzi) is a novel drug that acts on δ-, κ-, and μ-opioid receptors.
    - Eluxadoline was found to be more effective than placebo with response rates of 27% versus 17% in a combined diarrhea-pain endpoint at 100 mg twice a day.[19]
    - Common side effects include constipation early in the course, with rare side effects of pancreatitis (0.3%), and sphincter of Oddi spasm (0.5%). This has led FDA to recommend against use in patients with alcohol dependence or pre-existing pancreaticobiliary disease. It is contraindicated in patients who are status-post cholecystectomy.
  - **Anticholinergic or "antispasmodic" agents** often are used in all classes of IBS, though probably are most useful in the setting of IBS-D.
    - Anticholinergic medications possess antidiarrheal properties via decreases in intestinal transit and modulation of bowel secretory function.
    - **Hyoscyamine** (Levsin) 0.125–0.25 mg orally or sublingual and **dicyclomine** (Bentyl) 10–20 mg orally, up to three times a day.
    - **Glycopyrrolate** (Robinul) 1–2 mg two to three times a day and **methscopolamine** (Pamine) 2.5–5 mg twice a day are also available and have decreased CNS side effect potential.
    - These agents are most useful in patients with postprandial symptoms of abdominal pain, bloating, diarrhea, or fecal urgency.
    - They should be prescribed to circumvent symptoms, such as before meals.
    - These agents often become less effective with long-term use.

- Limited data also exist, supporting the use of peppermint oil as an antispasmodic agent. A proprietary, triple-coated microsphere preparation has shown benefit over placebo in a small clinical trial.[4,20]
- The use of antibiotic regimens in IBS recently has generated considerable interest.
  - Gut-selective antibiotics such as rifaximin or neomycin have been proposed for use in patients with IBS for whom bacterial overgrowth is suspected, particularly in those with significant gas-bloat symptoms.
  - The results of two large, randomized, controlled studies recently demonstrated a benefit in global and individual symptom scores using **rifaximin (Xifaxan)** 550 mg three times daily for 2 weeks in non–IBS-C patients (the number needed to treat around 11).[21]
  - These benefits persisted past the period of time patients were on the drug, though relapse of symptoms does occur with a mean of 10 weeks. Retreatment with rifaximin upon recurrence of symptoms is an FDA-approved strategy for IBS-D management.[21]
- Emerging data support the use of **probiotics** in the management of IBS symptoms. All probiotics are not equally effective, however; the most benefit has been shown with *Bifidobacteria* spp. and little to no benefit shown using *Lactobacillus* spp.[4]

Centrally Acting Agents

- **Antidepressant medications** are most useful in patients with chronic, refractory symptoms.
  - They are particularly helpful with those who have concomitant psychiatric and somatic complaints, although their efficacy is independent of any direct influence on these comorbid conditions.
  - It is thought that antidepressants serve to interrupt or modulate the CNS interpretation of peripheral gut signaling.
  - Patient perceptions and expectations should be adequately addressed in using antidepressants in the management of IBS to optimize compliance.
- **Tricyclic antidepressants** (TCA), such as nortriptyline, amitriptyline, imipramine, and desipramine, are the best studied agents.
  - They are used in doses much lower than those traditionally used in depression management (starting dose, 10–25 mg at bedtime).
  - The anticholinergic properties of TCA may be beneficial in IBS-D but should not dissuade use in patients with IBS-C.
  - Side effects can include sedation, dry mouth, urinary difficulties, sexual dysfunction, and dizziness.
  - Individuals experiencing such side effects may tolerate use of agents with fewer anticholinergic effects such as desipramine.
- **Selective serotonin reuptake inhibitors (SSRIs)** increasingly are being used in IBS and appear to be nearly as effective as TCAs, with a number needed to treat of 3.5 in meta-analysis.
  - **Citalopram** may be a good option because of its low side effect profile and its effect on colonic tone and sensitivity.
  - **Paroxetine** may be useful in patients with IBS-D because of its anticholinergic effect.
- The serotonin–norepinephrine reuptake inhibitor (SNRI) **venlafaxine** has been shown to reduce colonic compliance and relax the colon in healthy volunteers, an effect not seen with citalopram or fluoxetine.[4]

Nonpharmacologic Therapies

- **Cognitive behavioral therapy (CBT)** and **hypnotherapy** may be useful in IBS management, particularly in patients who correlate an increase in severity of symptoms with life stressors.
- CBT has been demonstrated to be beneficial in IBS in randomized controlled trials, particularly in its positive influence on global well-being.[22,23]

- Although response is sporadic, factors favoring a good response include high patient motivation, diarrhea or pain as the predominant symptom, overt psychiatric symptoms, and intermittent pain exacerbated by stress.

REFERENCES

1. Drossman DA. Functional gastrointestinal disorders: history, pathophysiology, clinical features and Rome IV. *Gastroenterology.* 2016;150:1262–1279.
2. Mearin F, Lacy BE, Chang L, et al. Bowel disorders. *Gastroenterology.* 2016;160:1393–1407.
3. Russo MW, Gaynes BN, Drossman DA. A national survey of practice patterns of gastroenterologists with comparison to the past two decades. *J Clin Gastroenterol.* 1999;29:339–343.
4. Brandt LJ, Chey WD, Fox-Orenstein AE, et al. An evidence based systematic review on the management of irritable bowel syndrome. *Am J Gastroenterol.* 2009;104(Suppl 1):S1–S35.
5. Gralnek I, Hays RD, Kilbourne A, et al. The impact of irritable bowel syndrome on health-related quality of life. *Gastroenterology.* 2000;119:654–660.
6. Posserud I, Stotzer PO, Bjornsson ES, et al. Small intestinal bacterial overgrowth in patients with irritable bowel syndrome. *Gut.* 2007;56:802–808.
7. Gunnarson J, Simren M. Peripheral factors in the pathophysiology of irritable bowel syndrome. *Dig Liver Dis.* 2009;41:788–793.
8. Whitehead WE, Palsson O, Jones KR. Systematic review of the comorbidity of irritable bowel syndrome with other disorders: what are the causes and implications? *Gastroenterology.* 2002;122:1140–1156.
9. Koloski NA, Jones M, Weltman M, et al. Identification of early environmental risk factors for irritable bowel syndrome and dyspepsia. *Neurogastroenterol Motil.* 2015;27:1317–1325.
10. Saito YA, Zimmerman JM, Harmsen WS, et al. Irritable bowel syndrome aggregates strongly in families: a family-based case-control study. *Neurogastroenterol Motil.* 2008;20:790–797.
11. Van Rheenen PF, Van de Vijver E, Fidler V. Faecal calprotectin for screening of patients with suspected inflammatory bowel disease: diagnostic meta-analysis. *BMJ.* 2010;341:c3369.
12. Slattery SA, Niaz O, Aziz Q, et al. Systematic review with meta-analysis: the prevalence of bile acid malabsorption in the irritable bowel syndrome with diarrhoea. *Aliment Pharmacol Ther.* 2015;42:3–11.
13. Pimentel M, Morales W, Rezaie A, et al. Development and validation of a biomarker for diarrhea-predominant irritable bowel syndrome in human subjects. *PLoS One.* 2015;10(5):e0126438.
14. Drossman DA, Camilleri M, Mayer E, et al. AGA technical review on irritable bowel syndrome. *Gastroenterology.* 2002;123:2108–2131.
15. Ford AC, Moayyedi P, Lacy BE, et al. American College of Gastroenterology monograph on the management of irritable bowel syndrome and chronic idiopathic constipation. *Am J Gastroenterol.* 2014;109(Suppl 1):S2–S26.
16. Halmos EP, Power VA, Shepherd SJ, et al. A diet low in FODMAPs reduces symptoms of irritable bowel syndrome. *Gastroenterology.* 2014;146(1):67–75.e5.
17. Busby RW, Kessler MM, Bartolini WP, et al. Pharmacologic properties, metabolism, and disposition of linaclotide, a novel therapeutic peptide approved for the treatment of irritable bowel syndrome with constipation and chronic idiopathic constipation. *J Pharmacol Exp Ther.* 2013;344:196–206.
18. Vazquez-Roque MI, Bouras EP. Linaclotide, novel therapy for the treatment of chronic idiopathic constipation and constipation predominant irritable bowel syndrome. *Adv Ther.* 2013;30:203–211.
19. Lembo AJ, Lacy BE, Zuckerman MJ, et al. Eluxadoline for irritable bowel syndrome with diarrhea. *N Engl J Med.* 2016;374:242–253.
20. Spanier JA, Howden CW, Jones MP. A systematic review of alternative therapies in the irritable bowel syndrome. *Arch Intern Med.* 2003;163:265–724.
21. Pimentel M, Lembo A, Chey WD, et al. Rifaximin therapy for patients with irritable bowel without constipation. *N Engl J Med.* 2011;364(1):22–32.
22. Drossman DA, Toner BB, Whitehead WE, et al. Cognitive-behavioral therapy versus education and desipramine versus placebo for moderate to severe functional bowel disorders. *Gastroenterology.* 2003;125:19–31.
23. Lackner JM, Brasel AM, Quigley BM, et al. Rapid response to cognitive behavioral therapy predicts outcome in patients with irritable bowel syndrome. *Clin Gastroenterol Hepatol.* 2010; 8(5):426–432.

Acute Liver Disease

Michael J. Weaver and Kevin M. Korenblat

19

Introduction

- Acute liver disease encompasses a wide range of disorders from mild hepatitides to acute liver failure (ALF).
- Viral hepatitis and drug-induced liver injury (DILI) are the most frequent causes in adults.
- Histologic changes to the liver are typically those of acute inflammation with varying degrees of necrosis and collapse of the liver's architectural framework. These features contrast with changes of cirrhosis and development of portal hypertension that characterize the end stages of chronic liver disease.

Viral Hepatitis

- Hepatotropic viruses include hepatitis A (HAV), hepatitis B (HBV), hepatitis C (HCV), hepatitis D (HDV), and hepatitis E (HEV). Nonhepatotropic viruses known to cause liver injury include Epstein–Barr virus, Cytomegalovirus (CMV), herpes virus (HSZ), varicella zoster virus (VZV), adenovirus, Ebola virus, and others.
- Acute viral hepatitis is defined by the sudden elevation of aminotransferases.
- Clinical presentation is widely variable and often nonspecific.
- The condition may resolve or progress to ALF or chronic hepatitis.

Hepatitis A Virus

GENERAL PRINCIPLES

Hepatitis A is usually transmitted via the fecal–oral route and is an RNA virus that in unimmunized patients often results in self-limited icteric hepatitis. Fulminant hepatic failure occurs in less than 1% of cases.

Classification

HAV is an RNA virus within the *Picornaviridae* family.

Epidemiology

- The incidence of HAV has declined due to the implementation of vaccination.
- In 2015 there were 1390 reported cases of hepatitis A in the United States and an estimated 2800 cases in 2014.[1]
- It is associated with unsanitary living conditions, improper food handling techniques, household or sexual contact with a person with HAV, and illicit drug use.
- Morbidity and mortality (case-fatality rate) of infection are determined by age of onset and comorbid liver disease.
- Risk factors for ALF from HAV include age >40 years and coexisting chronic hepatitis (i.e., HCV).

- ALF is relatively rare, but risk increases with age: 0.1% in patients younger than 15 years to >1% in patients older than 40 years.

Pathogenesis

Hepatic injury is due to host response against HAV with viral replication occurring within the cytoplasm of the hepatocyte. An exaggerated response is associated with severe hepatitis.

Risk Factors

High-risk groups include people living in or traveling to developing countries (food and water contamination), men having sex with men, injection drugs users, patients with clotting factor disorders, persons working with nonhuman primates, staff and attendees at daycare centers, homelessness, and patients with chronic liver disease (increased risk for fulminant hepatitis A).

Prevention

Immunization programs are available (see Treatment section under Hepatitis A Virus).

DIAGNOSIS

- Diagnosis of acute HAV infection is made by the detection of **anti-HAV IgM antibodies** in serum.
- **Aminotransferase elevations** range from 10–100 times the upper limits of the reference range (ULR).
- Liver biopsy is typically not necessary for diagnosis but if pursued may demonstrate more portal inflammation than found in hepatitis B, but less parenchymal changes (i.e., focal necrosis, Kupfer cells, ballooning).
- Resolution of the illness is associated with emergence of **anti-HAV IgG antibodies**, and this change provides the basis for distinguishing acute from convalescent infection.

Clinical Presentation

- HAV can be silent (subclinical), especially in children and young adults. Symptoms vary from mild illness to ALF.[2]
- Malaise, fatigue, pruritus, headache, abdominal pain, myalgias, arthralgias, nausea, vomiting, anorexia, jaundice, and fever are common but nonspecific symptoms occur in >70% of patients.

History

History should include a review of symptoms, temporal course of illness, and assessment for any potential exposures from traveling to developing countries or food and water ingestion.

Physical Examination

Physical examination may reveal jaundice, hepatomegaly, and, in rare cases, lymphadenopathy, splenomegaly, or a vascular rash.

TREATMENT

- Treatment is **supportive**; however, careful attention should be paid to identifying those at risk for ALF.
- Liver transplantation may be an option for ALF.
- **Pre-exposure prophylaxis: Inactivated HAV vaccines** (containing the single HAV antigen) and **combination vaccines** (containing both HAV and hepatitis B antigens)

are available. Vaccinations should be administered intramuscularly in a two-dose regimen (single antigen HAV vaccine; first dose at time zero and second dose at 6–18 months) or in a three-dose regimen (combination vaccine; first dose at time zero, second dose at 1 month, and third dose at 6 months).

OUTCOME/PROGNOSIS

- Clinical and biochemical recovery is observed in 3 months in 85% of patients. Complete recovery is observed in nearly all patients at 6 months.
- Although there is no chronic phase of HAV infection, a polyphasic form of the disease can occur associated with relapse of symptoms. During relapse, symptoms are often milder than the initial episode and may be asymptomatic in 50% of patients. Extrahepatic manifestations can occur and include arthritis, vasculitis, nephritis, and cryoglobulinemia.

Hepatitis B Virus

GENERAL PRINCIPLES

HBV is a parenteral or sexually transmitted virus that is rarely associated with fulminant hepatic failure but can develop into chronic infection with progression to cirrhosis, end-stage liver disease, and hepatocellular carcinoma (HCC). At-risk populations are protected by administration of recombinant vaccine that confers hepatitis B surface antibody positivity.

Classification

- HBV is a DNA virus in the *Hepadnaviridae* family.
- Eight genotypes of HBV have been identified, designated A through H.

Epidemiology

- Two billion people worldwide have serologic evidence of past or present infection, and approximately 248 million people are chronic carriers. 600,000 die annually.
- Prevalence of HBV genotypes varies depending on the geographic location. Genotypes A, D, E, and H are the most prevalent in the United States.[3]
- HBV is the indication for 5–10% of cases of liver transplantation.

Pathophysiology

Modes of transmission include:
- **parenteral or percutaneous routes** (e.g., injection drug use, hemodialysis, transfusions, needle stick injury);
- **sexual contact** (e.g., men who have sex with men, intercourse with HBV-infected partners); and
- **vertical or perinatal transmission** (from mother to infant) in high prevalence areas.

Risk Factors

High-risk groups include individuals with a history of multiple blood transfusions, patients on hemodialysis, injection drug users, sexual promiscuity, men having sex with men, household and heterosexual contacts of hepatitis B carriers, residents and employees of residential care facilities, travelers to endemic regions, and individuals born in areas of high or intermediate prevalence.

Prevention

Immunization programs are available (see Treatment section under Hepatitis B Virus).

Associated Conditions

Extrahepatic manifestations occur in approximately 10–20% of patients with chronic hepatitis B and include polyarteritis nodosa, glomerulonephritis, cryoglobulinemia, serum sickness–like illness, and aplastic anemia.

DIAGNOSIS

Clinical Presentation

- The period from exposure to symptoms ranges from 30–120 days.
- In 70% of cases, the presentation can be subclinical, especially in children and young adults.
- Symptoms vary from mild illness to ALF (<1%). Malaise, fatigue, pruritus, headache, abdominal pain, myalgias, arthralgias, nausea, vomiting, anorexia, right upper quadrant pain, and fever are common but nonspecific symptoms.
- Most acute HBV infections are self-limited in adults.

Diagnostic Testing

Diagnosis of HBV often requires the combination of data obtained from liver chemistries, serology, and histology. With rare exceptions, the diagnosis of hepatitis B is made by the presence of hepatitis B surface antigen (HBsAg).

Laboratory Testing

- **Liver chemistries** typically abnormal in acute hepatitis include aspartate aminotransferase (AST), alanine aminotransferase (ALT), alkaline phosphatase (AP), and total bilirubin.
- Tests that measure cholestasis (AP, γ-glutamyltransferase [GGT], and total bilirubin) or liver synthetic function (albumin and prothrombin time (PT)/international normalized ratio [INR]) may be abnormal according to the disease stage.
- HBV contains two genes (s and core) that produce antigens that elicit a corresponding antibody response. **HBV antigens** detected in serum and used for diagnostic purposes in clinical practice include **HBsAg** and **hepatitis B e antigen (HBeAg)**.
- **HBV antibodies** are specific to their corresponding antigen and include: antibody against HBsAg **(anti-HBs)**, antibody against HBeAg **(anti-HBe)**, and IgM and IgG antibodies against HBcAg **(IgM and IgG anti-HBc)** (Table 19-1).
- **HBV viral DNA** (HBV DNA) is the **most accurate marker of viral replication**. It is detected by the polymerase chain reaction (PCR) and most commonly expressed as international units per milliliter (IU/mL).
- **Genotypic determination** is growing in clinical significance as data are emerging with respect to response to antivirals, disease progression, and risk of HCC.
- The presence of HBsAg for >6 months separates chronic from acute HBV infection.

Diagnostic Procedures

Liver biopsy is useful to assess the degree of necroinflammation and fibrosis in patients with chronic hepatitis. During acute flares of disease, liver biopsy may demonstrate an acute hepatitic pattern with lobular disarray, ballooning, apoptotic bodies, and lymphocyte-predominant portal inflammation. During the chronic phase there may be different degrees of lymphocyte-predominant portal inflammation with interface hepatitis. Inflammation is mild in the immune tolerant phase and in inactive carriers but is prominent in the immune reactive phase.

TREATMENT

Most cases of symptomatic, acute HBV infection in adults resolve with the development of antibodies to the surface protein (anti-HBs), the central neutralizing antibody to HBV.

TABLE 19-1 SEROLOGIC TESTING FOR ACUTE HEPATITIS B VERSUS CHRONIC HEPATITIS B

Diagnosis	HBsAg	Anti-HBs	Anti-HBc	HBeAg	Anti-HBe	HBV DNA
Acute Hepatitis	+		IgM	+		+
Window period			IgM	+/−	+/−	+
Recovery		+	IgG		+/−	
Immunization		+				
Chronic hepatitis (HBeAg+)	+		IgG	+		+
Chronic hepatitis (HBeAg−)	+		IgG		+	+

Anti-HBc, antibody against Hepatitis B core antigen; anti-HBe, antibody against Hepatitis B e antigen; anti-HBs, antibody against Hepatitis B surface antigen; HBsAg, Hepatitis B surface antigen; HBV DNA, Hepatitis B virus DNA.

Thus, generally no role exists for antiviral therapy with acute infection unless for ALF or in patients with a severe course (i.e., INR >1.5, bilirubin >10 mg/dL).

Medications

* Seven agents are currently available for the treatment of HBV infection. They are divided into three main groups:
  * **Interferon-based therapy** (interferon-α and pegylated interferon-α) should be avoided unless in young patients with compensated liver disease who desire finite treatment.
  * **Nucleoside analogs** (lamivudine, entecavir, and telbivudine).
  * **Nucleotide analogs** (adefovir and tenofovir). Tenofovir has two forms: tenofovir disoproxil fumarate (prodrug) and tenofovir alafenamide.
* Of the oral agents, **entecavir and tenofovir** are the two agents with the highest genetic barrier to resistance and therefore are **preferred if treatment of acute HBV infection is indicated**. Treatment can be discontinued after confirming clearance of HBsAg.
* **Pre-exposure prophylaxis**
  * **HBV vaccine** should be considered for everyone, but particularly for individuals at high risk (see Risk Factor section).
  * HBV vaccination schedule includes three intramuscular injections at 0, 1, and 6 months in infants or healthy adults. Protective antibody response is >90% after the third dose. Response to vaccination is measured by anti-HBs ≥10 IU/mL.
* **Postexposure prophylaxis**
  * **Infants born to HBsAg-positive mothers** should receive HBV vaccine and hepatitis B immune globulin (HBIG), 0.5 mL, within 12 hours of birth to prevent vertical transmission of the virus.
  * **Susceptible sexual partners** of individuals with HBV and **those with needlestick injury** should receive HBIG (0.04–0.07 mL/kg) and the first dose of HBV vaccine at different sites preferably within 48 hours but no >7 days after exposure. A second dose of HBIG can be administered 30 days after exposure, and the vaccination schedule should be completed.

Surgical Management

Liver transplantation is indicated for patients with ALF secondary to acute HBV infection.

OUTCOME/PROGNOSIS

- Depending on the age at infection, people may have spontaneous resolution or progression to chronicity.
  - Children younger than 5 years: 90% will develop chronic HBV infection.
  - Adults: 5–10% will develop chronic HBV.
- Screening for HCC is indicated in high-risk individuals (i.e., cirrhotics, Asian men >40, Asian women >50, African Americans, family history of HCC, high viral load, and active inflammation). The REVEAL-HBV study from Taiwan demonstrated a strong association between HBV-DNA level at study entry and risk of HCC over time. The risk of HCC begins to increase when the HBV-DNA level was >2000 IU/mL.[4]

Hepatitis C Virus

GENERAL PRINCIPLES

HCV is a parentally transmitted virus that in the acute phase is not frequently recognized; however, upon establishment of chronicity, it can lead to cirrhosis, end-stage liver disease, and HCC. It is the most frequent indication for liver transplantation in the United States.

Classification

- HCV is an RNA virus of the *Flaviviridae* family.
- Six to seven HCV genotypes are recognized worldwide with >50 subtypes.
- Genotype 1 is most common in the United States, Europe, and Latin America.

Epidemiology

HCV is a global health problem, with approximately 180 million carriers worldwide.[5]

Pathophysiology

- HCV infection occurs primarily through exposure from infected blood (see Risk Factors section).
- **Modes of transmission** include:
  - **parenteral** (e.g., transfusion, injection drug use, body piercing, needlestick injury);
  - **intranasal drug use**;
  - **sexual transmission**, especially associated with high-risk sexual practices.

Risk Factors

Risk factors for HCV infection include a history of multiple blood transfusions or clotting factors before the institution of screening in 1992, birth between 1945 and 1965, hemodialysis, injection drug use, multiple sexual partners, and occupational exposure with blood and blood-derived products.

Prevention

No pre-exposure prophylaxis or vaccine exists. Prevention of high-risk behavior should be emphasized.

Associated Conditions

- **Extrahepatic manifestations** include essential mixed (type II) cryoglobulinemia, glomerulonephritis, porphyria cutanea tarda, cutaneous necrotizing vasculitis, lichen planus, lymphoma, and autoimmune disorders such as thyroiditis.
- The frequency of extrahepatic manifestations is uncertain. In one series of 321 patients, extrahepatic manifestations were observed in 38% of patients.

DIAGNOSIS

Clinical Presentation

- Incubation period for HCV infection varies from 15–150 days.
- Acute HCV infection is typically subclinical.
- Symptoms vary from mild fatigue to ALF.
- Malaise, fatigue, pruritus, headache, abdominal pain, myalgias, arthralgias, nausea, vomiting, anorexia, and fever are common but nonspecific symptoms.

Diagnostic Testing

Laboratory Testing

- **Antibodies against HCV (anti-HCV)** may be undetectable for the first 8 weeks after infection. A **false-positive test** (anti-HCV positive with HCV RNA negative) may occur in the setting of prior cleared infection, autoimmune hepatitis (AIH), or hypergammaglobulinemia. A false-negative (anti-HCV negative with HCV RNA positive) test may occur in immunosuppressed individuals or in patients on hemodialysis.
- **HCV RNA** can be detected by PCR in serum as early as 1–2 weeks after infection.
- **HCV genotypes** can be detected by commercially available assays. HCV genotype influences the duration, dosage, and response to treatment.
- **Liver biopsy** can be used to score the degree of necroinflammation and fibrosis in the liver of chronically infected patients.
- **Noninvasive testing** includes serum-based biomarkers (e.g., Fibrosure, APRI, FIB-4, and others), elastography measurements (transient elastography, Shear Wave elastography, MR elastography) are increasingly used to assess fibrosis stage.

TREATMENT

Medications

- All patients with evidence of chronic HCV infection should be considered for antiviral treatment with a goal of sustained virologic response (see Chapter 19 for full details).
- Regimens vary by genotype and presence of cirrhosis. Some regimens include: Glecaprevir–pibrentasvir × 8–12 weeks, ledipasvir–sofosbuvir × 12 weeks, sofosbuvir–velpatasvir × 12 weeks, simeprevir and sofosbuvir × 12–24 weeks. HCVguidelines.org is a useful reference when determining treatment.[5]

OUTCOME/PROGNOSIS

- Acute hepatitis is frequently clinically silent.
- Chronic infection occurs in 50–85% of those exposed to HCV.
- In those with chronic infection, there is a 15–30% prevalence of cirrhosis 20 years after infection.

Hepatitis D Virus

GENERAL PRINCIPLES

Hepatitis D is a subviral particle that requires the hepatitis B virus for infectivity.

Classification

Hepatitis D virus (HDV) is considered a subviral particle with a circular RNA genome and is the only member of the genus *Deltavirus*.[6]

Epidemiology

- HDV is endemic to the Mediterranean basin, Asia, and portions of South America.
- Outside endemic areas, infections occur primarily either in individuals who have received transfusions, injection drug users or individuals who have emigrated from endemic countries.
- HDV requires the presence of HBV for infection and replication.

Pathophysiology

HDV infection clinically presents as a coinfection (acute hepatitis B and D), superinfection (chronic hepatitis B with acute hepatitis D), or as a latent infection (e.g., in the setting of liver transplantation).

Risk Factors

High-risk groups are similar to HBV (see HBV Epidemiology section).

Prevention

Although there is no vaccine to prevent HDV infection in carriers of HBV, both infections can be prevented by HBV vaccination.

DIAGNOSIS

Clinical Presentation

- In patients with **coinfection**, the course is transient and self-limited. The rate of progression to chronicity is similar to that reported for acute HBV infection.
- In **superinfection**, HBV carriers may present with a severe acute hepatitis exacerbation with frequent progression to chronic HDV infection.

Diagnostic Testing

Diagnosis is made by finding **HDV RNA** or **HDV antigen** in serum and by detecting **antibody to the HDV antigen**.

TREATMENT

Medications

There is no specific treatment for acute hepatitis D. In a small study, three patients treated with **foscarnet** for fulminant hepatitis recovered.[7] However, in vitro it has been shown to have a paradoxical stimulatory effect on HDV replication.[8]

Hepatitis E Virus

GENERAL PRINCIPLES

Hepatitis E is an **enterically transmitted RNA virus** that leads to acute hepatitis in special populations including pregnant women and immunosuppressed solid-organ transplant patients.

Classification

Hepatitis E virus (HEV) is an RNA virus belonging to the *Hepeviridae* family.

Epidemiology

- HEV is implicated in epidemics in India, Southeast Asia, Africa, and Mexico.[9]

- Hepatitis E is considered a zoonotic disease and reservoirs include pigs and potentially other species.
- There are five HEV genotypes, four of which are associated with human infection. Genotypes 1 and 2 are confined to humans, while genotypes 3 and 4 infect both humans and animals.[10]

Pathophysiology

Transmission is through the fecal–oral route and resembles that of HAV infection.

Prevention

No approved pre- or postexposure prophylaxis exists.

DIAGNOSIS

- Acute hepatitis E is clinically indistinguishable from other acute viral hepatitis.
- A **high fatality rate is seen in pregnant women** in the second and third trimesters.

TREATMENT

- Treatment is supportive in most patients as the disease is typically self-limited.
- Ribavirin should not be used in pregnant women as it is a teratogen.
- Small retrospective studies in patients with chronic liver disease and on immunosuppressive agents have suggested a possible benefit of ribavirin therapy for acute hepatitis E.[11]
- In patients with chronic hepatitis E (almost exclusively immunocompromised patients), a 12-week course of ribavirin can be used.
- Immunosuppressive agents should be reduced if possible.

OUTCOME/PROGNOSIS

Although generally considered an acute illness, chronic HEV infection has been detected in immunosuppressed organ transplant patients.

Herpes Simplex Virus Hepatitis

GENERAL PRINCIPLES

Herpes simplex virus (HSV) rarely causes ALF; however, liver involvement in immunosuppressed or pregnant women can cause severe anicteric hepatitis leading to fulminant hepatic failure prompting consideration of empiric treatment while the diagnosis is being established.[12]

Classification

Infection with both HSV-1 and HSV-2 can lead to visceral dissemination and hepatitis.

Epidemiology

- Commonly acquired infection, with 62% of adolescents testing positive for HSV-1 and 12% for HSV-2.
- Hepatitis is an uncommon manifestation of HSV.
- Hepatitis occurs in neonates or malnourished children; rare in adults.
- Most adult cases of hepatitis are in immunocompromised (most often deficiency of cell-mediated immunity) or pregnant; however, HSV hepatitis has been described in immunocompetent patients.

Pathophysiology

- Large HSV inoculum at the time of initial infection may result in dissemination.
- Activation of latent infection may occur.
- HSV strains have affinity to the liver ("hepatovirulent").

Risk Factors

High-risk groups include **neonates, pregnant women** (primarily in the third trimester), and those who are **immunosuppressed**.

DIAGNOSIS

- Diagnosis of acute HSV infection may be made by serologic tests, detection of viremia, or liver biopsy.
- **Aminotransferase elevations** range from 10–100 times the ULR. These elevations may be out of proportion to the degree of jaundice; thus, HSV hepatitis is often considered anicteric hepatitis.
- Biopsy may demonstrate multinucleated hepatocytes and areas of bland coagulative necrosis with minimal inflammatory response and punched-out necrosis.

Clinical Presentation

- Symptoms vary from mild illness to ALF.
- Malaise, fatigue, pruritus, headache, abdominal pain, myalgias, arthralgias, nausea, vomiting, anorexia, and fever are common but nonspecific symptoms.
- Classical oral and/or genital lesions occur in only 30% of patients.

History

History should include a review of symptoms, temporal course of illness, and any potential HSV exposures.

Physical Examination

- Hepatosplenomegaly. Jaundice is often mild.
- Oral mucocutaneous lesions in HSV infection are found in approximately 30% of cases.

TREATMENT

- Treatment is with **intravenous (IV) acyclovir 5–10 mg/kg IV q8h**; it can be initiated presumptively if there is any degree of clinical suspicion.
- Liver transplantation may be an option for ALF.

OUTCOME/PROGNOSIS

Cases may rapidly progress to fulminant hepatic failure; however, prompt administration of parenteral antiviral therapy may result in complete resolution of liver dysfunction.

Acetaminophen

GENERAL PRINCIPLES

When ingested at toxic levels, acetaminophen (APAP) and its metabolites may lead to hepatocellular damage and ALF. Recognition of potential toxic ingestions allows for prompt administration of its antidote *N*-acetylcysteine (NAC) which may prevent progression to ALF.

Epidemiology

- APAP toxicity is the most common cause of DILI in the United States.
- It is most frequently a consequence of intentional ingestion; however, unintentional overdoses do occur and can result in severe liver injury.

Pathophysiology

- Significant hepatic injury generally requires ingestions above a threshold value of 150 mg/kg body weight.
- APAP can be metabolized to a toxic metabolite (*N*-acetyl-*p*-benzoquinone imine [NAPQI]), which can induce toxic free radical damage to liver parenchymal cells.
- Chronic, excessive alcohol use may predispose to liver injury, although only with overdoses of APAP.

DIAGNOSIS

- Made with **measurement of APAP level** in the serum.
- **History is critical** to assess time of ingestion, as well as concurrent substances ingested, which effects treatment (see later).

TREATMENT

Medications

Antidote to treatment, **NAC** administered within 8 hours of ingestion, is indicated in those with APAP levels above the "possible" toxicity line on the **Rumack–Matthew nomogram** (line connecting 150 μg/mL at 4 hours with 50 μg/mL at 12 hours) (Fig. 19-1).[13]

- NAC can be given orally (loading dose of 140 mg/kg followed by 70 mg/kg every 4 hours for a total of 17 doses).
- IV dosing of NAC is acceptable: if no biochemical evidence of hepatic failure: 150 mg/kg loading dose over 60 minutes, followed by 50 mg/kg infused over 4 hours, with the final 100 mg/kg infused over the remaining 16 hours.
- If biochemical evidence of liver failure: 150 mg/kg loading dose over 60 minutes, followed by 50 mg/kg infused over 4 hours, followed by 100 mg/kg infused over the next 16 hours, followed by a continuous IV NAC infusion at 6.25 mg/kg/hr until INR is <2.
- For ingestions that present late (>8 hours), a longer duration of IV treatment is recommended (loading dose, 140 mg/kg IV over 1 hour followed by 14 mg/kg/hr for 44 hours).

Surgical Management

Liver transplantation can be considered in patients with ALF secondary to APAP.

PROGNOSIS/OUTCOME

- In addition to APAP's effects on the liver, acute renal failure can occur independently of hepatic injury.
- Prognosis is excellent with timely recognition and administration of NAC; however, complications from ALF can occur (see ALF section).

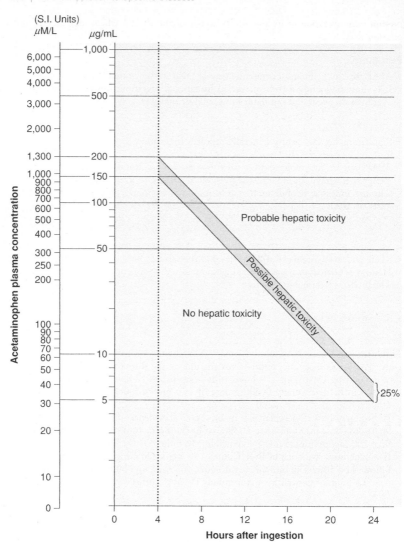

Figure 19-1. Acetaminophen toxicity nomogram. The area below the *lower line* represents nontoxic ingestion. The shaded area between the two lines is potentially toxic, and the area above the *upper line* is likely to be toxic. Treatment should be initiated for any level above the *lower line*. (Reprinted with permission from Kline-Tilford AM, Haut C. *Lippincott Certification Review: Pediatric Acute Care Nurse Practitioner.* Philadelphia, PA: Wolters Kluwer; 2015.)

Drug-Induced Liver Injury

GENERAL PRINCIPLES

Drug-induced liver injury (DILI) is a common cause of acute liver disease and over 1000 medications and herbal products have been implicated. Prognosis often depends upon the dose-dependent or idiosyncratic effect of the specific offending agent.

Classification

- **Three major patterns** of DILI occur as a result of both dose-dependent and idiosyncratic hepatotoxicity:
  - **Hepatocellular**
  - **Cholestatic**
  - **Mixed hepatocellular and cholestatic** injury
- Less common forms of DILI include granulomatous hepatitis and carcinogenesis.

Epidemiology

DILI causes approximately 50% of the cases of ALF in the United States, with APAP the most common agent.

Pathophysiology

- **Intrinsic hepatotoxicity** results from usually predictable and dose-dependent hepatotoxic effects of the drug or its metabolite.[14]
- **Idiosyncratic hepatotoxicity** can be divided into hypersensitivity (allergic) and metabolic (nonallergic) reactions. These reactions depend on multiple variables and are not predictable.
  - **Hypersensitivity responses** occur as a result of stimulation of the immune system by a metabolite of a drug alone or after haptenization (covalently binding) to a liver protein. Repeated challenge with the same agent leads to prompt recurrence of the reaction.
  - **Metabolic hepatotoxicity** occurs in susceptible patients as a result of altered drug clearance or accelerated production of hepatotoxic metabolites. The latency of this reaction is variable.

DIAGNOSIS

Clinical Presentation

- Acute presentation can be clinically silent. When symptoms are present, they are nonspecific and include nausea/vomiting, general malaise, fatigue, pruritus, jaundice, and abdominal pain.
- In the acute setting, the majority of patients will recover after cessation of the offending drug.
- Fever, rash, and eosinophilia may also be seen in association with hypersensitivity reactions.

Diagnostic Criteria

No diagnostic criteria are established, but diagnosis requires clinical suspicion, temporal relation of liver injury to drug usage, and resolution of liver injury after the suspected agent has been discontinued.

Diagnostic Testing

Laboratory Testing

Biochemical abnormalities include the following:

- **Hepatocellular injury:** AST and ALT elevation more than two times the upper limit of normal but can be >25 times the upper limit of normal.

- **Cholestatic injury:** AP and conjugated bilirubin elevation more than two times upper limit of normal.
- **Mixed injury:** Increases in all of these biochemical abnormalities to more than two times upper limit of normal.
- The **R value** is defined as the ratio of ALT/ULN (upper limit of normal): ALP/ULN. An R value >5 indicates hepatocellular injury, <2 cholestatic injury, and 2–5 mixed-type injury.

Diagnostic Procedures

Liver biopsy can be useful as part of the diagnostic workup and should be obtained if the diagnosis remains unclear.

TREATMENT

- Treatment includes **cessation of offending drug** and supportive measures.
- NAC is used for acetaminophen toxicity.
- The benefit of corticosteroids for most forms of DILI is unproven. Although, they may be of benefit for treating patients with hypersensitivity reactions with progressive cholestasis or who have features of autoimmune hepatitis on biopsy.
- Liver transplantation may be an option for patients with ALF.

OUTCOME/PROGNOSIS

- Prognosis of DILI if often unique to the offending medication.
- It is important to be attuned to the development of jaundice because this sign is associated with case fatality rates of 10–50%.[14]

Ischemic Hepatitis

GENERAL PRINCIPLES

Ischemic hepatitis is characterized by a transient and often dramatic rise in aminotransferases that results from cardiovascular collapse.

Definition

Ischemic hepatitis ("shock liver") results from liver hypoperfusion.

Etiology

Clinical scenarios associated include severe blood loss, cardiac failure, heat stroke and sepsis.[15]

DIAGNOSIS

Clinical Presentation

Ischemic hepatitis presents as acute and transient rise of liver enzymes to levels as high as >20 times the upper limit of normal range during or following a hypotensive episode.

Diagnostic Testing

Laboratory Testing

- Laboratory studies demonstrate a rapid rise and fall in levels of serum AST, ALT (>1000 mg/dL), and lactic dehydrogenase within 1–3 days of the insult, with subsequent slow decline in aminotransferases if the underlying cause is corrected.
- Total bilirubin, AP, and INR may initially be normal but subsequently rise even as the levels of aminotransferases improve.

Diagnostic Procedures

Liver biopsy is not usually needed for diagnosis. Centrilobular necrosis and sinusoidal distortion with inflammatory infiltrates in zone 3 (central areas) are classic histologic features.

TREATMENT

Correction of the underlying condition that caused circulatory collapse.

OUTCOME/PROGNOSIS

- Prognosis is determined by the rapid and effective correction of hemodynamics or treatment of the underlying cause.
- Ischemic hepatitis is almost always self-limited.

Budd–Chiari Syndrome

GENERAL PRINCIPLES

Budd–Chiari syndrome is characterized as hepatic venous outflow obstruction most often resulting from thrombosis, which can lead to an acute or subacute illness characterized by ascites, hepatomegaly, and jaundice.

Definition

Hepatic vein thrombosis (HVT; also known as Budd–Chiari syndrome) causes hepatic venous outflow obstruction. It has multiple etiologies and a variety of clinical consequences.

Etiology

- Thrombosis is the main factor leading to obstruction of the hepatic venous system, frequently in association with myeloproliferative disorders (polycythemia rubra vera) or hypercoagulable states (e.g., antiphospholipid antibody syndrome, paroxysmal nocturnal hemoglobinuria, factor V Leiden, protein C and S deficiency, and contraceptive use).
- HVT can occur during pregnancy and in the postpartum period.
- Less than 20% of cases are idiopathic.

DIAGNOSIS

Clinical Presentation

- Patients may present with acute, subacute, or chronic illness characterized by ascites, hepatomegaly, and right upper quadrant abdominal pain.
- Jaundice, encephalopathy, ascites, and lower extremity edema are variably present. Variceal bleeding may occur.

Diagnostic Testing

Laboratory Testing

- Serum to ascites albumin gradient is >1.1 g/dL. Serum albumin, bilirubin, AST, ALT, and PT/INR are mildly abnormal with aminotransferases in the range of 100–600 IU/L.
- Laboratory evaluation to identify a potential hypercoagulable state or myeloproliferative disorder should be performed.

Imaging

- Doppler ultrasound can be used to establish the diagnosis.
- CT or MRI can be used to confirm the diagnosis or can be used in patients with an unremarkable ultrasound.
- Hepatic venography can be used if noninvasive testing is negative and there is strong clinical suspicion.

TREATMENT

Medications

Nonsurgical treatment includes anticoagulation, thrombolytics, diuretics, angioplasty, stents, and transjugular intrahepatic portosystemic shunt (TIPS).[16]

Surgical Management

Both surgical shunts and liver transplantation have been used as therapeutic options.

Wilson Disease

GENERAL PRINCIPLES

Wilson disease is a genetic disorder in which ineffective excretion of copper results in hepatocellular damage; its presentations include fulminant hepatic failure, and progression of disease may lead to cirrhosis and end-stage liver disease.

Definition

Wilson disease is an autosomal recessive disorder (*ATP7B* gene on chromosome 13) that results in progressive copper overload.

Epidemiology

Prevalence is 1 in 10,000–30,000 live births worldwide. Females are more likely to develop ALF.

Pathophysiology

Absent or reduced function of ATP7B protein leads to decreased canalicular excretion of copper, resulting in hepatic copper accumulation and injury.

Associated Conditions

Extrahepatic manifestations include **Kayser–Fleischer rings** on slit-lamp examination (gold to brown rings due to copper deposition in the Descemet membrane in the periphery of the cornea), Coombs-negative hemolytic anemia, renal tubular acidosis, arthritis, neuropsychiatric manifestations, and osteopenia.[17]

DIAGNOSIS

Clinical Presentation

- Liver disease can be highly variable, ranging from asymptomatic with only biochemical abnormalities to ALF.
- The diagnosis of acute Wilson disease should be considered in patients with unexplained liver disease with or without neuropsychiatric symptoms, first-degree relatives with Wilson disease, or individuals with fulminant hepatic failure (with or without hemolysis).
- The average age at presentation of liver disease is 6–20 years, but it can manifest later in life.
- Neuropsychiatric disorders usually occur later, most of the time in association with cirrhosis. The manifestations include asymmetric tremor, dysarthria, ataxia, and psychiatric features.

Diagnostic Testing

Laboratory Testing

- **Low serum ceruloplasmin level** (<20 mg/dL), **elevated serum free copper level** (>25 µg/dL), and **elevated 24-hour urinary copper level** (>100 mg).
- Korman et al. demonstrated that an alkaline phosphatase to total bilirubin level <4 was highly sensitive and specific for the diagnosis of ALF due to Wilson disease. When combining this ratio to an AST:ALT ratio >2.2, there was 100% sensitivity and 100% specificity.[18]
- Most patients with the ALF presentation of Wilson disease have a characteristic pattern of findings including: Coombs-negative hemolytic anemia with features of acute intravascular hemolysis; rapid progression to renal failure; modest rise in serum aminotransferases (typically <2000 IU/L) from the beginning of clinical illness; normal or subnormal serum AP (typically <40 IU/L).

Diagnostic Procedures

- **Liver biopsy**
  - The liver histology (massive necrosis, steatosis, glycogenated nuclei, chronic hepatitis, fibrosis, cirrhosis) findings are nonspecific and depend on the presentation and stage of the disease.
  - Elevated hepatic copper levels of >250 µg/g dry weight (normal <40 µg/g) on biopsy are highly suggestive of Wilson disease.

TREATMENT

Medications

Treatment is with copper-chelating agents.

- **Penicillamine** Initial doses of 250–500 mg/day plus pyridoxine 25 mg/day. Indicated in patients with hepatic failure. Use may be limited by side effects (hypersensitivity, bone marrow suppression, and proteinuria, systemic lupus erythematosus, and Goodpasture syndrome). Penicillamine should not be given as initial treatment to patients with neurologic symptoms.
- **Trientine** at 20 mg/kg is a second-line agent. This has similar side effects as penicillamine but at a lower frequency. The risk of neurologic worsening with trientine is less than with penicillamine.

Surgical Management

Liver transplantation is the only therapeutic option in ALF or in progressive dysfunction despite chelation.

OUTCOME/PROGNOSIS

In the absence of neurologic symptoms, liver transplantation has a good prognosis and requires no further medical treatment.

Acute Liver Failure

GENERAL PRINCIPLES

ALF is the relatively rapid development of coagulopathy and encephalopathy in the absence of pre-existing liver disease; its etiologies are diverse and intensive monitoring is critical, as is timely referral for the evaluation of liver transplantation.

Definition

ALF is a rare condition that includes evidence of coagulation abnormalities (INR >1.5) and encephalopathy in a patient without pre-existing cirrhosis and with an illness of <26 weeks' duration.

Classification

Terms used signifying length of illness in ALF such as hyperacute (<7 days), acute (7–21 days), and subacute (>21 days to <26 weeks) are generally considered unhelpful, as they do not have prognostic significance distinct from the cause of illness.[19]

Epidemiology

Approximately 2000 cases of ALF occur in the United States yearly.

Etiology

- APAP hepatotoxicity and viral hepatitis are the most common causes of ALF.[20]
- Other causes include AIH, drug and toxin exposure, ischemia, acute fatty liver of pregnancy, Wilson disease, Budd–Chiari syndrome, veno-occlusive disease, and malignant infiltration.
- In about 20% of cases, no clear etiology of ALF is identified.

DIAGNOSIS

Clinical Presentation

- Patients may present with mild to severe mental status changes in the setting of moderate to severe acute hepatitis and coagulopathy.
- Jaundice may or may not be initially present.
- A history of APAP overdose, toxin ingestion, or risk factors for viral hepatitis may be obtained.
- Cardiovascular collapse, acute renal failure, cerebral edema, and sepsis may be part of the clinical presentation.

Diagnostic Testing

Laboratory Testing

- **Aminotransferases** are typically elevated and in many cases are >1000 IU/L.
- **INR ≥1.5.**
- **Initial workup** to determine the etiology of ALF should include:
  - Acute viral hepatitis panel;
  - Serum drug screen, which includes APAP;
  - Ceruloplasmin;
  - AIH serologies; and
  - Pregnancy test

Imaging

- **Right upper quadrant Doppler ultrasound** to evaluate for obstruction of venous inflow or outflow, evaluate hepatic parenchyma and liver architecture.
- **CT/MRI** can be used to assess for hepatic malignant infiltration as they are more sensitive than ultrasound.
- **Computed tomographic scan of the head** may be obtained to evaluate and track progression of cerebral edema; however, the radiologic findings may lag behind the development of cerebral edema.

TABLE 19-2 GRADES OF ENCEPHALOPATHY

I	Behavioral changes
II	Disorientation, drowsiness, inappropriate behavior
III	Confusion, somnolence but responds to painful stimuli, incoherent speech
IV	Comatose, unresponsive to noxious stimuli.

Diagnostic Procedures

Liver biopsy can be used if the etiology is indeterminate despite laboratory and imaging investigation. Liver biopsy may be helpful to help with diagnosis of malignant infiltration, Wilson disease, HSV hepatitis, and autoimmune hepatitis. Given the presence of coagulopathy, a transjugular biopsy is the preferred approach.

TREATMENT

- **Supportive therapy in the intensive care unit** at a center experienced with liver disease and liver transplantation is essential.
- **Precipitating factors should be identified** and treated if possible.
- **Sedation should be avoided** to allow for serial assessments of mental/neurologic status.
- Blood glucose, electrolytes, acid–base, coagulation parameters, and fluid status should be monitored serially.
- The **coagulopathy** of ALF need only to be corrected in the setting of active bleeding or when invasive procedures are required.
- **Cerebral edema and intracranial hypertension** are related to severity of encephalopathy (Table 19-2). In patients with grade III or IV encephalopathy, intracranial pressure monitoring should be considered (intracranial pressure should be maintained below 20–25 mm Hg, cerebral perfusion pressure should be maintained above 50 mm Hg). Therapies to decrease cerebral edema include mannitol (0.5–1 g/kg IV), hyperventilation (reduce $Paco_2$ to 25–30 mm Hg), hypothermia (32–34°C), and barbiturates.
- **Lactulose is not indicated for encephalopathy.** Its use may result in increased bowel distention, which may complicate liver transplantation.
- **Liver transplantation is the ultimate therapy** for those with ALF (see Chapter 21). Several criteria have been proposed to identify those unlikely to recover spontaneously and in whom liver transplantation would be lifesaving. The King's College criteria are most commonly used (Table 19-3). In the United States, patients with ALF are eligible to be listed for transplantation with the highest priority status.

OUTCOME/PROGNOSIS

- Prior to transplantation, survival was <15%; in the posttransplant era, survival is >65%.
- Death often results from progressive liver failure, GI bleeding, cerebral edema, sepsis, or arrhythmia.
- Poor prognostic indicators in APAP-induced ALF include arterial pH <7.3, INR >6.5, creatinine >2.3 mg/dL, and encephalopathy grades III–IV.

TABLE 19-3 KING'S COLLEGE CRITERIA

Acetaminophen Induced

Arterial pH <7.3
or
All three of the following:
    PT >100 sec (INR >6.5)
    Serum creatinine >3.4 mg/dL
    Grade III or IV encephalopathy

Nonacetaminophen Induced

INR >6.5 irrespective of coma grade
or
Three of the following five criteria:
    Patient age <10 or >40
    Serum bilirubin >17.5 mg/dL
    PT >50 sec (INR ≥3.5)
    Unfavorable cause (seronegative hepatitis or DILI)
    Jaundice >7 days before encephalopathy

PT, prothrombin time; INR, international normalized ratio.

REFERENCES

1. Centers for Disease Control and Prevention. Hepatitis A questions and answers for health professionals. http://www.cdc.gov/hepatitis/hav/havfaq.htm#general. Accessed July 13, 2018.
2. Cuthbert JA. Hepatitis A: old and new. *Clin Microbiol Rev*. 2001;14(1):38–58.
3. Lok AS, McMahon BJ. Chronic hepatitis B. *Hepatology*. 2007;45(2):507–539.
4. Chen CJ, Iloeje UH, Yang HI. Long-term outcomes in hepatitis B: the REVEAL-HBV study. *Clin Liver Dis*. 2007;11(4):797–816.
5. www.HCVguidelines.org. Accessed June 9, 2020.
6. Hughes SA, Wedemeyer H, Harrison PM. Hepatitis delta virus. *Lancet*. 2011;378(9785):73–85.
7. Hedin G, Weiland O, Ljunggren K, et al. Treatment of fulminant hepatitis B and D coinfection with foscarnet. *Prog Clin Biol Res*. 1987;234:309–320.
8. Rasshofer R, Choi SS, Wolf P, et al. Inhibition of HDV RNA replication in vitro by ribavirin and sumarin. *Viral Hepatitis and Liver Disease*. Baltimore: Williams & Wilkins; 1991:659.
9. Dalton HR, Bendall R, Ijaz S, et al. Hepatitis E: an emerging infection in developed countries. *Lancet Infect Dis*. 2008;8(11):698–709.
10. Lu L, Li C, Hagedorn CH. Phylogenetic analysis of global hepatitis E virus sequences: genetic diversity, subtypes and zoonosis. *Rev Med Virol*. 2006;16(1):5–36.
11. Dalton HR, Kamar N. Treatment of hepatitis E virus. *Curr Opin Infect Dis*. 2016;29(6):639–644.
12. Montalbano M, Slapak-Green GI, Neff GW. Fulminant hepatic failure from herpes simplex virus: post liver transplantation acyclovir therapy and literature review. *Transplant Proc*. 2005;37(10):4393–4396.
13. Kline-Tilford AM, Haut C. *Lippincott Certification Review: Pediatric Acute Care Nurse Practitioner*. Philadelphia, PA: Wolters Kluwer; 2015.
14. Navarro VJ, Senior JR. Drug-related hepatoxicity. *N Engl J Med*. 2006;354(7):731–739.
15. Weisberg IS, Jacobson IM. Cardiovascular diseases and the liver. *Clin Liver Dis*. 2011;15(1):1–20.
16. Plessier A, Valla DC. Budd-Chiari syndrome. *Semin Liver Dis*. 2008;28(3):259–269.
17. Roberts EA, Schilsky ML. AASLD position paper: diagnosis and treatment of Wilson disease: an update. *Hepatology*. 2008;47(6):2089–2111.
18. Korman J, Volenberg I, Balko J, et al. Screening for Wilson disease in acute liver failure: a comparison of currently available diagnostic tests. *Hepatology*. 2008;48(4):1167–1174.
19. Polson J, Lee WM. AASLD position paper: the management of acute liver failure. *Hepatology*. 2005;41(5):1179–1197.
20. Lee WM. Etiologies of acute liver failure. *Semin Liver Dis*. 2008;28(2):142–152.

Chronic Liver Disease

Yeshika Sharma and
Mauricio Lisker-Melman

20

Chronic Viral Hepatitis

GENERAL PRINCIPLES

- **Chronic viral hepatitis** is defined by the persistence of viral infection for longer than 6 months, resulting in liver necroinflammatory and fibrotic changes which can lead to cirrhosis and hepatocellular carcinoma (HCC).
- Histopathologic classification of chronic liver disease is based on etiology, grade, and stage; a grade score is used to measure the severity of necroinflammation and a stage score measures the severity of fibrosis.
- The two most frequent viruses that result in chronic hepatitis are the hepatitis B (HBV) and C (HCV) viruses. The hepatitis D virus (HDV) is an infrequent cause of chronic hepatitis in the United States. In rare occasions, and when associated with liver transplantation, the hepatitis E virus can also cause chronic hepatitis.

Chronic Hepatitis B

GENERAL PRINCIPLES

Epidemiology

- There are about 2 billion people worldwide infected with HBV and more than 200 million chronic carriers with positive hepatitis B surface antigen (HBsAg).[1,2]
- Hepatitis B positive mothers can infect their newborns with a 90% risk of acute to chronic hepatitis B progression. The risk of progression to chronic HBV decreases to 25% in infected infants/children, and to 5–10% in adults.
- Approximately 0.5% of chronic HBsAg carriers will clear the infection yearly. Spontaneous clearance of hepatitis B e antigen (HBeAg) reaches about 8–12% annually, and it is affected by age, baseline alanine aminotransferase (ALT) levels, and HBV genotype.
- Patients with chronic HBV have <1% per annum risk of developing HCC before or after the development of cirrhosis.

Etiology

- HBV is a DNA virus that belongs to the *Hepadnavirus* family.
- In endemic regions, such as Asia and sub-Saharan Africa, hepatitis B infection is frequently transmitted from mother to child (vertical transmission) or early in life; whereas in the Western world, where chronic hepatitis B is relatively rare, infection is transmitted from adult to adult (horizontal transmission).
- Infection is **acquired through sexual contact, parenteral routes** (e.g., needlestick, injection drug use, and blood transfusions), or **perinatal transmission**.
- **Chronic hepatitis B** is defined by HBsAg positivity for longer than 6 months.
- The **clinical phenotypes or phases** of chronic hepatitis B infection are immune-tolerant (IT), immune-active (IA), and low replicative phase. The IA phase is divided into wild

type or HBeAg positive and precore/basal core promoter mutation or HBeAg-negative chronic hepatitis B. See Table 20-1 for further understanding of the HBV clinical phenotypes.
- Patients with hepatitis B can have a fluctuating disease course and may progress from one phase to another.

Risk Factors

- **High-risk groups for chronic hepatitis B infection** include individuals with a history of homosexual or heterosexual promiscuity, intravenous (IV) drug users, patients on hemodialysis (HD), healthcare workers, children of chronic HBV–infected mothers, recipients of multiple blood transfusions or blood products, travelers to endemic areas, and natives of Alaska, Asia, or the Pacific Islands.
- **Risk factors for developing** HCC include family history of HCC, age >40 years, male sex, high viral replication, coinfection (i.e., HIV, HCV, HDV), aflatoxin exposure, and alcohol use.

Prevention

- **Screening** is recommended for people born in high or intermediate endemic areas, unvaccinated US-born adults whose parents are from countries with high or intermediate HBV prevalence, patients with chronically elevated liver function tests, those receiving immunosuppression/chemotherapy or multiple blood transfusions, men with homosexual partners, history of sexually transmitted diseases, history of sexual promiscuity, prison inmates, IV drug users, patients on HD, HIV/HCV patients, pregnant women, and household and sexual contacts of patients with HBV infection.
- **Pre-exposure prophylaxis with HBV vaccine** should be considered for everyone, but particularly for individuals with the above-mentioned risk factors.
  - The Centers for Disease Control and Prevention recommends universal vaccination programs for infants and sexually active adolescents in the United States.
  - Vaccination is administered as a three-shot series at 0, 1, and 6 months. For patients who require rapid immunity, vaccination can be administered at 0, 1, and 2 months with a follow-up booster shot at 6 months for long-lasting immunity.
  - Additional doses, higher doses, booster doses, and alternative vaccine routes can be considered in nonresponders, immunocompromised individuals, and hyporesponders (<10 IU/mL of anti-hepatitis B surface antibody [anti-HBs]) to elicit protective anti-HBs levels and long-lasting immunity.
- **Postexposure prophylaxis**
  - This should be considered in infants born to HBsAg-positive mothers. Newborns should receive HBV vaccine and hepatitis B immune globulin (HBIG) within 12 hours of birth. This strategy has been shown to be 95% efficacious in preventing vertical transmission of HBV; to increase prophylaxis efficacy, mothers in the third trimester should be treated with appropriate antivirals to diminish HBV high viral load (VL).
  - Susceptible sexual partners of HBV-infected individuals and individuals with HBV-contaminated needlestick injuries should receive HBIG followed by the first dose of HBV vaccine at different body sites as soon as possible. A second dose of HBIG should be administered 30 days postexposure and the vaccine series should be completed.
  - Those who remain susceptible to HBV infection, including healthcare workers, patients on dialysis, and sexual partners of carriers should be tested for vaccination response 1–2 months after the last dose of the vaccine.
  - HBIG and antiviral therapy is indicated in HBV-seronegative recipients of HBV-infected organs.

All chronic HBV patients should receive the HAV vaccine 6–12 months apart, if not immune to HAV.

Associated Conditions

Patients with chronic hepatitis B may develop **immune-mediated extrahepatic manifestations**, including polyarteritis nodosa, glomerulonephritis, cryoglobulinemia vasculitis, serum sickness-like illness, papular acrodermatitis (predominantly in children), and aplastic anemia.

DIAGNOSIS

Clinical Presentation

The clinical presentation of chronic viral hepatitis varies significantly from asymptomatic to manifestations of advanced liver disease (cirrhosis or HCC). Frequently, patients manifest vague symptoms like **malaise, fatigue and weakness, abdominal pain, myalgias, arthralgias, nausea, and anorexia**.

History

Clinical history should include details about place of birth, family history of HBV infection and liver cancer, personal history of smoking, ETOH use, tattooing, IV drug abuse, drug transfusions, sexual habits, travel to endemic countries, and employment.

Physical Examination

* Physical examination findings of chronic viral hepatitis vary according to the stage of the disease at diagnosis. In early phases, the patient may not show physical examination abnormalities.
* **Findings of cirrhosis** include jaundice, parotid gland enlargement, gynecomastia, ascites, abdominal collateral circulation, peripheral edema, telangiectasia, muscle wasting, palmar erythema, and mental status abnormalities.

Diagnostic Criteria

Chronic hepatitis B infection is generally defined by the following characteristics: HBsAg positive for more than 6 months, presence or absence of HBeAg, elevated levels of serum HBV DNA (levels vary depending on the phase of the infection), persistently elevated, intermittently abnormal or normal ALT and aspartate aminotransferase (AST) levels, and liver biopsy showing chronic hepatitis with different grade and stage.

Diagnostic Testing

Laboratory Testing

Patients with chronic HBV infection are evaluated for the presence or absence of markers of infection, as follows:

* **Hepatitis B surface antigen (HBsAg)** is detectable in serum or hepatocyte cytoplasm (immunoperoxidase staining) in acute or chronic HBV infection. This marker disappears when the virus is cleared. The persistence of HBsAg is the diagnostic hallmark of chronic HBV infection.
* **Antibody against HBsAg (anti-HBs)** appears after the disappearance of HBsAg and after vaccination. The presence of anti-HBs demonstrates clearance or immunity to the disease.
* **Hepatitis B core antigen (HBcAg)** is not detectable in serum but can be found in the hepatocyte nuclei by immunoperoxidase staining during active viral replication.
* **IgM antibody against HBcAg (IgM anti-HBc)** is present during acute infection and in periods of high viral replication in chronic disease (flares).

- **IgG antibody against HBcAg (IgG anti-HBc)** is usually present in patients with chronic disease and in conjunction with anti-HBs in patients who cleared the disease. In some cases, patients with isolated IgG anti-HBc can be infected (occult hepatitis B) or develop reactivation of the HBV infection after immunosuppression or chemotherapy.
- **Hepatitis B e antigen (HBeAg)** appears in the serum shortly after HBsAg. It is indicative of active viral replication and high infectivity. Patients harboring HBV infection with precore or basal core promoter mutations cannot synthesize or secrete this marker despite high viral replication.
- **Antibody against HBeAg (anti-HBe)** usually indicates low-level replication and lower degree of infectivity. The best-known exception is the patient infected with precore or basal core promoter mutations (HBeAg negative and anti-HBe positive).
- **HBV DNA is the most accurate and sensitive marker of viral replication.** It is detected by polymerase chain reaction and reported as international units per milliliter (IU/mL).
- **For interpretation of laboratory tests, please see** Table 20-1.
- Patients with chronic HBV infection may progress through these clinical phases:
  - **Immune-tolerant phase:** It is usually seen with perinatally acquired infection. Patients generally have subclinical or mild disease with normal ALT levels. HBV is actively replicating (HBV DNA $>10^7$ IU/mL). HBeAg is present. The liver biopsy is generally normal or with mild inflammatory changes. Some of these patients may develop active liver disease later in life.
  - **Immune-active phase:** It is characterized by elevated HBV DNA levels ($>20,000$ IU/mL), positive (wild type) or negative (precore or basal core promoter mutation) HBeAg, elevated ALT and abnormal biopsy with different degrees of inflammation and fibrosis.

TABLE 20-1 USE OF LABORATORY TESTS IN CHRONIC HBV

Test	Immune Tolerant	Immune Active/High Replicative Chronic HBV	Low Replicative Chronic HBV	Precore/BCP Mutation	Occult HBV Infection
HBsAg	+	+	+	+	−
HBeAg	+	+	−	−	−
Anti-HBs	−	−	−	−	−
Anti-HBe	−	−	+	+	−
IgM anti-HBc	−	−	−	−	−
IgG anti-HBc	−	+	+	+	+
HBV DNA	$>10^7$ IU/mL	$>10^5$ IU/mL	$<10^3$ IU/mL	$>10^4$ copies/mL	$<10^3$ IU/mL
ALT/AST	Normal	+++	Normal	+/++	Normal

ALT, alanine transaminase; AST, aspartate transaminase; BCP, basal core promoter; HBc, hepatitis B core antigen; HBeAg, hepatitis B e antigen; HBsAg, hepatitis B surface antigen; HBV, hepatitis B virus.

Low replicative or inactive phase: These patients have few or no symptoms. There is low replicative activity with low HBV DNA levels (<2000 IU/mL), negative HBeAg, and normal ALT. The liver biopsy shows mild or no inflammation and different degrees of fibrosis. Inactive carriers may flare to active replication even after years of quiescent disease.

Occult HBV infection: It is characterized by negative HBsAg with positive HBV DNA. Immunosuppression/chemotherapy may lead to HBV reactivation.

- Additional tests
   - **Genotype determination** of HBV has growing clinical significance and is becoming a standard marker in clinical practice.
   - Patients with genotypes A and B are more likely to have spontaneous HBeAg seroconversion at an earlier age, have slower progression to cirrhosis, have less hepatic inflammation, and are more responsive to interferon treatment.

Diagnostic Procedures

Liver biopsy is useful in determining the degree of inflammation (grade) and fibrosis (stage) in patients with chronic hepatitis B. Noninvasive methods are available to assess liver fibrosis. (See Diagnostic Procedures under the NAFLD section.)

TREATMENT

- Treatment of chronic HBV infection has the following goals: clearance/suppression of HBV DNA, HBeAg clearance to anti-HBe seroconversion, HBsAg clearance to anti-HBs seroconversion, normalization of serum ALT, and normalization of liver histology.[3]
- Treatment is indicated for patients with:
   - Decompensated cirrhosis despite low HBV-DNA levels (<2000 IU/mL),
   - Compensated cirrhosis with HBV DNA >2000 IU/mL, regardless of ALT level,
   - HBeAg-positive and HBeAg-negative patients with elevated HBV DNA (VL >20,000 IU/mL and >2000 IU/mL, respectively) and ALT > 2× ULN regardless of degree of fibrosis.
- Patients with mildly elevated ALT levels (< 2× ULN) or persistently elevated HBV DNA levels should be evaluated for possible treatment on a case-by-case basis. Liver biopsy evaluation of inflammatory changes and fibrosis may help determine treatment. Patients with moderate or severe inflammation or significant fibrosis may benefit from treatment.

Medications

Current treatment options include **pegylated-interferon alpha therapy (peg-IFNα), nucleotide, and nucleoside analogs (NA)** (Table 20-2).

First-Line Treatments

- **Interferon therapy**
   - Interferons are glycoproteins with antiviral, immunomodulatory, and antiproliferative actions. The addition of polyethylene glycol to the standard IFN (α2a or α2b) molecule results in prolonged half-life with improved bioavailability.
   - Peg-IFNα is administered as weekly subcutaneous injections. No antiviral-resistance mutations are induced by IFN.
   - Interferon therapy is contraindicated in patients with decompensated liver disease. Side effects include flu-like syndrome (headache, fatigue, myalgias, arthralgias, fever, and chills), neuropsychiatric symptoms (depression, irritability, and concentration impairment), reversible bone marrow suppression, and other effects (alopecia, thyroiditis, and injection site reactions).

TABLE 20-2 THERAPEUTIC AGENTS IN CHRONIC VIRAL HEPATITIS

	Indication	Side Effects	Contraindications
Ribavirin	Chronic hepatitis C	Teratogenicity, hemolytic anemia, hyperuricemia, itching, rash, pulmonary symptoms, renal disease. Severe anemia and lactic acidosis when used with didanosine or AZT in HIV patients.	Pregnancy Renal insufficiency Inability to tolerate anemia Erythrocyte membrane enzymatic defects
Pegylated-IFN	HBeAg+ patients HBeAg– patients	Flu-like symptoms, neuropsychiatric symptoms, bone marrow suppression, autoimmune phenomena	Advanced liver disease with complications
Nucleotide inhibitors (TDF)	HBeAg+ patients HBeAg– patients Cirrhotics LAM-resistant patients	Tolerable medication with few important side effects: renal failure, bone loss, Fanconi syndrome, and hypophosphatemia. Few common side effects include nausea, diarrhea, muscle pain, and weakness	Caution if concurrent nephrotoxic agents. Dose adjust in patients with renal disease Pregnancy category B
Nucleoside inhibitors (ETV, TAF)	HBeAg+ patients HBeAg– patients Cirrhotics	Tolerable medication with few important side effects. Lactic acidosis has been reported as a serious reaction to ETV. TAF is the best alternative to prevent renal damage or bone density abnormalities. Common side effects include headaches, fatigue, dizziness, nausea.	Caution if concurrent nephrotoxic agents. Dose adjust in patients with renal disease. Pregnancy category B (TBD) and category C (ETV).

AZT, zidovudine; ETV, entecavir; LAM, lamivudine; TBD, timely birth dose; TDF, tenofovir disoproxil fumarate; TAF, tenofovir alafenamide.

- **Nucleotide and nucleoside analogs (NA)**
  - NA are orally administered agents that are better tolerated than IFN therapy; the concern for long-term use of these agents is the selection of antiviral-resistant mutations.
  - First-line agents are tenofovir and entecavir. These analogs have robust antiviral activity and are associated with lower rates of drug-resistance mutations. Both should be dose adjusted in patients with renal disease.
- **Tenofovir disoproxil fumarate (TDF) and tenofovir alafenamide (TAF)**
  - TDF is a nucleotide analogue and TAF is an NA. Both effectively suppress the HBV DNA with low rates of HBsAg loss or seroconversion. HBeAg-positive patients are frequently treated until they achieve HBeAg loss and seroconversion to anti-HBe, normal ALT, and negative HBV DNA. HBeAg-negative patients are treated indefinitely.
  - The daily dose for TDF is 300 mg with adjustment required once the eGFR is <50 mL/min. TDF has an excellent safety profile. Resistance mutations are not yet known to this agent. TAF dosage is at 25 mg until the eGFR is <15 mL/min. TAF has less renal or bone mineral density adverse events.
- **Entecavir (ETV)** is an NA that effectively suppresses HBV DNA. Just like TDF and TAF, ETV has a low rate of HBsAg loss or seroconversion. ETV has an excellent safety profile at a dose of 0.5–1 mg daily. In lamivudine-resistant patients, 51% develop ETV-resistant mutants and 43% develop virologic breakthrough.
- **Adefovir, lamivudine**, and **telbivudine** are rarely used due to their low barrier against HBV resistance.

Surgical Management

Liver transplantation is indicated in patients with advanced cirrhosis caused by HBV. Immunoprophylaxis with HBIG combined with a nucleoside or nucleotide analog is used to diminish the possibility of postliver transplantation recurrence and fibrosing cholestatic hepatitis.

MONITORING/FOLLOW-UP

Patients with chronic HBV should be screened with imaging studies (abdominal ultrasound, computed tomography [CT], magnetic resonance imaging [MRI]) every 6–12 months for early detection of HCC.

Chronic Hepatitis C

GENERAL PRINCIPLES

Epidemiology

- About 180 million people are infected throughout the world with the HCV.
- In the United States, HCV is the most frequent blood-borne infection; between 3 and 7 million people are positive for antibodies against HCV (anti-HCV).
- HCV infection is the main cause of liver disease–related deaths and the primary indication for liver transplantation in the United States.

Etiology

- HCV is an RNA virus that belongs to the *Flaviviridae* family. There are seven HCV genotypes with multiple subtypes.
- HCV is transmitted parenterally via transfusion, injection drug use, or needlestick injury. It is rarely acquired through sexual or vertical transmission.

- Acute hepatitis progresses to chronicity in 60–80% of HCV patients and results in cirrhosis in about 15–20% of patients. Cirrhotic patients are at increased risk for the development of HCC.
- The incubation period for the virus is 15–150 days.
- Chronic HCV has an indolent clinical course over many years to decades. Patients with immunosuppression, alcoholism, and obesity may have a faster progression to cirrhosis.

Risk Factors

- Risk factors for HCV infection include patients who received **blood transfusions before 1991, history of IV drug use** (leading mode of transmission in the United States), **patients on hemodialysis, tattooing or body piercing, monogamous sexual partners of HCV-infected people** (quite rare), and **healthcare workers with occupational exposure to needlesticks.**
- Risk factors for rapid development of cirrhosis include male gender, older age, alcohol consumption (more than 50 g/day), obesity with hepatic steatosis, and HIV coinfection.

Prevention

There is no available vaccine for HCV prevention.

Associated Conditions

Extrahepatic manifestations of HCV include mixed cryoglobulinemia vasculitis (10–25% of patients with HCV), glomerular diseases (mixed cryoglobulinemia syndrome, membranous nephropathy), porphyria cutanea tarda, cutaneous necrotizing vasculitis, lichen planus, and lymphoma.

DIAGNOSIS

Clinical Presentation

Chronic HCV symptoms and physical examination are similar to those described in other forms of chronic viral hepatitis (see Chronic Hepatitis B, Clinical Presentation).[4]

Diagnostic Testing

Laboratory Testing

- Diagnosis of HCV infection is suspected by the presence of anti-HCV antibodies and confirmed with the detection of HCV RNA. **Anti-HCV antibodies** may be undetectable for the first 8–12 weeks after infection; **acute HCV** can be diagnosed by the presence of **HCV RNA** during this time.
- A **false–positive anti-HCV test** can be seen in the setting of hypergammaglobulinemia or autoimmune hepatitis (AIH). A **false–negative anti-HCV test** may be seen in immunocompromised patients, patients on hemodialysis, and solid-organ transplant recipients. **The presence of anti-HCV antibodies does not confer immunity.**
- **HCV RNA** is detected in serum as early as 1–2 weeks after infection. This test is useful both for diagnosis and for assessment of sustained virologic response (**SVR**) after treatment.
- **HCV genotype** determination influences the duration, dosage, and susceptibility to treatment. Genotype 1 (subtypes 1a and 1b) accounts for majority of infections in the United States. Genotypes 2 and 3 account for 20% of HCV infection in the United States. Treatment sensitivity varies according to the different genotypes.

Diagnostic Procedures

Liver biopsy is useful in determining the grade and stage of liver disease and serves as a prognostic factor. Noninvasive markers of fibrosis are increasingly being used as an alternative.

TREATMENT

The goal of treatment is to clear the HCV and to modify the natural history of the infection toward complications of chronic HCV infection, including cirrhosis and HCC.[5]

- **Treatment response** is defined by achievement of **SVR**. SVR is defined as absence of detectable HCV RNA, 12 weeks after completion of therapy.
- **Nonresponders** are patients who fail to achieve SVR. **Virologic breakthrough** is defined as reappearance of HCV RNA after clearance while on treatment. **Relapse** is defined as reappearance of HCV RNA after the end of treatment.

Medications

First Line

- Chronic HCV infection is treated with direct-acting antivirals (DAAs). The selection of treatment regimen is frequently based on history of prior treatment (naïve vs. experienced), HCV VL, genotype/subtype, cirrhosis status (compensated vs. decompensated), coinfections (HIV, HBV), drug–drug interactions, and renal function.
    - DAAs target specific nonstructural proteins of the virus, resulting in disruption of viral replication.
    - Current treatment regimens include the combination of more than one DAA for 8–16 weeks (depending on the HCV infection variables). Current DAAs have an eradication efficacy (SVR) that fluctuates between 95% and 99% with a very tolerable side effect profile, with several agents having a pan-genotypic spectrum.
        - **Nonstructural proteins 3/4A (NS3/4A) protease inhibitors (PIs):** Currently approved NS3/4A PIs include simeprevir, grazoprevir, glecaprevir, paritaprevir, and voxilaprevir. These drugs are contraindicated in decompensated cirrhosis.
        - **NS5A complex inhibitors** include ledipasvir, ombitasvir, daclatasvir, velpatasvir, elbasvir, and pibrentasvir.
        - **NS5B polymerase inhibitors** include sofosbuvir and dasabuvir.
- **Genotype 1** treatment options: sofosbuvir/ledipasvir, sofosbuvir/velpatasvir, grazoprevir/elbasvir, glecaprevir/pibrentasvir.
- **Genotype 2** treatment options: sofosbuvir/velpatasvir, glecaprevir/pibrentasvir.
- **Genotype 3** treatment options: sofosbuvir/velpatasvir, sofosbuvir/daclatasvir, glecaprevir/pibrentasvir.
- **Genotype 4, 5**, and **6** are less frequently found genotypes in the United States and are treated effectively with pan-genotypic regimens.
- **Nonresponders to prior treatments** with interferon, ribavirin and some DAAs, can be treated with a dual regimen containing glecaprevir/pibrentasvir or triple regimen containing sofosbuvir/velpatasvir/voxilaprevir.
- **HCV patients with renal failure** are treated (based on genotype) with grazoprevir/elbasvir (genotype 1) or glecaprevir/pibrentasvir (pan-genotypic). Sofosbuvir containing regimens should not be used with eGFR <30 mL/min.
- No optimal treatment is available for decompensated cirrhosis. Sofosbuvir/velpatasvir with ribavirin is a good option for some of these patients. Patients with advanced cirrhosis are referred to liver transplant programs. In these patients, HCV is treated effectively after liver transplantation with sofosbuvir/ledipasvir and ribavirin.
- If concurrent HBsAg or anti-HBc positivity is found, patient should have HBV DNA and ALT measured. Consider simultaneous HBV treatment if appropriate, to avoid DAA-induced HBV flares, fulminant hepatitis, or death.

Surgical Management

Liver transplantation is indicated in patients with advanced cirrhosis. HCV recurrence is almost universal after transplantation; patients should be treated to promote SVR and cure.

SPECIAL CONSIDERATIONS

Patients with cryoglobulinemia with mild/moderate proteinuria and slowly progressive renal disease should be treated with DAA combination therapy.

Alcoholic Liver Disease

GENERAL PRINCIPLES

Classification

Liver toxicity induced by alcohol generates a spectrum of liver damage that fluctuates from: **simple steatosis to alcoholic steatohepatitis, progressive fibrosis, cirrhosis**, and development of **HCC**.

Epidemiology

- Steatosis, the most common manifestation of alcoholic liver disease, is present in 90% of chronic intense alcohol users.
- Progression to cirrhosis is seen in 5–15% of these patients despite abstinence, and in 30–37% if alcohol use continues.
- Despite the high prevalence of fatty liver disease in heavy drinkers, only 10–35% will develop alcoholic hepatitis.

Risk Factors

- Risk factors for liver disease in alcoholics include higher doses (i.e., more than 60 g/day), longer alcohol use, obesity, iron overload, concomitant viral hepatitis, genetic factors, malnutrition, metabolic syndrome, ethnicity, and female gender.
- Consumption of approximately 30–40 units (one unit is equal to 8 g of alcohol, one glass of wine, or one 240 mL can of 3.5–4% beer) of alcohol per week results in cirrhosis in 3–8% of patients with more than 12 years of alcohol use.
- Rates of alcohol-related cirrhosis are higher among blacks and Hispanics.

Associated Conditions

Associated conditions induced by alcohol include **cardiomyopathy, skeletal muscle wasting, pancreatic dysfunction, and neurotoxicity**.

DIAGNOSIS

Clinical Presentation

- Patients with evidence of liver disease should be screened for alcohol dependency by obtaining a thorough social history and sometimes random alcohol levels.
- The **CAGE questionnaire** has high sensitivity and specificity for identification of alcohol dependency. It consists of four questions: (1) Have you ever felt you needed to **C**ut down on your drinking? (2) Have people **A**nnoyed you by criticizing your drinking? (3) Have you ever felt **G**uilty about drinking? (4) Have you ever felt you needed a drink first thing in the morning (**E**ye-opener) to steady your nerves or to get rid of a hangover? Answering "yes" to two questions indicates need for further evaluation.
- Physical examination findings in patients with alcoholic liver disease vary according to the stage of the disease at diagnosis.
- Patients with **steatosis/fatty liver disease** are usually asymptomatic.
- **Alcoholic hepatitis** has a spectrum of clinical presentations and severity. Patients may have clinically silent disease or severe hepatitis with rapid development of hepatic failure and death.

- Patients with **alcoholic cirrhosis** may show classic signs and symptoms of advanced liver disease (see Hepatitis B section).

Diagnostic Testing

Laboratory Testing

- Alcoholic hepatitis should be suspected in patients with elevated aminotransferases when the **AST to ALT ratio is >2:1.**
- A cholestatic picture characterized by **elevated alkaline phosphatase (AP), total bilirubin (predominantly conjugated)**, and **abnormal coagulation parameters** may also be found.
- Poor prognosis is indicated by: elevated creatinine levels, leukocytosis, marked cholestasis, and coagulopathy (not improving despite parenteral vitamin K administration).
- **Discriminant function** (DF) can be determined to assess in-hospital mortality. DF = 4.6 × (PT patient − PT control) + serum total bilirubin. DF >32 is associated with poor prognosis.

Imaging

Abdominal ultrasound, MRI, and/or CT are used to investigate other liver diseases including obstructive biliary pathology and infiltrative and neoplastic disease.

Diagnostic Procedures

- **Liver biopsy** is rarely indicated during the acute phase of alcoholic hepatitis. In later stages, it may be used to assess the stage and severity of liver damage.
- **Histology** includes Mallory hyaline bodies, ballooning degeneration, neutrophilic infiltrate, confluent parenchymal necrosis of hepatocytes, megamitochondria, intrasinusoidal and pericentral collagen deposition, lobular inflammation, nuclear vacuolation, bile duct proliferation, fatty change, and perivenular and perisinusoidal fibrosis.

TREATMENT

Nonpharmacologic Treatment

- **Abstinence from alcohol is the cornerstone of treatment.**
- Treatment of alcoholic liver disease also includes **nutritional support**.
  - In the absence of hepatic encephalopathy or with a functioning gastrointestinal tract, enteral feeding should be considered if the patient is not eating appropriately.
  - In patients with hepatic encephalopathy or with ileus, total parenteral nutrition should be considered; it confers a mortality benefit.
  - In patients with alcoholic cirrhosis, a regular oral diet with multiple feedings and high protein and caloric content improve survival.

Medications

Corticosteroids: Treatment of alcoholic hepatitis with corticosteroids is controversial.[6] Evidence suggests, however, that patients with a DF >32 or hepatic encephalopathy may benefit from steroid therapy. Prednisolone is started at 40 mg/day orally for 4 weeks and then tapered-down over 2–4 weeks. After 7 days of steroid therapy, a *Lille score* is calculated to predict response to therapy. If the patient has a Lille score >0.45 (poor response), treatment should be stopped.[7]

Surgical Management

Liver transplant is indicated in patients with advanced alcoholic liver disease. A minimum of 6 months of abstinence and active participation in a rehabilitation program are required to be considered a candidate for liver transplantation.

Nonalcoholic Fatty Liver Disease

GENERAL PRINCIPLES

Definition

Nonalcoholic fatty liver disease (NAFLD) is a clinicopathologic syndrome that encompasses several clinical entities, including liver steatosis, steatohepatitis, fibrosis, and end-stage liver disease in the absence of significant alcohol consumption.

Classification

- **Nonalcoholic steatohepatitis (NASH)**, which is part of the spectrum of NAFLD, is defined by the presence of steatosis, hepatocellular ballooning, lobular inflammation, and pericellular or perisinusoidal fibrosis. It accounts for about one-fifth of NAFLD and has the risk for progression to cirrhosis.[8]
- **Nonalcoholic fatty liver (NAFL)** consists of "simple" liver steatosis without significant inflammation and is characterized by more stable disease with lesser risks for progression to cirrhosis.

Epidemiology

- A worldwide condition, NAFLD is a common liver condition in the United States affecting 20–30% of the adult population. The prevalence of NASH is about 2–3%.
- NAFLD affects both children and adults; its incidence increases with age.
- Approximately 30% of patients with NASH will progress to fibrosis over 5 years and 15–20% progress to cirrhosis over time. About 37% of patients with fibrosis will progress to cirrhosis.
- Mortality among NASH patients is more often from cardiovascular disease rather than cirrhosis.

Pathophysiology

- The mechanism by which NAFLD progresses to NASH is not completely clear.
- Decreased lipid output from the liver, increased peripheral lipolysis, and increased hepatic uptake of fatty acids lead to the development of macrovesicular steatosis which is worsened by insulin resistance. In addition, hyperinsulinemia induces mitochondrial dysfunction which causes increased hepatic oxidative stress and development of steatohepatitis.
- Secondary causes of NASH include hepatotoxic drugs (amiodarone, nifedipine, estrogens), surgical procedures (jejunoileal bypass, extensive small bowel resection, pancreatic and biliary diversions), and miscellaneous conditions (total parenteral nutrition, hypobetalipoproteinemia, environmental toxins).

Risk Factors

Risk factors for NAFLD include female gender, insulin resistance, and metabolic syndrome.

DIAGNOSIS

Clinical Presentation

- Disease presentation can vary from asymptomatic to advanced disease and HCC.
- Significant alcohol use (defined as more than two drinks per day for males and more than one drink per day for females) must be ruled out by history.

- A thorough review of patients' medications is essential, including over-the-counter medications, herbal remedies, and vitamin supplements.

Diagnostic Criteria

Diagnosis is suspected clinically and confirmed by imaging and liver biopsy.

Diagnostic Testing

Laboratory Testing

Liver enzyme elevations are generally mild. Up to 80% of patients have normal liver enzymes.

Imaging

- Imaging studies, such as ultrasonography, CT, and MRI may detect liver steatosis.[9]
- Magnetic resonance spectroscopy offers a quantitative measurement of liver fat content, but is not commonly available in US medical centers.

Diagnostic Procedures

- **Liver biopsy is the gold standard for diagnosis; however, newer noninvasive measures of liver fibrosis are being used.**
  - Histologic lesions necessary for diagnosis of NASH include macrosteatosis, hepatocyte ballooning, and mixed lobular inflammation. More severe injury on initial biopsy is found in patients who are older, have elevated body mass index, and have diabetes.
  - Several noninvasive methods for the assessment of liver fibrosis are now widely used. These methods cannot accurately differentiate the stages of fibrosis but are good in differentiating early from advanced fibrosis. The likelihood of fibrosis on these tests can be used to guide treatment decisions and to predict which patients are at risk for adverse outcomes, including HCC, complications of portal hypertension and death.
  - Indirect serologic markers of liver fibrosis include, the **NAFLD Fibrosis score** and **Fibrosis-4 score**, which uses laboratory values (AST, ALT, platelet, albumin), comorbid conditions (insulin resistance or diabetes, BMI), and demographic information (age). A score of >0.675 on the NAFLD Fibrosis score and >3.25 on the Fibrosis-4 score predicts the presence of significant fibrosis. The **FibroSure assay** assesses circulating markers of fibrogenesis, fibrinolysis, or both. It analyzes the results of six blood serum tests to generate a score that is correlated with the degree of fibrosis.
  - Imaging modalities to assess liver stiffness include vibration-controlled transient elastography (VCTE) and magnetic resonance elastography (MRE). Both VTCE and MRE are also useful in assessing if liver steatosis is present in addition to fibrosis, which can be calculated by the proton-density fat fraction or spectroscopy.

TREATMENT

Medications

- **There is no specific medical therapy proven for NASH.** However, pioglitazone and vitamin E have shown to improve liver histology and liver function tests and can be used in biopsy-proven NASH patients.[10]
- **Correction of associated conditions** such as hyperlipidemia, diabetes, and insulin resistance is warranted. It is imperative to discontinue potential hepatotoxic agents.

Nonpharmacologic Therapies

Weight loss and exercise should be recommended to improve insulin resistance and other parameters of the metabolic syndrome.[11]

Surgical Management

- **Bariatric surgery** can be considered in obese individuals (BMI >40) with NAFLD or NASH. However, if cirrhosis is present, bariatric surgery may be considered on a case-by-case basis.
- **Liver transplantation** should be considered in patients with advanced cirrhosis. Recurrence of NAFLD may occur after transplantation.

MONITORING/FOLLOW-UP

Since NASH is associated with increased risk of HCC, annual screening with abdominal imaging studies and α-fetoprotein is warranted.

Autoimmune Liver Disease

GENERAL PRINCIPLES

Autoimmune liver disease encompasses a spectrum of illnesses, including AIH, primary sclerosing cholangitis (PSC), primary biliary cholangitis (PBC), and overlap syndromes. These diseases have different clinical presentations and the diagnosis is often challenging to the physician (Table 20-3). Patients with autoimmune liver disease may have concurrent nonhepatic autoimmune illnesses.

Definition

AIH is a chronic inflammatory disease of the liver associated with circulating antibodies and hypergammaglobulinemia which, if untreated, can result in progressive fibrosis and cirrhosis.

Classification

There are two main types of AIH: Type 1 and Type 2.
- **Type 1** affects predominantly females with a peak incidence in the second through fourth decades of life. It accounts for 90% of AIH cases.
- **Type 2** predominantly affects children with elevated serum IgG levels.
- Both types are commonly associated with other autoimmune diseases, can progress to cirrhosis, and differ in their diagnostic markers (see Diagnosis section).

Epidemiology

- AIH occurs worldwide and in all age groups; it most commonly affects women aged 10–30 years and older than 60 years (20% of all cases).
- Cirrhosis is more often the initial clinical presentation in African Americans than Caucasian patients.
- Patients older than 60 years generally have greater degree of fibrosis, cirrhosis, and a higher frequency of portal hypertension at presentation.
- Incidence of HCC is about 1.1% per year.
- There are also cases of drug-induced AIH (e.g., nitrofurantoin and minocycline) which can be difficult to differentiate from drug-induced liver injury (DILI).

Pathophysiology

- Environmental and genetic factors, along with regulatory T-cell dysfunction, cause dysregulation of immune responses to autoantigens resulting in a loss of immune tolerance.
- Genetic studies have demonstrated different HLA antigen alleles in the AIH of adults (Type 1) compared with the AIH of children (Type 2), indicating that genetic factors may influence the presentation in different age groups.

	Liver Test Pattern	Serologies	Liver Biopsy	"Clinical Pearls"
Autoimmune Liver Diseases				
Autoimmune hepatitis	Hepatocellular	Type 1: Anti-SMA Type 2: Anti-LKM-1 Elevated IgG	Interface hepatitis and plasma cell infiltrate	Responsive to steroids
PBC	Cholestatic	90% AMA positive Elevated IgM	Destructive cholangitis affecting interlobular and septal bile ducts. Lymphocyte and mononuclear infiltrate. Several stages	Decreases morbidity and mortality in those treated with ursodeoxycholic acid (UCDA). In refractory UCDA cases the combination of UDCA and obeticholic acid is indicated.
PSC	Mixed, predominantly, cholestatic	50–80% p-ANCA +	Ductular proliferation, obliterative fibrous cholangitis, inflammation and fibrosis. Several stages	Associated with IBD. ERCP diagnostic method of choice.
Metabolic Liver Diseases				
Hemochromatosis	Hepatocellular	HFE-gene mutation, high transferrin sat.	Iron deposition in hepatocytes. HII 1.9>; High iron per µg/g dry weight	If treated appropriately mortality/morbidity equal to the general population
Wilson Disease	Hepatocellular	Low ceruloplasmin High copper levels in the liver	Fatty infiltration, glycogenic nuclei. Orcein stain positive	Chelating therapy is the cornerstone of treatment
α_1-Antitrypsin deficiency	Hepatocellular	Low α_1-antitrypsin levels	PAS +, diastase + resistant periportal globules	No medical therapy for early stages. Liver transplantation ideal option for end-stage liver disease

AMA, antimitochondrial antibody; ERCP, endoscopic retrograde cholangiopancreatography; IBD, inflammatory bowel disease; anti-LKM, anti-lower-kidney microsomal antibody; p-ANCA, perinuclear antineutrophil cytoplasmic antibody; PBC, primary biliary cholangitis; PSC, primary sclerosing cholangitis; SMA, smooth muscle antibody.

Associated Conditions

- Extrahepatic manifestations may be found in 30–50% of patients. They include celiac sprue, Coombs-positive hemolytic anemia, Hashimoto thyroiditis, Graves disease, rheumatoid arthritis, ulcerative colitis (UC), type 1 diabetes, lupus, and vitiligo.
- Patients with AIH may have concurrent autoimmune liver diseases (e.g., PBC, PSC, autoimmune cholangitis) giving rise to "variant" syndromes.

DIAGNOSIS

Clinical Presentation

- AIH has a range of clinical presentations. In approximately 30% of cases, the presentation is acute with fever, abdominal pain, jaundice, and malaise. Some of these patients may progress to fulminant hepatic failure.
- AIH may have an indolent course with 25–30% of patients progressing to cirrhosis over time.
- About 40% of patients are asymptomatic (usually men with lower serum ALT levels).
- Careful history should be obtained to investigate the use of excessive alcohol, viral hepatitis risk factors, use of hepatotoxic agents, and risk factors for metabolic disorders to rule out overlapping conditions and confounding variables.

Diagnostic Criteria

Diagnosis is made by detection of elevated serum aminotransferases, circulating autoantibodies, elevated immunoglobulin levels, and liver biopsy abnormalities.

Diagnostic Testing

Laboratory Testing

- The most commonly elevated biomarkers include **antinuclear antibody (ANA), antismooth muscle antibody (ASMA), anti–liver-kidney microsomal antibody (LKM-1), and IgG**. In type 1 AIH, ANA and ASMA are positive, whereas in type 2, anti-LKM-1 antibody is positive.
- **Other causes of liver disease should be excluded** such as Wilson disease (WD), α_1-antitrypsin (α_1-AT) deficiency, viral hepatitis, alcohol-mediated liver disease, PBC, PSC, and other infections or medications that could cause liver disease.

Diagnostic Procedures

- **Liver biopsy** is essential for the diagnosis of AIH.
- Pericentral necrosis and interface hepatitis with lobular/panacinar inflammation along with lymphocytic and plasmacytic infiltration are the histologic hallmarks. Bridging necrosis, fibrosis, or well-developed cirrhosis is found in advanced stages.

TREATMENT

- **Treatment is directed at achieving disease remission:** normalization of serum bilirubin, AST, ALT, and immunoglobulin levels; disappearance of symptoms; resolution of histologic changes and preventing further progression of liver disease. Remission should be achieved for 2–4 years to decrease the likelihood of relapse.
- Other treatment outcomes include **incomplete response** defined as no remission after 3 years of treatment and **relapse** defined as increase in serum AST to more than three times the ULN or increase in serum γ-globulin to >2 g/dL with redevelopment of interface hepatitis.
- Symptomatic patients with AST levels at least 5× ULN with serum IgG more 2× ULN, hepatic activity index (HAI) >4/18 and those with bridging fibrosis or multilobular

necrosis have a high mortality rate and should be treated promptly. In addition, treatment can also be considered in advanced fibrosis and cirrhosis with active disease.[12]

Medications

- Therapy is initiated with **prednisone** (0.5–1 mg/kg/day) alone, followed by the addition of **azathioprine** (1–2 mg/kg/day) after 2 weeks. Prednisone is tapered down by 5–10 mg every week to 2 weeks when biochemical and clinical improvement is noted. Incomplete responders require lifelong low-dose prednisone and/or azathioprine therapy.
- **Relapses** should be retreated with prednisone and azathioprine, with eventual weaning of prednisone and continuation of azathioprine at 2 mg/kg daily chronically. An alternative treatment includes low-dose prednisone to maintain ALT level less than three times upper limit of normal.
- **Refractory disease** occurs in about 20% of patients and may require "salvage" therapy with mycophenolate mofetil, cyclosporine, or tacrolimus.
- **Budesonide**, a synthetic steroid with high affinity for glucocorticoid receptors and high first-pass metabolism in the liver, can be used as a safer alternative to prednisone.[13] Budesonide in conjunction with azathioprine may be effective in causing biochemical remission of disease in noncirrhotic AIH patients after 6 months of treatment with less steroid-specific side effects compared to prednisone. However, follow-up data on histology and long-term data are not available.
- **Side effects** associated with azathioprine include cholestatic hepatitis, pancreatitis, nausea, rash, bone marrow suppression, malignancy, teratogenicity, and diarrhea. Side effects associated with corticosteroids include diabetes, psychosis, cataracts, glaucoma, and severe osteoporosis.
- AIH patients should be **vaccinated against HBV and HAV prior to treatment**.[14]

Surgical Management

Liver transplantation is considered for patients with advanced cirrhosis and treatment failure. Five-year patient and graft survivals exceed 80%. Recurrent AIH posttransplant is seen in about 25% of patients and responds well to augmentation of existing immunosuppression with steroids and calcineurin inhibitors. *De novo* AIH (AIH in patients with liver transplant for nonautoimmune disease) can be treated with prednisone and azathioprine.

Primary Sclerosing Cholangitis (PSC)

GENERAL PRINCIPLES

Definition

- PSC is a cholestatic liver disorder characterized by chronic inflammation and fibrosis resulting in progressive destruction of the extrahepatic and intrahepatic biliary ducts which can progress to cirrhosis.[15]
- Variants of PSC
  - **Small duct PSC:** A variant in which the main bile ducts are normal on imaging studies but with cholestatic and histologic features of PSC due to damage of small biliary ducts; it has a more favorable prognosis.
  - **Overlap syndrome (AIH-PSC):** A variant in which patient exhibits both clinical and histologic features of hepatocellular and cholestatic liver damage with the presence of autoimmune markers (ANA +, ASMA +/− and AMA—antibodies.)
  - **Secondary sclerosing cholangitis:** A nonautoimmune variant in which the destruction of bile ducts and resulting fibrosis/cirrhosis are a consequence of long-term biliary obstruction, chemotherapy-induced, immunodeficiency-induced, infection and ischemia of the biliary ducts.

IgG4-associated sclerosing cholangitis is a poorly defined entity in which patients have increased levels of serum IgG4 and bile ducts infiltrated with IgG4-positive plasma cells.

Epidemiology

- The prevalence of PSC is about 10 per 100,000 in Northern European descendants.
- PSC occurs mainly in the fourth or fifth decade of life with no clear gender predilection.
- Most patients have involvement of both the intra- and extrahepatic ducts. At a lower frequency, the disease involves only the intrahepatic or the extrahepatic biliary ducts.
- The lifetime risk of cholangiocarcinoma in patients with PSC varies from 7–15%. Gallbladder neoplasms are also associated with PSC, but at a lower frequency.
- PSC median survival depends on the stage at diagnosis.

Risk Factors

Genetic associations in PSC and complex family inheritance patterns have been demonstrated. A significant increased risk of PSC exists among siblings.

Associated Conditions

- PSC is frequently associated with **ulcerative colitis** (UC) although their clinical courses have no correlation.[16] In the United States, 70% of patients with PSC have UC and approximately 2–4% of patients with UC have PSC.
- **Other autoimmune diseases**, such as autoimmune pancreatitis and AIH, can coexist with PSC.

DIAGNOSIS

Clinical Presentation

- Many patients are initially asymptomatic with normal physical examinations and isolated elevation of liver enzymes. Presentation with cholestatic syndrome with jaundice and pruritus is also common.
- **Acute cholangitis** manifested by fever or rigors, right upper quadrant pain, and jaundice may be a clinical emergency. Usually, these patients have bacteremia and require IV antibiotics.
- Patients may present to the physician in late stages with cirrhosis.

Diagnostic Criteria

Diagnosis is supported by liver chemistry, biliary tree imaging, and rarely a liver biopsy.

Differential Diagnosis

The differential diagnosis for PSC includes postoperative biliary strictures, choledocholithiasis, chronic bacterial cholangitis, HIV-related cholangiopathy, biliary malignancy, Caroli disease or other types of ductal plate malformations, ischemic and medication-induced biliary injuries, metabolic liver diseases, viral hepatitis, and primary biliary cholangitis.

Diagnostic Testing

Laboratory Testing

- **AP** is the most commonly elevated liver test. **ALT and AST** are often elevated up to 2–3× ULN. **Serum IgG levels** are elevated to 1.5× ULN in about 60% of patients.
- **ANA** is often positive and **perinuclear antineutrophil cytoplasmic antibody (p-ANCA)** is positive in about 50–80% of the cases.

Imaging

- **Abdominal ultrasound** may be normal or may show bile duct wall thickening or dilation. Gallbladder pathology including gallbladder dilation or wall thickening, gallstones, cholecystitis, and mass lesions can also be present.
- **Abdominal CT** may show thickening and enhancement of biliary ducts, duct dilation, evidence of portal hypertension, and lymphadenopathy.
- PSC is confirmed by demonstration of multiple strictures, segmental dilations, or irregularities of the intrahepatic and/or extrahepatic bile ducts ("beaded" pattern) by **magnetic resonance cholangiopancreatography (MRCP) or** endoscopic retrograde cholangiopancreatography **(ERCP)**. Given its noninvasive nature, MRCP is the gold standard in the diagnosis of PSC. ERCP is used in patients who require a therapeutic or diagnostic intervention.
- The finding of a "dominant stricture" (stenosis <1.5 mm in the common bile duct or <1 mm in the hepatic duct) should raise concern for cholangiocarcinoma. Brush cytology, fluorescent in situ hybridization (FISH), and biopsies should be obtained to rule out malignancy.

Diagnostic Procedures

- **Liver biopsy** is usually unnecessary in the setting of classic MRCP findings for PSC, but it can be helpful in the diagnosis of small duct PSC, in excluding other diagnoses, and when overlap syndromes are suspected.
- Characteristic histologic findings of PSC include concentric periductal fibrosis ("onion-skinning") that progresses to narrowing and obliteration of biliary ductules.
- PSC patients should obtain a **screening colonoscopy with biopsies** to rule out inflammatory bowel disease even if asymptomatic.

TREATMENT

Medications

- **Pruritus** associated with PSC can be treated medically. Refer to the section Treatment of Chronic Cholestasis for treatment options.
- **IgG4-associated sclerosing cholangitis is steroid responsive.**
- **Ursodeoxycholic acid (UDCA)**, despite improving liver biochemistries, **has not shown survival benefit** and should not be used in the management of PSC.[17]

Nonpharmacologic Therapies

- **Dominant biliary duct strictures** can be treated with **balloon dilation and stenting**; prophylactic antibiotics should be administered before these endoscopic procedures. Endoscopic treatment of dominant strictures is associated with improved survival rates.
- **Episodes of acute cholangitis require antibiotics** and may require endoscopic therapy to treat biliary duct strictures. Rarely, surgical management of biliary strictures (biliary diversion) is indicated.
- **Liver transplantation** is an option for PSC patients with advanced disease. Unique indications include intractable pruritus, recurrent cholangitis, and cholangiocarcinoma.
  - 5-year survival rates postliver transplantation is about 85%.
  - Recurrent PSC after liver transplantation has been documented. Other causes of posttransplant biliary strictures should be ruled out before establishing the diagnosis of posttransplant PSC recurrence.
- **PSC patients with cholangiocarcinoma can undergo surgical resection** in the absence of cirrhosis and in particular cases be considered for adjuvant chemotherapy and liver transplantation.

MONITORING/FOLLOW-UP

- Patients are monitored for chronic complications of cholestasis and for fat-soluble vitamin deficiencies.
- Surveillance for cholangiocarcinoma is conducted every 6–12 months with abdominal MRCP. ERCPs are done as needed.

Primary Biliary Cholangitis (PBC)

GENERAL PRINCIPLES

Definition

- PBC is a cholestatic liver disorder with autoimmune features. It is hypothesized that immunogenetic and environmental factors may play a role in its genesis.
- In PBC, granulomatous destruction of interlobular and septal bile ducts can result in progressive ductopenia, cholestasis, fibrosis, and cirrhosis.

Epidemiology

- PBC is seen worldwide but is more commonly described in North America and Northern Europe. It has a worldwide prevalence of <1:2000.
- PBC most commonly affects women in the fourth and fifth decades of life. It has a progressive course which may extend over many decades.

Associated Conditions

Extrahepatic manifestations associated with PBC include keratoconjunctivitis sicca (Sjögren syndrome), renal tubular acidosis, gallstones, thyroid disease, Raynaud phenomenon, celiac disease, and systemic progressive sclerosis (scleroderma).

DIAGNOSIS

Clinical Presentation

- Many patients are asymptomatic at the time of diagnosis.
- The most common clinical features of PBC include **fatigue** and **pruritus**. Patients with PBC can develop features of portal hypertension as the disease progresses.[18]
- Patients with PBC frequently develop clinical **complications from chronic cholestasis**.[19]
  - **Jaundice** and **pruritus** are the most common clinical manifestations associated with chronic cholestasis. Cholestasis increases the production of melanin in the skin resulting in hyperpigmentation.
  - Decreased secretion of bile acids and bile salts into the small bowel results in **malabsorption of fat and fat-soluble vitamins**, including vitamins A, D, E, and K. Lack of adequate vitamin absorption can lead to the development of vision loss, osteoporosis, osteomalacia, and increased bleeding risk.
  - Chronic cholestasis results in the development of **xanthomas** (nodules, plaques, or papules of the skin containing lipids) and **xanthelasma** (yellowish plaques near the inner canthus of the eyelid) as a result of **hypercholesterolemia**. Xanthomas and xanthelasma are more commonly seen in PBC than in other diseases with chronic cholestasis.
- Patients with PBC may develop cirrhosis after 10–15 years of disease progression.

Diagnostic Criteria

Diagnosis of PBC is based on laboratory tests. Liver biopsy shows cholestasis with nonsuppurative cholangitis, granulomas, and destruction of small and medium-sized bile ducts.

Differential Diagnosis

The differential diagnosis for PBC includes cholestasis due to drug reaction, biliary obstruction, sarcoidosis, AIH, and PSC.

Diagnostic Testing

Laboratory Testing

- Elevated **AP** is the most common abnormality seen in PBC. Hyperbilirubinemia, high cholesterol, elevated IgM, and elevated bile acids are also frequently found. AST and ALT are mildly elevated.
- **Antimitochondrial antibody (AMA)** is present in more than 90% of PBC patients and is the serologic hallmark for diagnosis.

Imaging

Abdominal ultrasound is initially done to rule out extrahepatic causes of cholestasis.

Diagnostic Procedures

Liver biopsy is usually not needed in classic cases of PBC. However, it can be used when the diagnosis is unclear or for staging purposes. Stages 1–3 are characterized by portal or periportal hepatitis with granulomatous destruction of bile ducts, bile duct proliferation, bridging necrosis, and fibrosis. Stage 4 is characterized by cirrhosis.

TREATMENT

Medications

- **UDCA** at a dose of 13–15 mg/kg/day may improve liver test abnormalities and delay disease progression with improvement in survival when given long term (>4 years). UDCA can be an effective treatment for any histologic stage of PBC. Side effects of UDCA include minimal weight gain, loose stools, and hair thinning.
- The bile acid analog **obeticholic acid (OCA)** is a selective farnesoid X receptor agonist and a treatment alternative in combination with UDCA for those with an inadequate response to UDCA. OCA can be used as monotherapy in those intolerant to UDCA. Main side effect of OCA is pruritus; it also decreases total cholesterol and high-density lipoproteins (HDL) and increases low-density lipoproteins (LDL).
- Symptom-specific therapy for pruritus, steatorrhea, and malabsorption can be added to treatment with UDCA.

Surgical Management

Liver transplantation is indicated in PBC patients with advanced cirrhosis. Recurrent PBC has been documented after transplantation.

Treatment of Chronic Cholestasis

NUTRITIONAL DEFICIENCIES

- Nutritional deficiencies result from fat malabsorption. Fat-soluble vitamin deficiency (vitamins A, D, E, and K) is often present in advanced cholestasis.
- **Vitamin A deficiency** can present as conjunctival xerosis, keratomalacia, follicular hyperkeratosis, and night blindness. **Vitamin E deficiency** is manifested as hemolytic anemia, posterior column degeneration, ophthalmoplegia, and peripheral neuropathy. **Vitamin K deficiency** is manifested as coagulopathy. **Vitamin D deficiency** can present as rickets/osteomalacia.

- Testing can be done to assess levels of these fat-soluble vitamins.
- Patients are supplemented with vitamin supplements to correct deficiencies.

OSTEOPOROSIS

- Osteoporosis is defined as a decrease in the amount of bone, leading to a decrease in structural integrity and increase in the risk of fractures.
- The relative risk of osteopenia in cholestasis is 4.4 times greater than the general population, matched for age and gender. Osteoporosis is more commonly seen in clinical cholestasis due to PBC.
- Bone mineral density should be measured by dual-energy x-ray absorptiometry (DEXA) in all patients at the time of diagnosis and during follow-up (every 1–2 years).
- **Treatment** of bone disease includes weight-bearing exercise, oral calcium and vitamin D supplementation and bisphosphonate therapy.

PRURITUS

- Pruritus results from impaired secretion of bile. It is most commonly seen in PBC and PSC.
- **Pruritus** associated with chronic cholestasis can be treated with anion exchange resins like **cholestyramine** or **colestipol**. In case of failure, rifampin, opiate antagonists, and serotonin antagonists can also be used. In refractory states, plasmapheresis, UV light, and liver transplantation should be considered.

Metabolic Liver Diseases

The most frequently encountered metabolic liver diseases include hereditary hemochromatosis (HH), α_1-AT deficiency, and WD (Table 20-3). These diseases generate different degrees of liver damage or progression to cirrhosis through different mechanisms.

Hereditary Hemochromatosis (HH)

GENERAL PRINCIPLES

Definition

HH is an autosomal recessive disorder of iron overload resulting in oxidative damage of hepatocytes.

Epidemiology

- HH is the most common inherited form of iron overload affecting Caucasians. HH is most common in middle-aged, Caucasian males, especially Northern Europeans.[20]
- The degree of iron overload has a direct impact on life expectancy in individuals with HH; thus, diagnosis is targeted at identifying individuals before they become symptomatic. Patients homozygous for HFE C282Y mutation can develop iron overload (38–50%) and HH-associated morbidity (10–33%).

Etiology

- HH is primarily caused by a missense mutation—C282Y—in the HFE gene located on chromosome 6. Other mutations—H63D and S65C—are not generally associated with iron overload unless they present as compound heterozygote with C282Y.

- **HFE gene mutation** causes deficient synthesis of the hormone hepcidin, causing increased iron entry into the bloodstream which exceeds the storage/binding capacity of ferritin/transferrin. This promotes increased iron accumulation in liver parenchymal cells leading to production of highly reactive oxygen species which damage intercellular structures. Furthermore, abnormal iron absorption in the duodenum, as well as increased release of iron from reticuloendothelial macrophages, leads to excessive and damaging iron deposition in the heart, pancreas, skin, and endocrine system.
- Approximately, 80% of patients with HH are of Northern European descent and homozygote for the C282Y mutation.

Risk Factors

- The major risk factor for development of this condition is **family history** of HH.
- Alcohol abuse is the main modifiable risk factor associated with disease progression to cirrhosis.
- Patients with cirrhosis caused by HH are at increased risk of HCC despite adequate iron depletion therapy.

Prevention

- Family members of patients with HH should be screened with fasting transferrin saturation and ferritin levels. Genetic testing may be performed if needed.
- Screening should also be considered in patients with liver disease of unknown etiology, porphyria cutanea tarda, testicular atrophy, and chondrocalcinosis.

Associated Conditions

Cardiomyopathies, hypogonadism, skin changes, and diabetes are frequently associated with HH.

DIAGNOSIS

Diagnosis is based on laboratory testing, imaging, and liver biopsy.[21]

Clinical Presentation

- Some patients are asymptomatic at presentation. Most common symptoms include fatigue, malaise, arthralgias, and hepatomegaly.
- Clinical manifestations include slate-colored skin, diabetes, cardiomyopathy, arthritis (esp. 2nd and 3rd metacarpophalangeal joints), and hypogonadism.
- Patients with progressive liver iron overload will develop fibrosis and clinical manifestations of cirrhosis.

Diagnostic Testing

Laboratory Testing

- **High fasting transferrin saturation** (>45%) is suggestive of the diagnosis.
- Other nonspecific laboratory tests include **elevated serum iron** and **ferritin** levels.
- The diagnosis is confirmed by the presence of **specific mutations in the HFE gene**.

Imaging

MRI is the imaging of choice for noninvasive assessment of iron storage in the liver.

Diagnostic Procedures

Liver biopsy is not required to establish the diagnosis of HH; however, it is helpful in staging the disease, especially in individuals at increased risk of advanced fibrosis/cirrhosis and in those with iron overload without typical HFE gene mutations.

TREATMENT

- Asymptomatic individuals homozygous for the HFE gene mutation with iron overload should be treated. Symptomatic individuals should also be treated to minimize extent of end-organ damage.
- Therapy consists of weekly **phlebotomy** until iron depletion is achieved (ferritin level <50 μg/L and transferrin saturation <30%). Maintenance phlebotomy of 2–4 units of blood yearly is continued for life, with goal ferritin levels between 50 and 100 μg/L.
- Treatment with phlebotomy before the onset of cirrhosis or diabetes significantly reduces the morbidity and mortality of HH.
- Phlebotomy can improve ALT/AST levels, skin pigmentation, hepatic fibrosis, daily insulin requirements, and symptoms of weakness, lethargy, and abdominal pain.
- HH-related hypogonadism, cirrhosis, destructive arthritis, and diabetes are usually irreversible.
- **Erythrocytapheresis** is a recent alternative that selectively removes RBCs and returns valuable blood components. It is useful in patients with hypoproteinemia and/or thrombocytopenia.

Medications

Deferoxamine, deferasirox, and deferiprone are iron-chelating agents used in the setting of HH, if phlebotomy is contraindicated secondary to severe anemia, cardiac failure, poor venous access, or poor tolerance.[22] They are usually used in secondary iron overload.

Surgical Management

- Liver transplantation may be considered in cases of HH with cirrhosis.
- Patients who undergo liver transplantation for HH tend to have poorer 1- and 5-year survival rates when compared with other liver transplant recipients.

Prognosis

Patients with appropriately treated HH without cirrhosis have survival rates identical to that of the general population.

α_1-Antitrypsin Deficiency

GENERAL PRINCIPLES

Definition

α_1-AT deficiency is an autosomal recessive disorder with codominant expression in which a mutant α_1-AT protein is formed. Retention of mutant α_1-AT protein in hepatocytes and decreased serum α_1-AT levels causes cirrhosis and panlobular emphysema.

Epidemiology

- PiZZ genotype has an incidence of about 1:3500 and occurs mostly in people of Northern European ancestry. More than 30% of patients with PiZZ genotype develop cirrhosis (more common in older males).
- The disease onset has a bimodal distribution from neonatal hepatitis and cholestatic jaundice in infants to chronic liver disease in adults (fifth decade of life).[23]
- There is an increased incidence of cholangiocarcinoma and HCC in PiZZ patients.

Pathophysiology

- α_1-AT is a serine protease inhibitor (prime inhibitor of neutrophil elastase). Accumulation of misfolded α_1-AT in the endoplasmic reticulum of the hepatocytes produces hepatic injury. Deficiency of serum α_1-AT causes lung injury because of uninhibited proteolytic damage to the lung connective tissue from unopposed action of elastase.
- The gene associated with this disorder is located on chromosome 14. The most common allele is M which gives rise to the normal protein protease inhibitor (PI) M.
- The most common deficiency alleles are S (expresses 50–60% of α_1-AT) and Z (expresses 10–20% of α_1-AT), with S being slightly more prevalent. Deficiency genotypes associated with liver disease include PiSZ, PiZZ, and possibly PiMZ. PiZZ genotype is associated with more severe disease manifestations.

Associated Conditions

Associated conditions include panniculitis, systemic vasculitis, interstitial fibrosis (in patients with rheumatoid arthritis), peripheral neuropathy, multiple sclerosis, intracranial aneurysms, and membranoproliferative glomerulonephritis.

DIAGNOSIS

Clinical Presentation

- Patients may present with clinical features of cholestasis or cirrhosis. Asymptomatic patients present with isolated abnormal aminotransferases.
- α_1-AT deficiency can present as emphysema in early adulthood.

Diagnostic Criteria

It includes quantification of the protease inhibitor and genotyping.

Diagnostic Testing

Laboratory Testing
- **Low serum α_1-AT level** (<10–15% of normal) is suggestive of the disease.
- Other suggestive tests include decreased α_1-globulin level (protein electrophoresis). Patients with proven enzyme deficiency should be tested for their α_1-AT genotype.

Diagnostic Procedures
Liver biopsy is essential for diagnosis. It shows characteristic periodic acid–Schiff-positive, diastase-resistant intracellular globules in the periportal hepatocytes.

TREATMENT

Medications

Currently, **no specific medical treatment** exists for the liver disease associated with α_1-AT deficiency. Gene therapy along with medications that stimulate autophagy is a potential future alternative for these patients. For patients with emphysema, "augmentation therapy" (IV purified pooled human plasma α_1-AT) raises serum α_1-AT levels but does not necessarily improve the rate of FEV1 decline.[24]

Surgical Management

- Liver transplantation is indicated in patients with α_1-AT deficiency and decompensated cirrhosis.
- Liver transplantation corrects the underlying disorder by normalizing α_1-AT production. It is unclear whether liver transplantation slows the onset of emphysema.

Wilson Disease

GENERAL PRINCIPLES

Definition

WD is an autosomal recessive disorder that results in progressive copper overload in the liver, kidney, brain, and cornea due to defective biliary excretion.[25]

Epidemiology

- The incidence of WD is 1:30,000.
- It usually presents primarily as hepatic disease in younger patients with neurologic or psychiatric symptoms in the second decade of life.

Pathophysiology

- WD is caused by a mutation in the ATP7B gene located on chromosome 13.
- Absence or reduced function of the ATP7B gene results in decreased hepatocyte excretion of copper, precipitating copper accumulation within the liver.
- Progressive copper buildup results in hepatocyte injury, fibrosis, and cirrhosis.
- Copper is subsequently released into the bloodstream and deposited into the brain, kidneys, and cornea.

Prevention

DNA testing for family members of affected individuals is becoming commercially available.
- The analysis requires identification of the patient's ATP7B gene mutation or haplotype; this same haplotype is screened for in first-degree relatives.
- Many patients are compound heterozygotes, making identification of mutations more difficult.
- To date, more than 500 mutations of the ATP7B gene have been identified.

DIAGNOSIS

Clinical Presentation

- WD can present as chronic hepatitis, cirrhosis, or rarely as fulminant hepatic failure.
- The diagnosis should be considered in patients with unexplained liver disease with or without neuropsychiatric symptoms, first-degree relatives with WD, or individuals with fulminant hepatic failure.
- **Neuropsychiatric manifestations** include asymmetric tremor ("wing-beating" appearance), dysarthria, ataxia, dystonia, and psychiatric features.
- **Other extrahepatic manifestations** include **Kayser–Fleischer rings** on slit-lamp examination (gold to brown rings caused by copper deposition in Descemet membrane in the periphery of the cornea), **hemolytic anemia, renal tubular acidosis, arthritis,** and **osteopenia**.

Diagnostic Testing

Diagnosis is based on laboratory studies, imaging, and liver biopsy.

Laboratory Testing

- Laboratory findings include **low ceruloplasmin levels** (<20 mg/dL), although normal values do not rule out the diagnosis. Low alkaline phosphatase levels and mild increase in transaminases can be seen.
- **Elevated serum free copper level (nonceruloplasmin bound)** (>200 µg/dL) and **elevated 24-hour urinary copper level** (>100 mg/24 hrs) may also be detected. These

laboratory tests are better used for monitoring treatment in patients with WD than for diagnostic purposes.

Imaging

Brain imaging can demonstrate basal ganglia changes due to copper accumulation.

Diagnostic Procedures

- Liver biopsy findings are nonspecific and depend on the presentation and stage of the disease.
- Liver histology can include steatosis, glycogenated nuclei, chronic hepatitis, fibrosis, and cirrhosis.
- Elevated hepatic copper levels >250 μg/g dry weight (normal <40 μg/g dry weight) on biopsy are highly suggestive of WD.

TREATMENT

Medications

- Treatment is with copper-chelating agents or zinc salts.[26] Chelating agents like trientine and penicillamine are used for initial and maintenance therapy, whereas zinc salts are used for maintenance therapy. Dietary restriction of copper containing food should be used in conjunction with drug treatment.
- Patients require lifelong therapy.
- **Chelating agents**
  - **Penicillamine**
    - Penicillamine 1–2 g/day PO in divided doses BID or QID plus pyridoxine 2.5 mg/day can be used in patients with hepatic failure.
    - Penicillamine should never be given as initial treatment to patients with neurologic symptoms.
    - Side effects include hypersensitivity rashes, bone marrow suppression, proteinuria, systemic lupus erythematosus, or Goodpasture syndrome.
  - **Trientine**
    - Trientine 1–2 g/day PO in divided doses BID or QID is also used.
    - Side effects are similar to those of penicillamine but occur in lower frequency. The risk of neurologic decompensation with trientine is less than with penicillamine.
  - **Tetrathiomolybdate**
    - Tetrathiomolybdate is both a chelating agent and inhibitor of copper absorption; the normal dose is 120 mg/day divided as 20 mg TID with meals and 60 mg at bedtime (without food). It can be given with zinc therapy.
    - Tetrathiomolybdate is the treatment of choice for patients presenting with neurologic symptoms. It has a good safety profile; possible side effects include anemia, leukopenia, and mild elevations of aminotransferases.
- **Zinc salts**
  - **Zinc salts** at a dose of 50 mg PO TID are indicated for treatment of WD in patients with chronic hepatitis and cirrhosis in the absence of hepatic failure.
  - It can be used in association with penicillamine and trientine.
  - Other than gastric irritation, zinc has a very good safety profile.
- **Other nonpharmacologic therapies**
  - Liver transplantation is the therapy of choice for fulminant hepatic failure and for progressive liver dysfunction despite chelation therapy.
  - Plasmapheresis and hemofiltration may help bridge patients to transplant by markedly reducing serum copper levels, thereby reducing hemolysis and second organ damage.
  - In the absence of neurologic symptoms, liver transplantation has a good prognosis and requires no further medical treatment.

REFERENCES

1. Lok AS, McMahon B. AASLD practice guidelines. Chronic hepatitis B: update 2009. *Hepatology.* 2009;50:1–36.
2. European Association for the Study of the Liver. Electronic address: easloffice@easloffice.eu; European Association for the Study of the Liver. EASL 2017 clinical practice guidelines on the management of hepatitis B virus infection. *J Hepatol.* 2017;67:370–398.
3. Yuen MF, Lai C. Treatment of chronic hepatitis B: evolution over two decades. *J Gastroenterol Hepatol.* 2011;26:138–143.
4. Ghany MG, Strader DB, Thomas DL, et al. Diagnosis, management, and treatment of hepatitis C: an update. *Hepatology.* 2009;49:1335–1374.
5. European Association for the Study of the Liver. Electronic address: easloffice@easloffice.eu. EASL recommendations on treatment of hepatitis C 2016. *J Hepatol.* 2017;66:153–194.
6. Rambaldi A, Saconato HH, Christensen E, et al. Systematic review: glucocorticoids for alcoholic hepatitis—a Cochrane Hepato-Biliary Group systematic review with meta-analyses and trial sequential analysis of randomized clinical trials. *Aliment Pharmacol Ther.* 2008;27:1167–1178.
7. European Association for the Study of Liver. EASL clinical practice guidelines: management of alcoholic liver disease. *J Hepatol.* 2012;57:399–420.
8. Neuschwander-Tetri B, Clark J, Bass N, et al. Clinical, laboratory and histological associations in adults with nonalcoholic fatty liver disease. *Hepatology.* 2010;52:913–924.
9. Tapper EB, Lok AS. Use of liver imaging and biopsy in clinical practice. *N Eng J Med.* 2017;377:756–768.
10. European Association for the Study of the Liver (EASL); European Association for the Study of Diabetes (EASD); European Association for the Study of Obesity (EASO). EASL-EASD-EASO clinical practice guidelines for the management of non-alcoholic fatty liver disease. *J Hepatol.* 2016;64:1388–1402.
11. Chalasani N, Younossi Z, Lavine JE, et al. The diagnosis and management of nonalcoholic fatty liver disease: practice guidance from AASLD. *Hepatology.* 2018;67:328–357.
12. Yeoman AD, Longhi MS, Heneghan MA. Review article: the modern management of autoimmune hepatitis. *Aliment Pharmacol Ther.* 2010;31:771–787.
13. Manns M, Woynarowski M, Kreisel W, et al. Budesonide induces remission more effectively than prednisone in a controlled trial of patients with autoimmune hepatitis. *Gastroenterology.* 2010;139:1198–1206.
14. European Association for the Study of the Liver. EASL clinical practice guidelines: autoimmune hepatitis. *J Hepatol.* 2015;63:971–1004.
15. European Association for the Study of the Liver. EASL clinical practice guidelines: management of cholestatic liver diseases. *J Hepatol.* 2009;51:237–267.
16. Gidwaney N, Pawa S, Das KM. Pathogenesis and clinical spectrum of primary sclerosing cholangitis. *World J Gastroenterol.* 2017;23:2459–2469.
17. Lindor KD, Kowdley KV, Luketic VA, et al. High-dose ursodeoxycholic acid for the treatment of primary sclerosing cholangitis. *Hepatology.* 2009;50:808–814.
18. European Association for the Study of the Liver. Electronic address: easloffice@easloffice.eu; European Association for the Study of the Liver. EASL clinical practice guideline. The diagnosis and management of patients with primary biliary cholangitis. *J Hepatol.* 2017;67:145–172.
19. Complications of Cholestasis. *The Washington Manual of Therapeutics.* 35th ed. Lippincott and Williams; 2016:597–599.
20. Rombout-Sestrienkova E, van Kraaij MG, Koek GH. How we manage patients with hereditary hemochromatosis. *Br J Hematol.* 2016;175:759–770.
21. Pietrangelo A. Hereditary hemochromatosis: pathogenesis, diagnosis, and treatment. *Gastroenterology.* 2010;139:393–408.
22. Phatak P, Brissot P, Wurster M, et al. A phase 1/2, dose-escalation trial of deferasirox for the treatment of iron overload in HFE-related hereditary hemochromatosis. *Hepatology.* 2010;52:1671–1679.
23. Fairbanks K, Tavill A. Liver disease in alpha 1-antitrypsin deficiency: a review. *Am J Gastroenterol.* 2008;103:2136–2141.
24. Lomas DA, Hurst JR, Gooptu B. Update on alpha-1 antitrypsin deficiency: new therapies. *J Hepatol.* 2016;65:413–424.
25. European Association for Study of Liver. EASL clinical practice guidelines: Wilson's disease. *J Hepatol.* 2012;56:671–685.
26. Roberts EA, Schilsky ML. Diagnosis and treatment of Wilson disease: an update. *Hepatology.* 2008;47:2089–2111.

21

Cirrhosis

Rajeev Ramgopal and Jeffrey S. Crippin

GENERAL PRINCIPLES

- Cirrhosis is the common endpoint of a multitude of insults to the liver, with myriad complications caused by progressive liver dysfunction and portal hypertension.
- Ascites, hepatic encephalopathy (HE), gastrointestinal (GI) bleeding, and renal dysfunction are the major sources of morbidity and mortality.
- Treatment of the underlying cause of cirrhosis as well as prevention of complications are the mainstays of treatment.
- Screening for hepatocellular carcinoma (HCC) and evaluation for liver transplantation are important steps in management.

Definition

- Cirrhosis is a pathologic diagnosis.
- The World Health Organization defines cirrhosis as a "diffuse process characterized by fibrosis and conversion of normal liver architecture into structurally abnormal nodules which lack normal lobular organization."[1]

Classification

- Classified by morphology, histology, and etiologic agent[1]:
  - Morphology may be classified as micronodular, macronodular, or mixed.
  - Histology may be classified as portal, postnecrotic, posthepatitic, biliary, or congestive.
  - Etiology corresponds to specific morphologic and histologic findings.
- Clinical classification using **Child–Turcotte–Pugh score (CTP)** (Table 21-1).[2]
  - This scoring system incorporates ascites, presence of encephalopathy, serum albumin, total bilirubin, and prothrombin time (PT).
  - It can be used to determine 1-year mortality.

Epidemiology

- According to the Summary Health Statistics from 2015, approximately 3.9 million adults suffer from chronic liver disease, including cirrhosis. However, this number may be an underestimate, as 2.2–3.2 million US adults have chronic hepatitis C infection.[3,4]
- Cirrhosis is the twelfth leading cause of death in the United States with 38,170 deaths/yr.[5]
- Cirrhosis is the fourth leading cause of death among both men and women of age 45–64 years.[5]

Etiology

- Cirrhosis is a common endpoint for many causes of liver disease (Table 21-2), with alcoholic liver disease and hepatitis C accounting for the majority of cases.[6]
- Other causes include autoimmune hepatitis, Wilson disease, hemochromatosis, nonalcoholic fatty liver disease, drug hepatotoxicity, and cryptogenic cirrhosis.[6]

TABLE 21-1 CHILD–TURCOTTE–PUGH SCORING SYSTEM

Criteria	1	2	3
Ascites	None	Slight	Moderate-severe
Encephalopathy	None	Mild	Moderate-severe
Bilirubin, mg/dL	<2	2–3	>3
Albumin, g/dL	>3.5	2.8–3.5	<2.8
Prothrombin time (seconds above normal prothrombin time)	1–3	4–6	>6

Child's class determined by adding scores from each of the five criteria together: class A, 5–6 points; class B, 7–9 points; class C, 10–15 points.

Pathophysiology

- The pathway to cirrhosis begins with hepatocellular damage. Fenestrated sinusoids with absent intercellular junctions and basement membranes ensure close interactions between the sinusoidal blood and hepatocytes; therefore, hepatocytes are sensitive to blood-borne toxins.[7]
- Hepatocellular injury leads to the initiation of an inflammatory cascade with the release of cytokines, which amplify and sustain the overall response.
- Cytokines activate effector cells, especially hepatic stellate cells, initiating an autocrine loop of inflammation and fibrosis.[7–9]
  - Stellate cells are transformed into myofibroblasts which have highly fibrinogenic, contractile, and proliferative properties. Due to this contractility, there is increased intrahepatic resistance and decreased sinusoidal blood flow.
  - Stellate cell transformation also leads to "capillarization" of the hepatic sinusoids with a shift from fenestrated sinusoids to "nonfenestrated" capillaries.
  - Capillarization induces a shift toward vasoconstriction, with increased production of endothelin and decreased production of nitric oxide.
- Thrombosis of the microvasculature occurs with formation of intrahepatic arterial shunts.[9]
- An erratic proliferation of hepatocytes takes place in hypoperfused areas, leading to a nodular pattern of regeneration within areas of fibrosis.

Risk Factors

- Cirrhosis is a common endpoint of chronic diseases that cause hepatic injury.
- These include chronic viral hepatitis, alcohol liver disease, iron overload, and chronic inflammatory conditions, such as nonalcoholic steatohepatitis.
  - **Alcohol:** men with intake of >168 g/wk; women with intake of >112 g/wk. A standard drink, as defined in the United States, contains roughly 14 g of alcohol.[10]
  - **Hepatitis C:** intravenous drug use or transfusion prior to 1992, and HIV infection.[11]

DIAGNOSIS

Many patients present with overt complications of cirrhosis; however, one must have a high clinical suspicion in patients with subtle or no symptoms. Manifestations of cirrhosis in different organ systems are presented in Table 21-3.

TABLE 21-2 EVALUATION OF CIRRHOSIS

Historical Factors	Laboratory Evaluation	Suspected Cause
Excessive alcohol use	Increased AST to ALT ratio	Alcoholic liver disease
Intravenous drug abuse, tattoos, multiple sexual partners, sharing of needles, transfusions before 1992	Positive hepatitis B or C serologies	Chronic viral hepatitis
Fatigue, jaundice, pruritus	Antimitochondrial antibody, elevated alkaline phosphatase	Primary biliary cholangitis/cirrhosis
Ulcerative colitis, bacterial cholangitis, or cholangiocarcinoma	Elevated alkaline phosphatase	Primary sclerosing cholangitis
Neuropsychiatric symptoms	Kaiser–Fleischer rings, low serum ceruloplasmin, high urinary copper	Wilson disease
Skin changes, arthritis, diabetes mellitus, hypogonadism	Ferritin, iron studies, hemochromatosis gene (HFE) mutations	Hemochromatosis
Autoimmune disease	ANA, increased serum quantitative immunoglobulins, smooth muscle antibody	Autoimmune hepatitis
Diabetes mellitus, obesity, dyslipidemia	Dyslipidemia, elevated levels of sugars	Nonalcoholic fatty liver disease
Emphysema without smoking history, positive family history	Emphysema, phenotype testing (PiZZ phenotype), α_1-antitrypsin level	α_1-Antitrypsin deficiency
Methotrexate or amiodarone use		Drug hepatotoxicity
History of anasarca, venous thromboembolism, or malignancy	Hypercoagulable state, nephrotic syndrome, paroxysmal nocturnal hemoglobinuria	Budd–Chiari syndrome
Stem cell transplant		Sinusoidal obstructive syndrome
Unknown factors		Cryptogenic cirrhosis

ALT, alanine aminotransferase; ANA, antinuclear antibody; AST, aspartate aminotransferase.

TABLE 21-3   MANIFESTATIONS AND PRESENTATION OF CIRRHOSIS

Constitutional	Fatigue, weight loss, anorexia, malaise, muscle wasting
Gastrointestinal	Hematemesis, melena, esophageal or gastric varices, portal hypertensive gastropathy, gastritis, ascites
Pulmonary	Shortness of breath, dyspnea on exertion, hypoxia, hepatopulmonary syndrome, respiratory alkalosis, hepatic hydrothorax, portopulmonary syndrome
Cardiovascular	Hypotension, hyperdynamic circulation
Renal	Hepatorenal syndrome, hyponatremia
Endocrine	Decreased libido, impotence, testicular atrophy, dysmenorrhea, gynecomastia
Neurologic	Confusion, short-term memory loss, hyperirritability, insomnia encephalopathy
Dermatologic	Jaundice, spider angioma, palmar erythema, Dupuytren contracture, caput medusae
Hematologic	Splenomegaly, thrombocytopenia, anemia, leukopenia, coagulopathy
Infectious	Spontaneous bacterial peritonitis, sepsis

Clinical Presentation

- **Subtle symptoms** include anorexia, nausea/vomiting, hyperirritability, pruritus, change in sleep pattern, decreased libido, shortness of breath.
- **Overt complications** of cirrhosis
  - Hematemesis/melena, abdominal distention, ascites, confusion, edema/fluid overload.
  - Complications can also include a myriad of infections, coagulopathy, acute on chronic liver failure, hepatopulmonary syndrome, and HCC.

History

- The history should focus on common causes of liver disease and cirrhosis.
- Duration and quantity of alcohol intake, intravenous/intranasal drug use, sexual activity, family history of liver disease, prescription medications, and over-the-counter drug use.
- Personal history of ulcerative colitis, metabolic syndrome, premature emphysema, and history of autoimmune disease places patients at risk for primary sclerosing cholangitis, nonalcoholic fatty liver disease, α_1-antitrypsin deficiency, and autoimmune hepatitis, respectively.
- A history of a hypercoagulable state or prior malignancy may lead to hepatic venous thrombosis (Budd–Chiari syndrome). A stem cell or bone marrow transplant increases the risk of sinusoidal obstructive syndrome.
- A constellation of skin changes, arthritis, diabetes mellitus, and hypogonadism is seen in individuals with hereditary hemochromatosis.

Physical Examination

Cirrhosis can lead to specific physical findings.

- These physical examination findings can include muscle wasting, jaundice, spider angiomata, gynecomastia, caput medusae, prominent venous collaterals, palmar erythema, Dupuytren contracture, testicular atrophy, and ecchymoses.

- Splenomegaly, a coarse liver edge, and evidence of ascites (fluid wave, dullness in flanks, and/or shifting dullness) may be present on abdominal examination.
- Rectal examination may reveal hemorrhoids, guaiac-positive stools, or melena.
- Confusion, agitation, asterixis, and hyporeflexia are signs of HE.

Diagnostic Testing

Etiology-specific testing for the cause of cirrhosis should be performed as outlined in Table 21-2; however, evaluation should begin with basic laboratory studies.

Laboratory Testing

- Complete blood cell count, basic metabolic panel, and hepatic function panel
  - **Complete blood cell count** may reveal macrocytic anemia due to liver disease or microcytic/normocytic anemia due to GI blood loss. Leukocytosis can be an indicator of underlying infection, especially spontaneous bacterial peritonitis (SBP) in the setting of ascites. Leukopenia and thrombocytopenia are markers of hypersplenism due to portal hypertension.
  - **Basic metabolic panel** may reveal hyponatremia in the setting of fluid overload or intravascular volume depletion. Blood urea nitrogen (BUN) and serum creatinine (SCr) may be acutely elevated because of the hepatorenal syndrome (HRS). Hypoglycemia may be present due to dysregulation of hepatic compensatory mechanisms.
  - **Hepatic function panel** may show hypoalbuminemia which reflects impaired hepatic synthetic function. Serum bilirubin may be elevated indicating an acute insult superimposed on chronic disease versus poor hepatic function. Transaminase elevations may indicate acute on chronic liver disease; however, the aspartate aminotransferase and alanine aminotransferase will often be normal to mildly elevated.
- Coagulation studies and ammonia
  - **Clotting factors** are synthesized in the liver. Therefore, clotting is often abnormal, with elevated PT/international normalized ratio (INR). PT/INR can be used as a marker for evaluating synthetic function.
  - **Ammonia level** is often used in the diagnosis and treatment of HE. However, ammonia levels have very poor specificity and are not particularly useful in the diagnosis of HE; some use ammonia levels to monitor treatment response, but no convincing data exist for reliability in monitoring a patient's course.

Imaging

- Imaging studies of the liver are useful in assessing the size and echotexture of the liver, the presence of ascites, biliary ductal dilation, and splenomegaly. Imaging can also be used to screen for liver masses such as HCC.
- Ultrasonography, computed tomography, and magnetic resonance imaging (MRI) are commonly used.
  - **Ultrasonography** has the added benefit of evaluating the hepatic vasculature and grading the severity of portal hypertension via color Doppler.
  - **MRI or magnetic resonance cholangiopancreatography (MRCP)** may be used to further characterize masses, assess the hepatic vasculature, and evaluate the biliary tree.
  - **Endoscopic retrograde cholangiopancreatography** allows direct imaging and intervention of the biliary tree.

Diagnostic Procedures

- **Paracentesis**
  - A diagnostic paracentesis should be performed on all patients admitted to the hospital with ascites as the prevalence of SBP among cirrhosis patients has been shown to be as high as 12%.[12] There is no need to correct coagulopathy prior to paracentesis unless the platelet count is <15,000/μL or INR is >2.5.[13]

Fluid sample should be obtained for cell count with differential albumin level, and protein level.

- An absolute ascites neutrophil count of >250 cells/μL suggests SBP. A bedside blood culture bottle inoculation with ascitic fluid should be performed if SBP is suspected.
- Serum ascites albumin gradient (SAAG) >1.1 suggests portal hypertension or heart failure while a SAAG <1.1 suggests peritoneal carcinomatosis or tuberculous peritonitis: See Chapter 10 for explanation of SAAG.
- An ascitic fluid total protein level >2.5 g/dL may suggest alternate etiologies such as heart failure, whereas a protein level <2.5 g/dL is consistent with portal hypertension due to cirrhosis.

- **Liver biopsy** is not necessary if imaging, laboratory, and clinical findings are consistent with cirrhosis. It may be useful if the specific etiology of cirrhosis needs to be determined.

TREATMENT

- Management focuses on treatment of the underlying cause of cirrhosis and management of complications. Complications of cirrhosis include GI hemorrhage, encephalopathy, ascites, SBP, and HRS.
- **GI hemorrhage**
  - Upper GI bleeding in cirrhotic patients is usually caused by variceal rupture, gastritis, portal hypertensive gastropathy, or peptic ulcer disease. Varices are present in 30–40% of patients with compensated cirrhosis and 60% of patients with ascites. The annual incidence of new varices is 5–10%.[14]
  - In addition to fluid resuscitation, octreotide infusion[14] (to lower portal pressure) and antibiotic therapy[15] with a third-generation cephalosporin (to reduce the risk of SBP, rebleeding, and mortality) are indicated early in the presentation. Endoscopic variceal ligation (EVL) is currently the mainstay of endoscopic therapy in acute variceal bleeding. See Chapter 6 for further details regarding treatment of GI hemorrhage.
  - Prevention and follow-up
    - **Periodic endoscopic evaluation** is essential to identify varices and prevent progression to variceal bleeding.
    - In patients with compensated cirrhosis with no varices on screening endoscopy, EGD should be performed every 2–3 years. In those with small varices (<5 mm), EGD should be repeated in 1–2 years.[14]
    - When cirrhosis is either decompensated or secondary to alcohol abuse, patients without known varices should undergo a yearly screening EGD.[14]
    - Patients who survive an episode of active bleeding should have repeat EVL until obliteration of varices. The first surveillance EGD is performed 1–3 months after obliteration and is repeated every 6–12 months to check for recurrence.[14]
    - Conventional **nonselective β-blockers** (nadolol, propranolol, or timolol) and carvedilol are used for prevention of variceal bleeding. β-Blockers decrease cardiac output and produce splanchnic vasoconstriction.
    - American Association for the Study of Liver Diseases (AASLD) does not recommend nonselective β-blocker use in patients with cirrhosis without varices.[14]
    - A trial comprising 200 patients followed for 55 months without evidence of prior varices showed no difference in the development of varices (39% vs. 40%) in patients on β-blockers versus placebo.[16]
    - AASLD recommends use of a nonselective β-blocker in patients with small varices with high-risk features, and in patients with medium and large varices. High-risk features include the red wale sign on endoscopy and CTP class C cirrhosis.[14]
    - Two separate meta-analyses comparing β-blockers with placebo showed a 40–50% reduction in the risk of bleeding.[17,18]

TABLE 21-4 GRADES OF ENCEPHALOPATHY

Grade	Characteristics
1	Sleep reversal pattern, mild confusion, irritability, tremor
2	Lethargy, disorientation, inappropriate behavior, asterixis
3	Somnolence/stupor, severe confusion, aggressive behavior, asterixis
4	Coma

- For secondary prophylaxis after a sentinel bleeding event, a combination of β-blockers and EVL should be used as the first-line therapy to prevent rebleeding.[14]
- β-Blockers should be dose reduced or discontinued in the setting of refractory ascites, severe hypotension, infection, and unexplained acute kidney injury (AKI).[14,19]
- **Proton pump inhibitors** should be considered in patients with peptic ulcer disease or other erosive findings on endoscopy; however, there is no recommendation for the use of a proton pump inhibitor in managing portal hypertensive gastropathy or esophageal varices.

- **Hepatic encephalopathy**
  - HE is a neuropsychiatric disorder associated with severe liver disease and is graded according to the West Haven criteria (Table 21-4).
  - Excess ammonia is central to the pathogenesis of this process due to the acceleration of astrocyte swelling and cerebral edema; however, the precise molecular mechanism is unclear.[20]
  - Despite its role in encephalopathy, ammonia levels have very poor specificity in the diagnosis and monitoring of HE.
  - HE is a **diagnosis of exclusion** and other causes of altered mental status *must* be ruled out.
  - The diagnosis is made on clinical grounds with altered mental status, asterixis, and hypo- or hyperreflexia. A precipitating cause for encephalopathy, such as sepsis, GI bleeding, constipation, dehydration, or electrolyte abnormality, should be identified and treated once the diagnosis of HE is made (Table 21-5).

TABLE 21-5 COMMON PRECIPITANTS OF HEPATIC ENCEPHALOPATHY

Gastrointestinal bleeding

Post-TIPS

Constipation

Spontaneous bacterial peritonitis and other infections

Narcotics or benzodiazepine use

Hepatocellular carcinoma

Worsening liver function

Diuretic use

Alkalosis

Hypokalemia

TIPS, transjugular intrahepatic portosystemic shunt.

Patients with grade 3 and 4 encephalopathy may require close monitoring in an intensive care unit setting with endotracheal intubation for airway protection. The risk of cerebral edema increases with progression of encephalopathy. Advanced cerebral edema can lead to uncal herniation and death. This is much more common in patients with acute liver failure; however, it can be seen in patients with chronic liver disease.

Medications:

- **Lactulose**, a disaccharide broken down by gut bacteria, is the mainstay of treatment due to its ability to reduce intraluminal pH, converting ammonia to ammonium, decreasing its absorption, and allowing it to be purged from the colon.[20]
    - Lactulose can be administered orally, rectally, or through a nasogastric tube, with a typical dose of 60–90 g/day, titrated to three to five loose bowel movements daily.
    - Abdominal bloating and diarrhea are the major side effects of lactulose; however, overtreatment with lactulose may lead to severe dehydration and hypernatremia.
- **Rifaximin** is a minimally absorbed oral antibiotic with FDA approval for the treatment of HE. It is recommended as an add-on therapy for preventing recurrent episodes of HE. A study published in 2010 demonstrated that remission of HE was prolonged in patients treated with rifaximin.[20] Rifaximin is administered orally at a dose of 550 mg twice daily.

Prevention and follow-up

- After resolution of HE, patients with cirrhosis tend to remain on empiric therapy with lactulose and rifaximin for an indefinite period of time or until they undergo transplantation.
- Patients should be educated on possible precipitants of HE such as dehydration, sedatives, opioid medications, poor compliance with lactulose therapy, and constipation.

- **Ascites**
    - Ascites is the most common complication seen in cirrhotic patients, with approximately 50% of patients with compensated cirrhosis developing ascites during 10 years of follow-up.
    - Approximately 85% of patients with ascites in the United States have cirrhosis.[13]
    - Ascites is caused by the activation of the renin–angiotensin–aldosterone system and sympathetic nervous system in response to splanchnic vasodilatation and arterial underfilling in the setting of portal hypertension. The activation of the renin–angiotensin–aldosterone system causes fluid retention and elevated hydrostatic pressure in the splanchnic microcirculation. Elevated hydrostatic pressure and low oncotic pressure cause increased lymph production, and once lymph production surpasses lymph return, ascites develops.
    - Patients present with increased abdominal girth, shortness of breath, and lower extremity edema. Common physical findings include dullness to percussion in the flanks, shifting dullness, pleural effusion, a fluid wave, and umbilical and inguinal hernias.
    - A paracentesis allows analysis of ascitic fluid (see Chapter 10).
    - Medications:
        - **Spironolactone**, an aldosterone antagonist, is first-line therapy for ascites due to cirrhosis. Hyperkalemia and breast tenderness are common side effects.[13]
        - **Furosemide**, a loop diuretic, is usually given with spironolactone.
        - Spironolactone and furosemide are prescribed at a ratio of 2.5:1, usually at a starting dose of 100 and 40 mg daily, respectively.[13]
            - This ratio often prevents hyperkalemia.
            - Dosage of each medication can be increased every 3–5 days to a maximum daily dose of 400 mg of spironolactone and 160 mg of furosemide.[13]

- Amiloride can be substituted for spironolactone in the setting of tender gynecomastia. Triamterene, metolazone, and hydrochlorothiazide may also be used in the treatment of ascites.
- The goal of diuretic therapy is the loss of 0.5 and 1 kg/day if peripheral edema is present.[13]
- Diuretic resistant or refractory ascites can be treated with large-volume paracenteses (LVP). If an LVP is required every 1–2 weeks, a TIPS may be needed, if there are no contraindications.
- In a meta-analysis, TIPS was more effective at decreasing ascites without a significant difference in mortality, GI bleeding, infection, and acute renal failure but with a significantly higher rate of HE.[21]

○ Dietary changes
- **Sodium restriction** to 2 g/day is an important component of the treatment of ascites. Salt restriction and diuretic therapy are effective in 90% of patients with ascites.
  □ Two grams of sodium is equivalent to 88 mmol/day. The body loses about 10 mmol/day of sodium chloride (NaCl) via sweat. Therefore, the kidney must excrete NaCl at a rate of 78 mmol/day to maintain homeostasis.[13]
  □ A spot urine study can determine which patient may respond to sodium restriction without diuretic therapy. If the urine sodium is greater than the urine potassium, the patient is excreting >78 mmol/day of NaCl and will respond to salt restriction alone.[13]
- **Hyponatremia** is often seen in the setting of ascites. A daily oral fluid restriction of 800–1200 mL/day can be utilized but efficacy data are lacking for this regimen. Current guidelines suggest daily fluid restrictions only when serum sodium is <125 mmol/L.[13]

● **Spontaneous bacterial peritonitis**
○ SBP is a common complication of cirrhosis and contributes to 25% of all bacterial infections seen in this population. It is caused by translocation of gut bacteria into the blood, causing transient bacteremia and seeding of ascitic fluid.
○ Presentation may be subtle, with abdominal pain, fever, chills, jaundice, or worsening encephalopathy. Up to half of patients with SBP are asymptomatic, and a diagnostic paracentesis with a 22- to 25-gauge needle is imperative, regardless of the reason for hospital admission.
○ A **diagnostic paracentesis is the gold standard diagnostic test**. Ascitic fluid should be sent for cell count with differential, Gram stain, and aerobic and anaerobic blood cultures. The presence of >250 polymorphonuclear cells/μL strongly suggests SBP and should be aggressively treated. A positive culture, regardless of the number of polymorphonuclear cells, should also be treated.
○ Medications:
  - A **third-generation cephalosporin administered for at least 5 days** is the standard of care.[13]
    □ **Cefotaxime** 1–2 g IV every 8–12 hours or **ceftriaxone** 1–2 g every 24 hours are effective therapies.
    □ If clinical deterioration is confirmed, coverage should be broadened to cover *Enterococcus,* methicillin-resistant *Staphylococcus aureus,* and anaerobic organisms.
  - Following repeated episodes of SBP, patients can be given **prophylactic antibiotic therapy,** such as norfloxacin 400 mg daily, ciprofloxacin 250 mg daily, or trimethoprim/sulfamethoxazole 800/160 five times per week.[13]
  - HRS is a feared complication of SBP and efforts to maintain adequate volume expansion are a necessity.
    □ Diuretics and LVP should be avoided in the setting of SBP.
    □ Albumin administration should be given to reduce the risk of HRS. A restricted approach to albumin administration can be utilized targeting patients with

high-risk features including a serum bilirubin >4 mg/dL, creatinine >1 mg/dL, or BUN >30 mg/dL.[22] In SBP patients treated with a third-generation cephalosporin, albumin administration at 1.5 g/kg on day 1 and 1 g/kg on day 3 is associated with a lower rate of renal failure (10% vs. 33%) and a lower hospital mortality rate (10% vs. 29%).[23]

- **Acute kidney injury and hepatorenal syndrome**
  - AKI is commonly encountered in cirrhotic patients. Based on recent modifications, AKI is now defined as an absolute increase in SCr of ≥0.3 mg/dL over 48 hours and/or an increase of ≥50% from baseline SCr. This change marks a shift from prior definitions that relied on an absolute SCr cutoffs (1.5 mg/dL).[24,25]
  - AKI in cirrhotic patients can be caused by **HRS**. Clinically HRS has been separated into two distinct types. **Type I HRS** is rapidly progressive and is often associated with a precipitating factor. Median survival is relatively short at 12 days, with >90% mortality at 10 weeks. **Type 2 HRS** is characterized by a steady and progressive reduction in GFR and recurrent, diuretic-resistant ascites. An identifiable precipitant may be difficult to find. Type 2 HRS is associated with a median survival of 3–6 months.
  - In patients with cirrhosis and ascites, the diagnosis of HRS is based on the following criteria[24]:
    - Diagnosis of AKI
    - No response within 48 hours to withholding diuretics and volume expansion with albumin
    - An absence of shock
    - No recent or current use of nephrotoxic agents
    - No other signs of kidney injury (absence of proteinuria >500 mg/day, absence of hematuria >50 RBC/HPF, normal findings on renal imaging)
  - Treatment of HRS can include a combination of vasoconstrictor therapy (terlipressin or octreotide and midodrine) with albumin, TIPS, liver transplantation, or a combination of these therapies.[26,27]

SPECIAL CONSIDERATIONS

- **HCC** is the second leading cause of death from cancer worldwide and the incidence in the United States is rapidly rising with an estimated 39,230 cases in 2016 alone.
- Surveillance with a liver ultrasound is recommended in specific populations with or without the use of serum α-fetoprotein (AFP) every 6 months.[28] Surveillance should be performed for the following populations:
  - Cirrhosis unless CTP class C and not on transplant list
  - Asian descendant with chronic hepatitis B (men >40 years, women >50 years)
  - Hepatitis B carrier with family history of HCC
  - African/North American blacks with chronic hepatitis B
- **Hepatopulmonary syndrome** can occur in up to 30% of cirrhotic patients and is defined by the triad of hypoxia, liver disease, and intrapulmonary shunting.[29]
  - Although patients are often asymptomatic, platypnea (shortness of breath with upright posture) and/or orthodeoxia (fall in arterial blood oxygen with upright posture) may be present.
  - Treatment options are limited to supplemental oxygen. Somatostatin analogs and inhaled nitric oxide inhibitors are possible strategies with uncertain efficacy.
  - Hepatopulmonary syndrome usually resolves following liver transplantation.
- **Portopulmonary hypertension** occurs in 2–5% of cirrhotic patients with portal hypertension and presents with dyspnea on exertion (most common), syncope, chest pain, fatigue, hemoptysis, or orthopnea. The prognosis is poor without treatment with a mean survival of 15 months.[29]

It is defined as precapillary pulmonary hypertension (mean pulmonary artery pressure >25 mm Hg) in the setting of portal hypertension.

Treatment is similar to primary pulmonary hypertension and consists of prostaglandin analogs, phosphodiesterase inhibitors, inhaled nitric oxide, and endothelin receptor antagonists.

- **Transplantation** is considered after the first episode of decompensation or worsening of liver function. The **Model for End-Stage Liver Disease (MELD) score** objectively evaluates liver function for patients listed for transplantation.[30]

It generates a number, ranging from 6–40, using SCr, total bilirubin, and INR in a complicated mathematical formula.

Higher scores are associated with a higher 90-day mortality.

MELD enables physicians to allocate donor livers to "sicker" patients, with higher scores given higher priority for allocated donor livers.

REFERENCES

1. Anthony PP, Ishak NG, Nayak NC. The morphology of cirrhosis: recommendations on definition, nomenclature, and classification by a working group sponsored by the World Health Organization. *J Clin Pathol.* 1978;31:395–414.
2. Child CG, Turcotte JG. Surgery and portal hypertension. In: Child CG, ed. *The Liver and Portal Hypertension.* Philadelphia, PA: Saunders; 1964:50–64.
3. Kochanek KD, Murphy SL, Xu JQ, et al. *Deaths: Final Data for 2014. National Vital Statistics Reports.* Vol 65, no 4. Hyattsville, MD: National Center for Health Statistics; 2016.
4. Denniston MM, Jiles RB, Drobeniuc J, et al. Chronic hepatitis C virus infection in the United States, National Health and Nutrition Examination Survey 2003 to 2010. *Ann Intern Med.* 2014;160:293–300.
5. National Center for Health Statistics. *Health, United States, 2016: With Chartbook on Long-Term Trends in Health.* Hyattsville, MD: Government Printing Office; 2017.
6. Bacon BR. Cirrhosis and its complications. In: Kasper DL, Fauci AS, Longo DL, et al., eds. *Harrison's Principle of Internal Medicine.* 19th ed. New York: McGraw-Hill; 2014.
7. Crawford JM. Liver and biliary tract. In: Vinay KV, Abbas AA, Fausto N, eds. *Robbins and Cotran Pathologic Basis of Disease.* 7th ed. Philadelphia, PA: Elsevier Saunders; 2005:877–927.
8. Rockey DC. Cell and molecular mechanisms of increased intrahepatic resistance and hemodynamic correlates. In: Sanyal AJ, Shah VH, eds. *Portal Hypertension: Pathobiology, Evaluation, and Treatment.* Totowa, NJ: Humana Press; 2005:37–50.
9. Pinzani M, Vizzutti F. Anatomy and vascular biology of the cells in the portal circulation. In: Sanyal AJ, Shah VH, eds. *Portal Hypertension: Pathobiology, Evaluation, and Treatment.* Totowa, NJ: Humana Press; 2005:15–36.
10. O'Shea RS, Dasarthy S, McCullough AJ. Alcoholic liver disease. *Hepatology.* 2010;51:307–328.
11. Ghany MG, Strader DB, Thomas DL, et al. Diagnosis, management and treatment of hepatitis C: an update. *Hepatology.* 2009;49:1335–1374.
12. Singal AK, Salameh H, Kamath PS. Prevalence and in-hospital mortality trends of infections among patients with cirrhosis: a nationwide study of hospitalised patients in the United States. *Aliment Pharmacol Ther.* 2014;40:105–112.
13. Runyon BA. Introduction to the revised American Association for the Study of Liver Diseases Practice Guideline management of adult patients with ascites due to cirrhosis 2012. *Hepatology.* 2013;57:1651–1653.
14. Garcia-Tsao G, Abraldes JG, Berzigotti A, et al. Portal hypertensive bleeding in cirrhosis: risk stratification, diagnosis, and management: 2016 practice guidance by the American Association for the Study of Liver Diseases. *Hepatology.* 2017;65:310–335.
15. Bernard B, Grange JD, Khac EN, et al. Antibiotic prophylaxis for the prevention of bacterial infections in cirrhotic patients with gastrointestinal bleeding: a meta-analysis. *Hepatology.* 1999;29:1655–1661.
16. Groszmann RJ, Garcia-Tsao G, Bosch J, et al. Beta-blockers to prevent gastroesophageal varices in patients with cirrhosis. *N Engl J Med.* 2005;353:2254–2261.
17. Hayes PC, Davis JM, Lewis JA, et al. Meta-analysis of value of propranolol in prevention of variceal haemorrhage. *Lancet.* 1990;336:153–156.

18. Vlachogiannakos J, Goulis J, Patch D, et al. Review article: primary prophylaxis for portal hypertensive bleeding in cirrhosis. *Alim Pharmacol Ther.* 2000;14(7):851–860.
19. Ge PS, Runyon BA. The changing role of beta-blocker therapy in patients with cirrhosis. *J Hepatol.* 2014;60:643–653.
20. Vilstrup H, Amodio P, Bajaj J, et al. Hepatic encephalopathy in chronic liver disease: 2014 practice guideline by the European Association for the study of the liver and the American Association for the Study of Liver Diseases. *J Hepatol.* 2014;61:642–659.
21. Saab S, Nieto JM, Lewis SK, et al. TIPS versus paracentesis for cirrhotic patients with refractory ascites. *Cochrane Database Syst Rev.* 2006;(4):CD004889.
22. Sigal SH, Stanca CM, Fernandez J, et al. Restricted use of albumin for spontaneous bacterial peritonitis. *Gut.* 2007;56:597–599.
23. Gines P, Tito L, Arroyo V, et al. Randomized comparative study of therapeutic paracentesis with and without intravenous albumin in cirrhosis. *Gastroenterology.* 1988;94:1493–1502.
24. Angeli P, Gines P, Wong F, et al. Diagnosis and management of acute kidney injury in patients with cirrhosis: revised consensus recommendations of the International Club of Ascites. *Gut.* 2015;64:531–537.
25. Wong F. Acute kidney injury in liver cirrhosis: new definition and application. *Clin Mol Hepatol.* 2016;22:415–422.
26. Salerno F, Gerbes A, Gines P, et al. Diagnosis, prevention and treatment of the hepatorenal syndrome in cirrhosis. *Gut.* 2007;56:1310–1318.
27. Cavallin M, Kamath PS, Merli M, et al. Terlipressin plus albumin versus midodrine and octreotide plus albumin in the treatment of hepatorenal syndrome: a randomized trial. *Hepatology.* 2015;62:567–574.
28. Heimbach J, Kulik LM, Finn R, et al. American Association for the Study of Liver Diseases guidelines for the treatment of hepatocellular carcinoma. *Hepatology.* 2018;67:358–380.
29. Surani SR, Mendez Y, Anjum H, et al. Pulmonary complications of hepatic diseases. *World J Gastroenterol.* 2016;22(26):6008–6015.
30. Malinchoc M, Kamath PS, Gordon FD, et al. A model to predict poor survival in patients undergoing transjugular intrahepatic portosystemic shunts. *Hepatology.* 2000;31(4):864–871.

Liver Transplantation

Saad Alghamdi and Avegail Flores

22

GENERAL PRINCIPLES

- Advances in immunosuppression, mainly with the introduction of calcineurin inhibitors (CNIs) (cyclosporine and tacrolimus), revolutionized liver transplantation from an experimental procedure to an accepted treatment for end-stage liver disease.
- Currently, the outcome of liver transplantation is excellent due to extensive pretransplant evaluation, early recognition and treatment of posttransplant complications, and long-term management of immunosuppression.
- Most recent data showed a total of 7127 adult liver transplants (6768 deceased donor and 343 living donor).[1] One-year allograft failure rate was 10.3% and the 5-year overall survival rate was 73.6%.[1] Limited donor supply remains a significant challenge to liver transplantation.
- The liver transplant allocation system is based upon the Model of End-Stage Liver Disease (MELD) score and allocates the organ preferentially to the patient with the highest MELD score (sickest) within a defined geographic region.
- The MELD score is calculated from the serum bilirubin, international normalized ratio (INR) of prothrombin time, and serum creatinine and accurately predicts the risk of short-term mortality from chronic liver disease.[2]
- The utilization of organs from extended criteria donors, including those with donation after cardiac death (DCD) had increased with improving preservation techniques and transplant center experience.
- Living donor liver transplantation has become an option for highly selected patients as an alternative way to decrease the waiting list.
- Combined liver–kidney transplantation comprises 9.4% of transplant in the United States.[1]

INDICATIONS

- Orthotopic liver transplantation (OLT) is indicated for acute or chronic liver failure from a variety of causes when limits of medical therapy had been reached (Table 22-1).
- Patients with cirrhosis without absolute contraindications should be considered for transplant referral with MELD score ≥15 or when they develop complications of end-stage liver disease (ascites, variceal bleeding, or encephalopathy).[3]
- Survival benefits of transplant increase with increasing MELD score. Transplant recipients with lower MELD score (<15) had reduced mean survival compared to matched candidates who remained on the waitlist.[4]
- Conditions associated with liver disease not served by MELD system of allocation (including hepatopulmonary syndrome, portopulmonary hypertension, hepatocellular carcinoma (HCC), and early-stage nonresectable cholangiocarcinoma) can prompt an expedited transplant evaluation regardless of hepatic synthetic dysfunction. These conditions may receive MELD exception points.
- Simultaneous liver–kidney transplantation is indicated for candidates with chronic kidney disease with glomerular filtration rate (GFR) <30 mL/min or prolonged need for dialysis (usually >8 weeks) or when extensive glomerulosclerosis is present on renal biopsy.[3]

TABLE 22.1 INDICATIONS FOR LIVER TRANSPLANTATION

Condition	Details
Acute liver failure	
Complications of cirrhosis	Severe synthetic dysfunction
	Refractory ascites, hepatic encephalopathy, and portal hypertension–related GI bleeding
	Hepatocellular carcinoma
	Cholangiocarcinoma
Metabolic conditions with systemic manifestations	Nonalcoholic fatty liver disease
	α_1-Antitrypsin deficiency
	Familial amyloid polyneuropathy hemochromatosis
	Primary hyperoxaluria
Systemic complications of chronic liver disease	Hepatopulmonary syndrome
	Portopulmonary syndrome
Rare conditions	Hereditary hemorrhagic telangiectasia
	Polycystic liver

- Other indications for liver transplant include decompensated liver disease from: α_1-antitrypsin deficiency (A1AT), hemochromatosis, and Wilson disease.
- Relatively rare liver diseases not served by the MELD allocation policy may receive MELD exception points: familial amyloid polyneuropathy (FAP), hereditary hemorrhagic telangiectasia (HHT), primary hyperoxaluria, and polycystic liver disease.
- The remainder of this section will discuss **disease-specific indications**.

Nonalcoholic Fatty Liver Disease

- Nonalcoholic fatty liver disease (NAFLD) encompasses a spectrum of fatty liver disease in the absence of significant alcohol use that include simple steatosis, nonalcoholic steatohepatitis (NASH), and NASH-related cirrhosis.
- NAFLD is strongly associated with obesity and the metabolic syndrome. The individual components of metabolic syndrome also increase the risk of developing NAFLD.
- The most common cause of death in patients with NAFLD is cardiovascular disease.
- Many cases of chronic liver failure previously reported as cryptogenic are likely a consequence of NAFLD. Although low level autoantibodies are frequently observed in NAFLD and considered an epiphenomenon.
- NAFLD has become one of the leading causes of liver transplantation in Unites States.
- The cornerstone of treatment remains lifestyle modification through diet, exercise, and weight loss.
- Patients with NAFLD undergoing liver transplantation require close monitoring for metabolic risk factors post transplantation given increased risk of cardiovascular events.
- Fatty liver disease may recur in an allograft liver, though this rarely leads to graft loss.[5]

Hepatitis C

- Since the widespread use of highly effective antiviral agents against hepatitis C virus (HCV) and the aging of persons born between 1945 and 1965 where the highest rate of HCV infection is seen, a decline in HCV waitlist candidates and HCV-related transplants were observed. While, there had been significant increases in transplants for alcoholic liver disease and nonalcoholic liver disease.[1]

- Several treatment options are currently available for post transplantation recurrence of HCV with excellent success rate.
- Monitoring and dose adjustment of immunosuppression should be performed when treating HCV in the post-transplant setting.
- Fibrosing cholestatic hepatitis C (FCH, the most aggressive form of recurrent HCV) and acute severe recurrent HCV are rapidly fatal post-transplant. Prompt HCV treatment is indicated and therapy is highly effective.[6,7]

Alcohol-Related Liver Disease

- Alcohol-related liver disease remains one of the most common indications for liver transplantation in the United States.
- Abstinence is the only effective treatment and can be associated with dramatic survival improvement, even in patients with decompensated cirrhosis.
- A period of abstinence before providing transplantation may have salutary effects on liver function that obviate the need for transplant.[8] Most US transplant centers require 6 months of abstinence prior to OLT listing.
- Early liver transplantation for first episode severe alcoholic hepatitis performed in highly selected patients with supportive family showed improved survival.[9]
- Routine follow-up and alcohol abuse counseling should be undertaken in the pre- and postoperative period to reduce rates of recidivism.
- Excellent long-term outcomes are common for patients transplanted for alcohol-related liver disease.
- Recent estimates of recurrent alcoholic cirrhosis after transplant is <6%. However, one-third of severe alcoholic relapse develop cirrhosis of the allograft in <5 years with a very poor prognosis.[10]

Hepatitis B

- It is estimated that approximately 248 million persons are HBV chronic carriers worldwide.[11]
- Prior to routine use of hepatitis B immune globulin (HBIG), hepatitis B infection in liver transplant patients was associated with poor outcomes and considered a contraindication to liver transplantation.[12]
- Peri- and posttransplant HBIG has dramatically decreased the rate of allograft hepatitis B infection and permitted transplantation of hepatitis B virus (HBV)-infected patients.
- Nucleos(t)ide analogs therapy for HBV has an excellent safety profile after liver transplantation. This allowed for a shorter duration (1 year) of HBIG treatment in low recurrence risk patients (fulminant HBV hepatitis, no HCC and hepatitis B e antigen–negative cirrhotic patients with HBV DNA levels <300 copies/mL).[13]
- The remains no consensus on the duration of HBIG treatment needed post-transplant.[14]

Autoimmune Hepatitis

- Corticosteroid and immunosuppressive therapy is largely effective in maintaining clinical and biochemical remission of autoimmune hepatitis (AIH).
- Usefulness of corticosteroid in AIH leading to fulminant liver failure is controversial and best reserved for less severe disease (MELD <28).[15]
- A fraction of patients with cryptogenic cirrhosis may have had long-standing unrecognized AIH.
- Long-term outcome after liver transplantation for AIH is excellent, with 5- and 10-year survival rates of >75%.[1]

- Recurrent disease can occur but is usually mild and managed with conventional immunosuppression.
- The development of de novo AIH post liver transplantation for other conditions has been described in the literature. This generally responds to immunosuppression.

Primary Biliary Cholangitis (Formerly Primary Biliary Cirrhosis)

- Patients with primary biliary cirrhosis (PBC) who present late in the course of their disease or respond inadequately to ursodeoxycholic acid may progress to cirrhosis requiring transplantation.
- Obeticholic acid is an available option for patients with inadequate response to ursodeoxycholic acid.[16]
- Occasional patients with PBC and stable liver function may be considered for transplant if they have severe pruritus, leading to sleep deprivation and emotional disturbances.
- Recurrence of PBC after transplantation has been documented, but has not had major impact on long-term postoperative survival.[17]

Primary Sclerosing Cholangitis (PSC)

- No specific medical therapy has been shown to improve survival in patients with PSC.
- PSC is associated with an increased risk of cholangiocarcinoma, gallbladder cancer, and colon cancer in patients with concurrent inflammatory bowel disease (IBD).
- Transplant outcomes for PSC are excellent.[1]
- Concurrent IBD may worsen post-transplant outcomes. Moreover poorly controlled IBD may result in diminished allograft survival.[18]
- IBD management should be optimized prior to transplant.

α_1-Antitrypsin (A1AT) Deficiency

- Only a minority of patients may present with mildly abnormal liver tests.
- An autopsy study in adults with severe A1AT deficiency showed 50% had cirrhosis and 28% had hepatocellular carcinoma.[19]
- After transplantation, donor A1AT phenotype is expressed and serum levels of A1AT return to normal ranges within weeks. Its impact on pulmonary disease is unknown.
- Careful assessment of lung disease should be performed in cirrhosis secondary A1AT deficiency, although coexistent disease is uncommon.

Wilson Disease

- Hepatic manifestations include acute on chronic hepatitis, cirrhosis, and acute liver failure.[20]
- Urgent liver transplantation is the only effective option for patients with fulminant hepatic failure (FHF) and those with decompensated cirrhosis.
- Transplant outcome for hepatic Wilson's is excellent.
- In patients receiving liver transplantation for chronic Wilson disease, copper chelation and zinc therapy are not needed after transplantation.

Hereditary Hemochromatosis (HH)

- Alcohol intake and HCV may accelerate HH-related liver disease.
- Patients with cirrhosis secondary to HH should be screened regularly for HCC.
- Early experience after transplant in HH showed inferior survival due to cardiovascular events (notably arrhythmias) and infections.[21]
- Careful patient selection with cardiac evaluation, pretransplant iron reduction therapy, and improvement in immunosuppressive therapy have resulted in improved outcome with similar survival in comparison to other indications for transplant.[22]

Hepatocellular Carcinoma

- Patients with chronic HBV infection and cirrhosis of any kind are at risk for HCC.
- Patient prognosis in HCC is dependent upon the stage of the tumor and the degree of liver function impairment.
- Liver transplant in small, unresectable HCC demonstrated a 4-year survival rate of 75% and recurrence-free survival of 83%.[23]
- The **Milan criteria** are used to identify patients with HCC who are expected to benefit from liver transplantation. Transplantation can be considered in patients with:
  - A single lesion 2 cm or larger but smaller than 5 cm, *or*
  - No more than three lesions, the largest of which is smaller than 3 cm, *and*
  - No evidence of vascular invasion or extrahepatic metastases.[23]
- Transplant may be an option for HCC in excess of Milan after successful downstaging procedures within Milan criteria.
- Enhanced priority or MELD exception points of 28 can be awarded to patients with HCC within Milan criteria after 6 months with 10% increment in score every 3 months and a MELD cap of 34.

Fulminant Hepatic Failure

- FHF is the rapid development of encephalopathy and coagulopathy within 56 days in a patient without pre-existing liver disease.
- Status 1A (highest priority) is assigned to adult candidates in the intensive care unit (ICU) with life expectancy without a liver transplant of <7 days and with at least one of the following conditions:
  - Ventilator dependence
  - Dialysis requirement
  - INR >2.0[24]
- Etiology is the most important predictor of outcome in acute or fulminant liver failure.
  - Acetaminophen toxicity represents at least half of the acute liver failure cases in the United States.
  - Nonacetaminophen-related FHF may result from drug-induced liver injury, hepatitis A and B, acute fatty liver of pregnancy, Wilson disease, immune-mediated liver disease, Budd–Chiari syndrome, and other causes.
  - Patients with FHF should be **promptly transferred to a transplant center and cared for in an ICU setting** until clinical improvement or transplantation. Brain edema, infection, and renal failure may occur and require intensive management while awaiting transplant.[3]

ORGAN ALLOCATION

- The growing need for liver transplantation with a limited donor supply has generated a waiting list of >14,000 patients in the United States.[1]
- The disparity between organ supply and demand mandates allocation policies to prioritize scarce donor organs to patients most in need.
- The national transplant list where patients are ranked according to their MELD score is managed through an independent nonprofit organization called United Network for Organ Sharing (UNOS) which also serves as the only Organ Procurement and Transplantation Network (OPTN) in the United States.
- UNOS and OPTN operate by grouping states into 11 geographic regions. There are regional differences in organ access.
- Since the implementation of MELD in 2002, there had been allocation policy changes to address the issues of equity and access. Most recent changes include:

- 2013. Regional Share 35. Organs be offered to candidates with a MELD ≥35 in the region before being considered for local candidates with a MELD <35.
- 2015. HCC cap and delay. Candidates must wait 6 months before receiving MELD exception points. Score is capped at 34.
- 2016. MELD-Sodium (Na). More accurate measure of waitlist mortality in patients with low MELD and hyponatremia.[25] Hyponatremia is a poor prognostic indicator in cirrhosis.
- 2016 to current. Ongoing proposal and discussion to change the number of geographic regions and redesign the liver distribution.[26]

PATIENT EVALUATION

- Liver transplant evaluation includes a comprehensive physical, physiologic, and psychosocial patient assessment. This involves a multidisciplinary approach including transplant hepatologists, surgeons, radiologists, psychiatrists, pharmacists, social workers, and case coordinators.
- **Important considerations for candidate evaluation**
  - Can the patient survive the operation and the immediate postoperative period?
  - Can the patient comply with a complex medical regimen and follow-up after the transplant?
  - Does the patient have comorbid conditions that require modification prior to transplant or that preclude transplant?
- **Components of the transplant evaluation**
  - A thorough history and physical examination.
  - Cardiopulmonary assessment including evaluation for structural and ischemic heart disease with pharmacologically induced stress echocardiography and pulmonary function testing.
  - Abnormalities identified on noninvasive cardiopulmonary testing warrant further evaluation with left or right cardiac catheterization.
  - Laboratory studies to confirm the etiology of liver disease and to evaluate for previously undetected medical conditions.
  - Assessment of creatinine clearance.
  - Serologic evaluation to determine the status of viral infections including hepatitis B and C virus, Cytomegalovirus, Epstein–Barr virus, and HIV.
  - Cross-sectional abdominal imaging to determine the liver volume, presence of HCC, as well as patency of hepatic inflow (portal vein and hepatic artery) and outflow (hepatic veins).
  - Age-matched cancer screening.

SPECIAL CONSIDERATIONS

- **Age.** There is no specific age limitation to successful OLT, and candidacy is determined on an individual basis.
- **Pulmonary hypertension.** This condition is often identified on echocardiography (pulmonary artery systolic pressure [PASP], >45 mm Hg) and requires more precise measurement with right heart catheterization. Pulmonary hypertension may preclude liver transplantation and should, at a minimum, be optimally controlled with medical therapy prior to transplantation.
- **Morbid obesity.** This is generally considered a relative contraindication to transplantation. Attention should be directed to improving body mass index prior to transplantation.
- **Renal insufficiency.** The etiology of the renal insufficiency should be investigated prior to transplantation and, in some cases, consideration given to combined liver–kidney transplantation.

- **Previous malignancy.** Given the increased risk for recurrence of cancer with systemic immunosuppression, consultation from the treating oncologist regarding the risk of posttransplant recurrence should be obtained.
- **HIV.** Although previously regarded as a contraindication to transplantation, improved medical therapies have allowed HIV-positive individuals to be successfully transplanted. There are numerous interactions between highly active antiretroviral therapy (HAART) and immunosuppressant medications requiring monitoring of serum drug levels.
- **Surgical issues.** Thrombosis of the main portal vein may be bypassed; however, more extensive thrombosis of the mesenteric vasculature or cavernomatous transformation of the portal vein may preclude adequate graft venous inflow.
- **Psychosocial issues.** Issues related to depression and previous alcohol or illicit substance abuse need to be explored and counseling offered.

CONTRAINDICATIONS TO LIVER TRANSPLANTATION

- Severe cardiopulmonary disease
- Extrahepatic malignancy without adequate survival
- Uncontrolled sepsis
- Anatomic abnormalities that precludes liver transplantation
- Poor social support and medical compliance
- Ongoing illicit substance abuse

TREATMENT

Surgical Considerations

- During transplantation, the liver is placed in the natural position in the right upper quadrant.
- Most OLTs are performed using a whole donor liver.
- Split-liver transplantation involves utilizing a portion of the left lobe of the donor liver for transplantation into a child and utilizing the remaining donor organ for transplantation into an adult.
- Living donor transplantation is performed at some centers in the United States but mostly used in countries without a national system of organ donation and allocation.
- Vascular reconstruction of the hepatic artery, portal vein, and hepatic venous drainage system to the inferior vena cava is undertaken to provide adequate vascular inflow and outflow to the allograft.
- Biliary reconstruction is accomplished using an end-to-end anastomosis of the proximal donor common bile duct to the distal recipient common bile duct.
- In transplant recipients with diseased ducts (i.e., PSC), a Roux-en-Y hepaticojejunostomy is performed. This ensures removal of the entire native biliary tree and, in the case of PSC, decreases the risk of future biliary strictures and neoplasia.

Medications

- The goal of posttransplant immunosuppression is to prevent allograft rejection while allowing physiologic defenses against infection.
- Although mechanisms are incompletely understood, the liver appears to be less susceptible to rejection than other transplanted organs.
- In general, currently used immunosuppressants deplete T cells or inhibit T-cell activation.
- **CNIs** (cyclosporine, tacrolimus, tacrolimus extended release) are the most commonly used maintenance immunosuppressive medicines.
  - CNI binds to cyclophilin, and inhibits T-cell activation and proliferation.
  - CNI requires monitoring of 12-hour trough levels.

- Because CNIs are metabolized by the cytochrome P450 system, drug levels can be significantly affected by commonly prescribed medications, requiring close monitoring of drug levels.
- Side effects of CNI include nephrotoxicity, neurotoxicity, hypertension, hyperlipidemia, and posttransplant diabetes. Additionally, patients taking cyclosporine may experience gingival hyperplasia and hirsutism.

- **Antimetabolites** include mycophenolate mofetil and mycophenolate sodium.
  - Mycophenolate mofetil and mycophenolate sodium are metabolized to mycophenolic acid (MPA), which inhibits guanosine synthesis and lymphocyte proliferation.
  - MPAs are generally not used as monotherapy but as supplements to CNIs.
  - The side effects of MPA include gastrointestinal disorders (primarily diarrhea) and bone marrow suppression.
  - MPAs carry an increased risk of spontaneous abortions and birth defects.

- **mTOR inhibitors** include sirolimus and everolimus.
  - mTOR inhibitors bind to FK506-binding protein inhibiting T-cell proliferation.
  - Sirolimus has been associated with hepatic artery thrombosis in the first few weeks of transplant and delayed wound healing. mTOR inhibitor is generally not used in the immediate posttransplant period.
  - Everolimus is a derivative of sirolimus and works similarly. It is increasingly used after a boxed warning on sirolimus of early hepatic artery thrombosis leading to allograft loss and death.
  - Common side effects of everolimus include stomatitis, diarrhea, peripheral edema, anemia, hypertriglyceridemia, and lymphopenia.

- **Corticosteroids** reduce cytokine release and lymphocyte activation.
  - Corticosteroids are used in the immediate posttransplant period, though efforts are made to wean steroids within a few months post transplantation to avoid side effects caused by prolonged corticosteroid use (diabetes, hypertension, osteoporosis, etc.).
  - Intravenous and oral steroids are commonly used to treat episodes of mild to moderate acute cellular rejection.

POSTTRANSPLANT COMPLICATIONS

- **Early posttransplant complications** may relate to allograft function, surgical anatomic issues, infections, and other causes; please see Table 22-2.
  - Early allograft dysfunction usually prompts liver biopsy, an assessment of the hepatic vasculature, and biliary system.
  - Early rejection may be treated with steroids and other immunosuppressants. Outcome is favorable if completely treated.
  - Biliary tract disease (bile leaks, stones, strictures, hemobilia) leading to graft dysfunction may require radiographic or endoscopic intervention.
  - Early hepatic artery thrombosis often requires retransplantation. If this occurs within 7 days of transplantation, the patient is relisted for transplantation as status 1A.
  - Primary nonfunction is the most severe type of allograft damage after transplant. Features include hepatocellular necrosis, rapidly rising transaminases, absence of bile production, severe liver-related coagulation deficit, high lactate levels, systemic hemodynamic instability, and acute renal failure. The patient is relisted for transplantation as status 1A.
  - Early hepatic venous outflow obstruction is a serious complication causing acute Budd–Chiari syndrome and may result in allograft loss. This is mostly due to technical problems of tight anastomosis, twisting of hepatic veins, or malpositioning of the allograft. Endovascular treatment by interventional radiology is often successful.

- **Late post-transplant complications** include chronic allograft rejection, recurrence of hepatic disease in the allograft, anatomic complications (biliary duct anastomotic and nonanastomotic stricture), infections, and malignancy.

TABLE 22-2	EARLY AND LATE COMPLICATIONS AFTER DECEASED DONOR LIVER TRANSPLANTATION
Early Complications After Liver Transplantation (<6 mo)	**Late Complications After Liver Transplantation (>6 mo)**
Acute cellular rejection	Chronic rejection
Biliary disease (bile leaks, hemobilia, biloma, casts/sludge)	Biliary strictures (anastomotic and nonanastomotic)
Hepatic artery thrombosis	Post-transplant lymphoproliferative disorder (PTLD)
Hepatic venous outflow obstruction	Malignancy (e.g., skin and cervical cancer)
Infection	Infection

○ Evidence of worsening hepatic function generally prompts biopsy of the allograft.
○ If no clear hepatic parenchymal cause is found on biopsy (i.e., rejection), a prompt evaluation of the allograft vasculature and biliary system is necessary.
○ Nonanastomotic strictures also known as ischemic cholangiopathy has been associated with the use of allografts from DCD, prolonged ischemia time, and ABO-incompatible allografts.
○ Anastomotic strictures or extrahepatic biliary strictures are usually treated by endoscopic retrograde cholangiopancreatography (ERCP) and in some cases by percutaneous transhepatic cholangiography (PTC) if the stricture is at the hepaticojejunostomy.
○ Posttransplant immunosuppression leads to increased risk for a variety of malignancies (skin cancer, cervical cancer, etc.) as well as adverse cardiometabolic risk factors (diabetes, hyperlipidemia, hypertension).
○ Posttransplant lymphoproliferative disorder (PTLD) ranges from polymorphic lymphoproliferation to high-grade monoclonal lymphoma. Risk factors include recipient Epstein–Barr virus status, young age, and intensity of immunosuppression.[27]

LONG-TERM MANAGEMENT

* Low-dose CNI in combination with mycophenolate mofetil (MMF) or everolimus should be considered in posttransplant patients who are found to have moderate kidney impairment.[28]
* Recipients should be counseled on sun protection and an increase risk in nonmelanoma skin cancers. They should see a dermatologist after transplantation and with annual evaluation at least every year after 5 years or more after transplant.[29]
* Recipients should receive annual influenza vaccination. They should avoid live vaccines.[29]
* Careful attention to cardiovascular risks and/or new-onset cancers especially in smokers.[29]

REFERENCES

1. Kim WR, Lake JR, Smith JM, et al. OPTN/SRTR 2015 annual data report: liver. *Am J Transplant.* 2017;17(Suppl 1):174–251.
2. Freeman RB Jr, Wiesner RH, Harper A, et al. The new liver allocation system: moving toward evidence-based transplantation policy. *Liver Transpl.* 2002;8:851–858.
3. Martin P, DiMartini A, Feng S, et al. Evaluation for liver transplantation in adults: 2013 practice guideline by the American Association for the Study of Liver Diseases and the American Society of Transplantation. *Hepatology.* 2014;59:1144–1165.

4. Merion RM, Schaubel DE, Dykstra DM, et al. The survival benefit of liver transplantation. *Am J Transplant*. 2005;5:307–313.

5. Charlton MR, Burns JM, Pedersen RA, et al. Frequency and outcomes of liver transplantation for nonalcoholic steatohepatitis in the United States. *Gastroenterology*. 2011;141:1249–1253.

6. Forns X, Charlton M, Denning J, et al. Sofosbuvir compassionate use program for patients with severe recurrent hepatitis C after liver transplantation. *Hepatology*. 2015;61:1485–1494.

7. Leroy V, Dumortier J, Coilly A, et al. Efficacy of sofosbuvir and daclatasvir in patients with fibrosing cholestatic hepatitis C after liver transplantation. *Clin Gastroenterol Hepatol*. 2015;13:1993-2001.e1–e2.

8. O'Shea RS, Dasarathy S, McCullough AJ. Alcoholic liver disease. *Hepatology*. 2010;51:307–328.

9. Mathurin P, Moreno C, Samuel D, et al. Early liver transplantation for severe alcoholic hepatitis. *N Engl J Med*. 2011;365:1790–1800.

10. Dumortier J, Dharancy S, Cannesson A, et al. Recurrent alcoholic cirrhosis in severe alcoholic relapse after liver transplantation: a frequent and serious complication. *Am J Gastroenterol*. 2015;110:1160–1166; quiz 1167.

11. Schweitzer A, Horn J, Mikolajczyk RT, et al. Estimations of worldwide prevalence of chronic hepatitis B virus infection: a systematic review of data published between 1965 and 2013. *Lancet*. 2015;386:1546–1555.

12. Lok AS. Prevention of recurrent hepatitis B post-liver transplantation. *Liver Transpl*. 2002;8:S67–S73.

13. Fernandez I, Loinaz C, Hernandez O, et al. Tenofovir/entecavir monotherapy after hepatitis B immunoglobulin withdrawal is safe and effective in the prevention of hepatitis B in liver transplant recipients. *Transpl Infect Dis*. 2015;17:695–701.

14. Saab S, Chen PY, Saab CE, et al. The management of hepatitis B in liver transplant recipients. *Clin Liver Dis*. 2016;20:721–736.

15. Ichai P, Duclos-Vallee JC, Guettier C, et al. Usefulness of corticosteroids for the treatment of severe and fulminant forms of autoimmune hepatitis. *Liver Transpl*. 2007;13:996–1003.

16. Nevens F, Andreone P, Mazzella G, et al. A placebo-controlled trial of obeticholic acid in primary biliary cholangitis. *N Engl J Med*. 2016;375:631–643.

17. Heathcote EJ. Management of primary biliary cirrhosis. The American Association for the Study of Liver Diseases practice guidelines. *Hepatology*. 2000;31:1005–1013.

18. Joshi D, Bjarnason I, Belgaumkar A, et al. The impact of inflammatory bowel disease post-liver transplantation for primary sclerosing cholangitis. *Liver Int*. 2013;33:53–61.

19. Elzouki AN, Eriksson S. Risk of hepatobiliary disease in adults with severe alpha 1-antitrypsin deficiency (PiZZ): is chronic viral hepatitis B or C an additional risk factor for cirrhosis and hepatocellular carcinoma? *Eur J Gastroenterol Hepatol*. 1996;8:989–994.

20. Roberts EA, Schilsky ML. Diagnosis and treatment of Wilson disease: an update. *Hepatology*. 2008;47:2089–2111.

21. Kowdley KV, Brandhagen DJ, Gish RG, et al. Survival after liver transplantation in patients with hepatic iron overload: the national hemochromatosis transplant registry. *Gastroenterology*. 2005;129:494–503.

22. Dar FS, Faraj W, Zaman MB, et al. Outcome of liver transplantation in hereditary hemochromatosis. *Transpl Int*. 2009;22:717–724.

23. Mazzaferro V, Regalia E, Doci R, et al. Liver transplantation for the treatment of small hepatocellular carcinomas in patients with cirrhosis. *N Engl J Med*. 1996;334:693–699.

24. Slaughter JC, Goutte M, Rymer JA, et al. Caution about overinterpretation of symptom indexes in reflux monitoring for refractory gastroesophageal reflux disease. *Clin Gastroenterol Hepatol*. 2011;9:868–874.

25. Kim WR, Biggins SW, Kremers WK, et al. Hyponatremia and mortality among patients on the liver-transplant waiting list. *N Engl J Med*. 2008;359:1018–1026.

26. McDonald-Haile J, Bradley LA, Bailey MA, et al. Relaxation training reduces symptom reports and acid exposure in patients with gastroesophageal reflux disease. *Gastroenterology*. 1994;107:61–69.

27. Kamdar KY, Rooney CM, Heslop HE. Posttransplant lymphoproliferative disease following liver transplantation. *Curr Opin Organ Transplant*. 2011;16:274–280.

28. Levitsky J, O'Leary JG, Asrani S, et al. Protecting the kidney in liver transplant recipients: practice-based recommendations from the American Society of Transplantation Liver and Intestine Community of Practice. *Am J Transplant*. 2016;16:2532–2544.

29. Lucey MR, Terrault N, Ojo L, et al. Long-term management of the successful adult liver transplant: 2012 practice guideline by the American Association for the Study of Liver Diseases and the American Society of Transplantation. *Liver Transpl*. 2013;19:3–26.

Pancreatic Disorders

Koushik K. Das

23

Introduction

- The pancreas is a mixed endocrine and exocrine gland consisting of lobular subunits composed of acini.[1,2]
- The exocrine pancreas consists of acinar, centroacinar, and ductal cells.
  - The acinar cells secrete approximately 20 digestive enzymes (in zymogen granules) into the central ductule of the acinus.[1,2]
  - The central ductule of the acinus connects with the intralobular ducts to form the interlobular ducts, which join to form the main pancreatic duct (MPD).[1,2]
  - The MPD empties into the duodenum through the ampulla of Vater.[1,2]
- The pancreas lies in the retroperitoneal space of the upper abdomen, with the head located abutting the duodenal sweep, the body located at the level of the L1–L2 vertebra and the tail adjacent to the splenic helium. Due to its retroperitoneal location and intimate associations with the luminal GI tract and biliary tree, diseases of the pancreas can be more difficult to manage than those of other abdominal viscera.
  - Lymphatic drainage of the pancreas occurs along several major routes. These include the splenic, hepatic, and superior mesenteric nodal systems, as well as the aortocaval and other posterior abdominal wall lymphatic vessels.[2]
  - Blood vessels in close proximity to the pancreas include major vessels of the epigastrium, such as the superior mesenteric vein, the portal vein (PV), and the celiac axis. Thus, local invasion of malignant pancreatic tumors often involves these vessels, and can potentially make such tumors unresectable and/or incurable.[2]
  - If the pancreas is resected, the need to excise the vessels and lymph nodes associated with it often necessitates resection of the duodenum, gallbladder, distal bile duct, spleen, upper jejunum, and part of the stomach.[2]

Acute Pancreatitis

GENERAL PRINCIPLES

Definition

- Acute pancreatitis is an autodigestive process that occurs when the proteolytic enzymes are prematurely activated within the pancreas rather than in the intestinal lumen. The active enzymes digest membranes within the pancreas, which leads to inflammation, edema, vascular damage, cellular injury, and possibly death.[3]
- Revised Atlanta Classification requires that the diagnosis of acute pancreatitis is established by at least two of the following three features:
  - Abdominal pain consistent with acute pancreatitis (acute onset of a persistent, severe, epigastric pain often radiating to the back)
  - An elevation of the amylase and/or lipase >3 times the upper limit of normal, and/or
  - Imaging confirmation of the diagnosis with contrast-enhanced computed tomography (CT) or magnetic resonance imaging (MRI).[4]

Classification

- In an effort to standardize clinical assessments, to identify patients who may benefit from ICU level of care or early/aggressive interventions, and to stratify patients for research/clinical trials, there have been numerous schema suggested for classifying the degree and severity of pancreatitis including: APACHE, bedside index of severity in acute pancreatitis (BISAP), Glasgow, HAPS, JSS, Panc 3, POP, Ranson, SIRS scores. Please see Table 23-1.[5,6]
- **Ranson score**[5]
  - At presentation: age >55, WBC >16,000/μL, glucose >200 mg/dL, LDH >350 UL, AST >250 U/L
  - At 48 hours: hematocrit decline by >10%, BUN increase by >5 mg/dL despite fluids, serum calcium <8 mg/dL, pO$_2$ <60 mm Hg, base deficit >4 mEq/L, fluid sequestration >6 L
  - Utilizing the above, mortality can be predicted with 1–2 criteria associated with <1% mortality, 3–5 criteria associated with 15% mortality, 6–8 criteria associated with 60% mortality, and 9–11 criteria associated with >75% mortality.
- **BISAP score**[6]:
  - 1 point for each of the following calculated at presentation and at 48 hours:
    - BUN >25 mg/dL

TABLE 23-1 COMPARISON OF SEVERITY SCORING SYSTEMS FOR ACUTE PANCREATITIS

Ranson Criteria[a]		BISAP Score
On Admission	Within 48 hrs	On Admission and at 48 hrs
WBC >16,000/μL	Hematocrit decrease by 10%	BUN >25 mg/dL
Age >55 yrs	BUN increase by >5 mg/dL	Abnormal mental status with Glasgow coma score <15
	Calcium <8 mg/dL	Evidence of SIRS (Systemic inflammatory response syndrome)
	Arterial po$_2$ <60 mm Hg	Age >60 years old
AST >250 IU/L	Base deficit >4 mEq/L	Imaging study revealing pleural effusion
LDH >350 IU/L	Fluid sequestration >6 L	
Glucose >200 mg/dL		
Mortality rate of ≤4 criteria is <15% and considered mild disease. Mortality rate rises greatly with more than four criteria		1 point for each criteria at presentation and at 48 hours. 0–2 points associated with <2% mortality, 3–5 points associated with >15% mortality

[a]Applies to nonbiliary causes of pancreatitis. Criteria are adjusted with biliary pancreatitis. Ranson JH, Rifkind KM, Roses DF, et al. Prognostic signs and the role of operative management in acute pancreatitis. *Surg Gynecol Obstet.* 1974;139:69–81; and Wu BU, Johannes RS, Sun X, et al. The early prediction of mortality in acute pancreatitis: a large population-based study. *Gut.* 2008;57:1698–1703.

AST, aspartate aminotransferase; BISAP, bedside index of severity in acute pancreatitis; BUN, blood urea nitrogen; LDH, lactate dehydrogenase; WBC, white blood cell count.

- Abnormal mental status with Glasgow coma score <15
- Evidence of systemic inflammatory response syndrome (SIRS)
- Age >60 years old
- Imaging study revealing pleural effusion
- 0–2 points associated with <2% mortality, 3–5 points associated with >15% mortality
- Please see Table 23-1 for the BISAP score
- **Revised Atlanta classification**[4]
  - *Organ Failure:*
    - Respiratory—PaO_2/FiO_2 <300
    - Renal—Cr >1.9
    - Cardiovascular—SBP <90, not fluid responsive
  - *Local Complications*
    - Acute peripancreatic fluid collections—Peripancreatic, homogeneous fluid associated with interstitial edematous pancreatitis with no associated necrosis without a definable wall encapsulating the collection. These occur within the first 4 weeks after onset of pancreatitis.
    - Pancreatic pseudocysts—A fully encapsulated collection of homogenous fluid with a well-defined inflammatory wall usually outside the pancreas with minimal or no necrosis occurring usually >4 weeks after the onset of pancreatitis.
    - Acute necrotic collections—A collection containing variable amounts of both fluid and solid necrosis associated with necrotizing pancreatitis. These collections are heterogeneous, have no definable wall encapsulating the collection, and may involve the parenchyma and/or the extrapancreatic tissue.
    - Walled-off necrosis (WON)—A mature, well-encapsulated collection of pancreatic and/or peripancreatic necrosis that has developed a well-defined inflammatory wall, usually >4 weeks after onset of necrotizing pancreatitis.
    - Gastric outlet obstruction.
    - Splenic/portal vein thrombosis.
    - Colonic necrosis.
  - *Mild acute pancreatitis:* Absence of organ failure and absence of local complications
    - These account for the majority (80%) of cases of pancreatitis.
    - Vascular supply is maintained and there is no progression to necrosis.
    - Recovery usually occurs within 7–14 days. Death or significant morbidity is uncommon.
  - *Moderately severe acute pancreatitis:* Local complications and/or transient organ failure (<48 hrs)
  - *Severe acute pancreatitis:* Persistent organ failure >48 hrs.
    - These account for the minority of cases of pancreatitis.
    - Vascular supply is often lost and there is progression to necrosis.
    - Morbidity and mortality is much more common, especially in the context of persistent organ failure and late (>2 weeks) infected necrosis.

Epidemiology

- Acute pancreatitis accounts for 275,000 hospital admissions in the United States each year, costing $2.5 billion.[3,7]
- The yearly incidence of acute pancreatitis ranges from 5–30 per 100,000, and has been rising over the past several years, in part possibly due to the relationship between obesity and gallstone disease.[7]
- As critical care has improved considerably, mortality associated with acute pancreatitis has reduced significantly and is now estimated at 2%, but is much higher in the elderly, the obese, those with comorbidities, and those with severe acute pancreatitis.[3]

Etiology

Gallstones

- Gallstone disease and excessive alcohol use account for 80% of cases of acute pancreatitis in Western countries. It is important to note, however, that pancreatitis develops in only a small percentage of patients with gallstones.[2,3]
- While the precise pathogenesis is unclear, gallstones are thought to cause pancreatitis by mechanically obstructing the pancreatic duct where it joins the common bile duct and/or by allowing the reflux of bile or duodenal contents into the pancreatic duct after passage across the sphincter of Oddi. Both of these mechanisms can lead to increased intraductal pressure which lead to activation of trypsin and subsequent activation of downstream enzymes including chymotrypsinogen, elastase, phospholipase A1, complement, kinins, and trypsinogen itself.[8]

Alcohol

- Prolonged alcohol use (4–5 drinks daily) over a period of more than 5 years is generally required for alcohol-associated pancreatitis, though the overall lifetime risk of pancreatitis even among heavy drinkers is only 2–5%.[3]
- As a minority of chronic heavy alcohol users develop pancreatitis, other hereditary or environmental risk factors (including smoking) likely play a role.[9]
- The pathogenesis of alcohol-induced pancreatitis has not fully been elucidated but appears to be in part due to direct sensitization of the acinar cells to cholecystokinin stimulation.[10]

Drugs

- Hundreds of drugs have been implicated as possibly causing pancreatitis, though definitively proving this can be very challenging. There has been some attempt to create an evidence-based classification of drugs and their likelihood of causing recurrent pancreatitis.[11] This schemata have labeled Class I drugs as those with one case report with positive rechallenge, Class II drugs with at least four cases in the literature, Class III drugs with at least two cases in the literature with no consistency in latency or data on rechallenge, and Class IV single reports in the literature.
- Commonly implicated agents include azathioprine, 6-mercaptopurine, L-asparaginase, pentamidine, didanosine, valproic acid, furosemide, angiotensin-converting enzyme inhibitors, sulfonamides, tetracyclines, mesalamine, estrogens, metronidazole, and erythromycin.[11]

Trauma

- Acute pancreatitis can be seen after blunt or penetrating abdominal trauma, and is the leading cause of pancreatitis in children.[12]
- Presentations are frequently seen after a motor vehicle accident, gunshot wound, or cardiothoracic surgery, often with delayed recognition after the development of pancreatic ascites or fluid collections.

Iatrogenic

- Acute pancreatitis may occur as a complication of endoscopic retrograde cholangiopancreatography (ERCP), pancreaticobiliary surgery, or cardiopulmonary bypass.[2]
- Post-ERCP pancreatitis (PEP) is more frequently seen in patients of female gender, younger age, with suspected sphincter of Oddi dysfunction, with prior PEP, with recurrent pancreatitis, and/or with pancreatic duct manipulation.[13]

Hypertriglyceridemia

- Chylomicrons are present in circulation when triglycerides are >900 mg/dL. These are thought to be large enough to occlude pancreatic capillaries, leading to local tissue ischemia and acinar release of lipase/trypsin. Lipolysis then leads to increased concentration of free fatty acids, reactive oxygen species, and inflammation.[2]
- Although triglyceride levels of >2000–3000 mg/dL are usually required for pancreatitis to develop, pancreatitis can also occur when serum levels are only 1000 mg/dL.[3]

- Hypertriglyceridemia sufficient to cause pancreatitis can occur in inherited disorders of lipoprotein metabolism (type I, II, and V hyperlipidemia), seen especially in children. In adults, there is often a mild form of type I/V disease with concomitant obesity, poorly controlled diabetes, hypothyroidism, pregnancy, and/or alcoholism.[8]
- The typical hypocaloric regimen (nothing by mouth) recommended during acute pancreatitis results in rapid decline in triglyceride levels. Treatment also includes fibrate therapy, fluids, insulin (as appropriate), and consideration of plasma exchange/lipid apheresis where appropriate. Consultation with endocrinology should be concurrently obtained.

Infection

- Infection is thought to be a rare cause of acute pancreatitis.
- The most common viral infections that involve the pancreas are mumps, Cytomegalovirus, and Coxsackie B virus.[9]
- Viral hepatitis, especially hepatitis B, has also been associated with pancreatitis.[14]
- Patients with HIV infection develop pancreatitis at a higher rate than the general population.
  - The virus itself appears to be the cause in some cases, but other factors (antiretroviral medications, alcohol abuse, dyslipidemia) may also play a role.[14]
  - Asymptomatic hyperamylasemia and hyperlipasemia have been reported in up to 40% of patients with acquired immunodeficiency syndrome (AIDS).[14]
- Bacteria associated with acute pancreatitis include *Salmonella, Shigella, Campylobacter,* hemorrhagic *Escherichia coli, Legionella, Leptospira,* and *Brucella* species. Pancreatitis associated with these infections is most likely toxin mediated and improves with clearance of the organisms. Parasites associated with acute pancreatitis include *Ascaris lumbricoides.*[14]

Miscellaneous Causes

- Other less common causes of pancreatitis include tumors (both benign and malignant), autoimmune disorders, hypercalcemia, celiac disease, SLE, hereditary pancreatitis, pancreas divisum, and, possibly, papillary stenosis (sphincter of Oddi dysfunction).[3,9]
- **Pancreas divisum** is the most common congenital abnormality of the pancreas, which is found in approximately 5–7% of subjects in autopsy series.[2] Although pancreas divisum has been implicated in the etiology of acute and chronic pancreatitis, more than 95% of patients with pancreas divisum are asymptomatic and it is unclear why symptoms develop in the minority of patients. There is likely a selection bias in the identification of divisum in patients with abdominal pain syndromes as these are the patients that undergo exhaustive workup with MRI, CT, and ERCP.
- In patients with proven recurrent acute pancreatitis and no evidence of chronic pancreatitis on dorsal duct pancreatography, there is a high likelihood of responding to ERCP with minor papillotomy and temporary stent placement. In some series, 50–70% of such patients will experience symptomatic improvement.[15,16]
- **Autoimmune pancreatitis**
  - Type 1 autoimmune pancreatitis (AIP) is the most common form worldwide accounting for more than 80% of cases in the United States.[17] It has a peak incidence in the sixth or seventh decades of life and tends to affect men twice as often as women. Type 1 AIP has a characteristic histology known as lymphoplasmacytic sclerosing pancreatitis. It is characterized by a periductal lymphoplasmacytic infiltrate, storiform fibrosis, obliterative phlebitis, and abundant IgG4 immunostaining (>10/high-power field IgG4-positive cells).[17] Type 1 AIP is a multiorgan disease termed "IgG4-related disease" as more than 60% of individuals have clinical and histologic involvement of other organs including the biliary tree, retroperitoneum, lacrimal and salivary glands, lymph nodes, periorbital tissues, kidneys, thyroid, lungs, meninges, aorta, breast, prostate, pericardium, and skin.[18] Type 2 AIP presents at a younger age, and

does not have an association to IgG4. The histologic hallmark of type 2 AIP is the presence of the granulocyte epithelial lesion (GEL) in pancreatic ducts with scant to no IgG4-positive cells.[17]

○ Response rates to glucocorticoid therapy are 92–99% but there can be a relapse rate of up to 62% when steroids are tapered, especially in type 1 patients.[19–21]

Idiopathic

Despite an extensive workup, the cause will not be identifiable in up many cases of acute pancreatitis.[3]

Pathophysiology

- Processes that contribute to the initiation of pancreatitis include pancreatic duct obstruction, pancreatic ischemia, and the premature activation of zymogens within the pancreatic acinar cells.[8]
- Subsequent digestion of pancreatic membranes causes tissue injury. This leads to release of inflammatory cytokines (tumor necrosis factor, interleukin-1, platelet-activating factor) that recruit inflammatory cells and increase vascular permeability.[8,9]
- This cascade of events leads to the development of acute pancreatitis and its systemic manifestations. If the resulting inflammation and tissue injury causes areas of the pancreas to become devitalized, necrotizing pancreatitis occurs.

DIAGNOSIS

Clinical Presentation

History

- The hallmark of acute pancreatitis is abdominal pain located in the epigastric and peri-umbilical areas, radiating to the back.[4]
- The abdominal pain typically is more intense when the patient is supine or ingests food and may be relieved if the patient leans forward or assumes a fetal position.
- Nausea, emesis, and abdominal distention are also frequently reported.

Physical Examination

- Systemic features may include fever and tachycardia, depending on the severity of disease. Patients may present with shock and/or in coma.
- Abdominal tenderness ranges from mild epigastric tenderness and distension to rigidity with rebound tenderness.
- Scleral icterus may be seen because of biliary obstruction or accompanying liver disease.
- A faint bluish discoloration around the umbilicus (Cullen sign) or flank (Turner sign), secondary to hemorrhage, is rarely seen.
- An epigastric mass due to pseudocyst formation may become palpable over the course of the disease.
- Less common features include polyarthritis, thrombophlebitis of the lower extremities, and panniculitis (subcutaneous nodular fat necrosis).[3,8,9]

Diagnostic Testing

Laboratory Testing

- **Lipase**
  ○ Lipase is produced by the pancreas, liver, intestine, tongue, stomach, and several other cells.
  ○ The main function of the pancreatic lipase is to hydrolyze triglycerides into glycerol and free fatty acids. Like amylase, lipase is a relatively small molecule that can be filtered by the kidney but unlike amylase, lipase can be reabsorbed in the renal tubules, which increases its half-life.[2]

Compared with amylase, lipase has slightly superior sensitivity and specificity for acute pancreatitis.[9] A level three times the upper limit of normal is required for the diagnosis of pancreatitis[4]; however, this can be seen in patients with renal insufficiency, malignant tumors, cholecystitis, and esophagitis.[22]

- **Amylase**
  - Amylase is primarily produced by the pancreas and salivary glands, but it can be found in other tissues. Patients with severe gastroenteritis may have serum amylase levels up to 2.2 times the upper limit of normal[23] and symptoms may be nonspecific and mimic those of pancreatitis.
  - Plasma levels of both enzymes peak at 24 hours of symptoms, but amylase has a shorter half-life.[9]

Imaging
- **Abdominal ultrasonography:** This is of limited utility in visualizing the pancreas or assessing for complications, but is very useful in establishing gallstones as the etiology of pancreatitis.
- **Computed tomography**
  - Not necessarily required for the initial diagnosis of pancreatitis in patients with typical symptoms and corresponding elevations of pancreatic enzymes.
  - May be normal in up to 30% of patients with mild pancreatitis, but almost always abnormal in patients with moderate or severe pancreatitis.[9]
  - CT can be particularly helpful if the diagnosis is in doubt or if initial clinical response was followed by sudden clinical deterioration. Scans should be performed using a pancreatic protocol, which involves thin cross-sectional images ("slices") through the pancreas during several contrast phases, sensitive for subtle signs of necrosis.[9]
  - Severity of pancreatitis can also be staged on the basis of CT findings such as pancreatic edema, peripancreatic infiltrates, peripancreatic fluid collections, vascular thrombosis, and areas of nonenhancement due to necrosis; please see Figure 23-1.

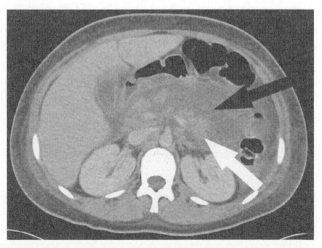

Figure 23-1. Computed tomography scan demonstrating pancreatic edema and necrosis in an 18-year-old man with gallstone pancreatitis. Note the large areas of low attenuation (*dark gray*) within the pancreatic bed (*black arrow*) compared with the areas with relatively preserved blood flow (*white arrow*). Normally, the pancreas has similar attenuation as the adjacent liver.

- **Magnetic resonance cholangiopancreatography (MRCP)** is highly sensitive for pancreatic inflammation and peripancreatic collections. This can be particularly useful when renal insufficiency or dye allergies preclude the use of CT. Due to the cost and complexity these are not routinely used in the initial evaluation of pancreatitis, but with the addition of MRCP, this study can be extremely useful for evaluating for persistent choledocholithiasis in cases of gallstone pancreatitis or potentially for pancreatic duct leaks/fistulas.
- **Endoscopic ultrasound (EUS)**
  - EUS is highly sensitive and specific for the evaluation of suspected choledocholithiasis/microlithiasis in patients with pancreatitis. In the absence of cholangitis and/or jaundice, MRCP/EUS is recommended to screen for choledocholithiasis if highly suspected.[24]
  - In patients >40 years of age with an idiopathic episode of acute pancreatitis, pancreatic tumors should be ruled out. EUS is extremely sensitive for small (<2 cm) or subtle pancreatic lesions including small neuroendocrine tumors; however, its sensitivity is highly limited in the setting of pancreatic edema/acute pancreatitis. As such, EUS should be considered in these cases after the resolution of inflammation (4–6 weeks at least).

Predictors of Severity

Please see above under Classification.

- **Hemoconcentration**—Acute pancreatitis results in extensive third spacing due to the inflammatory cascade that is activated. As a result, hemoconcentration is frequently seen. Studies have demonstrated that admission HCT >44% is accurate in predicting persistent organ failure and necrosis (OR 3.4/3.1).[25] However, a subsequent study that randomized patients to rapid hemodilution or slow hemodilution (goal HCT <35%) found that rapid hemodilution was associated with a higher rate of sepsis and slow hemodilution was associated with better survival.[26]
- **BUN**—Similar to hemoconcentration, elevated BUN reflects increasing third spacing and intravascular volume depletion. Elevated BUN levels were associated with mortality in acute pancreatitis.[27] A BUN >20 mg/dL was associated with an OR 4.6 for mortality and increase within 24 hours was associated with increased mortality (OR 4.3).[28] However, a small study using goal-directed therapy utilizing BUN as a trigger for further fluid resuscitation showed no difference with standard of care.[29]
- **CRP**—Serial CRP measurements demonstrated that CRP peaks in serum 3 days after symptom onset and high elevations were a good potential biomarker for prognosticating severe acute pancreatitis, pancreatic necrosis, and inhospital mortality.[30]

TREATMENT

Treatment is supportive with bed rest, oral intake when it is tolerable, intravenous hydration with LR, electrolyte replacement, antiemetics, and analgesics, minimizing narcotic use.

Medications

- **Fluids:** Hypovolemia, vomiting, and third spacing in the setting of profound vasodilation contribute to renal failure and acute tubular necrosis. Fluids prevent capillary microthrombi which may contribute to local tissue ischemia/necrosis.
  - **Lactate ringers (LR) versus normal saline (NS)**
    - NS can lead to acidosis and premature zymogen activation in acute pancreatitis. Lactate has been found to reduce liver and pancreatic injury in toll like receptor (TLR) and inflammasome-mediated inflammation via GPR81-mediated suppression of innate immunity.[31]
    - Lactated Ringers should not be used in hypercalcemia-associated pancreatitis as it contains 3 mEq/L calcium.

- In a randomized controlled trial of 40 patients, there was a significant reduction in systemic inflammatory markers (CRP) and SIRS at 24 hours in those receiving LR versus NS.[29]
  - **Rate**
    - Early fluid deficit has been shown to be associated with the development of pancreatic fluid collections, pancreatic necrosis, and persistent organ failure.[32]
    - However, conflicting studies exist weighing the risks of preserving tissue perfusion with precipitating pulmonary edema, congestive heart failure, and abdominal compartment syndrome. Primarily, early hydration studies (within 6–12 hours) have shown mortality benefit.
    - Based on original surviving sepsis guidelines, 5–10 mL/kg/hr has been suggested as an initial rate versus 250–500 mL/hr per ACG guidelines.[24]
    - No reliable biomarker (BUN, CVP, HCT) has emerged to guide fluid resuscitation (see above) and thus this should be driven by careful, frequent clinical assessments of intravascular and total body volume status, vital signs (HR <120 beats/min, MAP 65–85), oxygen requirements, and urine output (>0.5–1 cc/kg/hr).
- **Antibiotics**
  - The issue of prophylactic antibiotics in pancreatitis remains controversial as mortality in pancreatitis continues to be driven by infection.
  - Clinically, decision making is often clouded by the severe inflammatory reaction associated with acute pancreatitis and fluid collections which can frequently be associated with fevers, leukocytosis, and SIRS without a septic etiology. We do not recommend the sampling of fluid collections in these settings as this likely only propagates the risk of superinfection, but rather the use of empiric antibiotics if there is high clinical suspicion of infected necrosis.
  - Various antibiotic regimens have been trialed in a prophylactic setting; however, they have not been shown to be beneficial in reducing infected necrosis or mortality.[33]
  - Antibiotics should be given for biliary pancreatitis with suspected cholangitis, catheter-associated infections, bacteremia, urinary tract infections, or pneumonia.[24]

Nonpharmacologic Therapies

- Withholding oral intake has been a traditional mainstay of initial therapy for acute pancreatitis. This was thought to serve to minimize stimulation of the exocrine pancreas, thereby minimizing abdominal pain, nausea, and vomiting.[3,24] It was felt to also possibly mitigate pancreatic inflammation.
- However, enteral feedings are thought to maintain the health and barrier function of the bowel wall, reducing the probability of bacterial translocation and subsequent superinfection of pancreatic fluid collections.
- Options
  - Oral low-fat diet
  - **Enteral feedings (pre-/postpyloric):** A meta-analysis of nasogastric versus nasojejunal feeding demonstrated no difference in mortality nor in outcomes of aspiration, pain, or diarrhea.[34]
  - **Total parental nutrition (TPN)** requires central venous access, imparting a significant risk of infection. Also, TPN is financially costly and requires monitoring of key metabolic parameters. Enteral nutrition is always preferable to TPN which associated with increased mortality, infection, organ failure, and need for operative intervention.
- **Timing of feeding**
  - A meta-analysis of outcomes of acute pancreatitis with enteral nutrition initiated within 48 hours versus after 48 hours of hospital admission demonstrated that early nutrition was associated with significant reductions in infections (OR 0.38), pancreatic infection (OR 0.49), hyperglycemia (OR 0.24), length of stay, and mortality (OR 0.31). Importantly there was no increase in aspiration/pulmonary complications.[35]

More recently, a large, multicenter Dutch randomized trial of 209 patients with predicted severe acute pancreatitis was performed that randomized patients to enteral feeding within 24 hours versus attempted oral diet at 72 hours (dictated by clinical tolerance). Importantly, 69% in the oral diet group tolerated oral nutrition and there were no differences in clinical outcomes.[36]

Procedures

- **ERCP** has both diagnostic and therapeutic utility in biliary causes of pancreatitis. Given the risks associated with ERCP, however, this should be limited to cases of high clinical suspicion for choledocholithiasis with MRCP/EUS utilized to adjudicate low-risk/indeterminate risk cases.
- Very strong clinical predictors of choledocholithiasis include common bile duct (CBD) stone seen on transabdominal ultrasound, bilirubin >4 mg/dL, or cholangitis (right upper quadrant abdominal pain and tenderness, temperature >39°C, leukocyte count >20,000).[37] Strong predictors include a dilated CBD on ultrasound (>6 mm) or a bilirubin level of 1.8–4 mg/dL.
- Once identified, impacted gallstones can be extracted and infected bile can be drained via endoscopic sphincterotomy during ERCP.
- PEP may be reduced through the utilization of: guidewire cannulation, prophylactic pancreatic duct stenting (OR 0.22),[38] and pharmacologic intervention with indomethacin (relative risk reduction 46%).[39]

COMPLICATIONS

- **Pseudocyst**
  - **Asymptomatic pseudocysts** do not warrant intervention regardless of size, location, and or extension.[24]
  - In patients with **enlarging or symptomatic noninfected pseudocysts,** endoscopic or radiologic drainage is an attractive option. Radiologic placement of drainage catheters is often successful but can result in pancreatocutaneous fistulas.[40] However, transluminal endoscopic approaches to cyst-gastrostomy creation with the placement of plastic double-pigtail stents or metallic lumen–apposing metal stents (LAMS) under EUS guidance have been increasingly adopted to treat symptomatic fluid collections.[41] This allows for decompression and drainage of the pseudocyst contents directly into the bowel through the cystenterostomy; please see Figure 23-2.
  - For endoscopic drainage to be successful, the fluid collection should be mature (>4 weeks after acute episode of pancreatitis), well circumscribed, and within 1 cm of the lumen.[24,41] The absence of pseudoaneurysms in the wall of the cyst should be confirmed with CT and EUS before attempting endoscopic drainage.
  - Following drainage, patients are followed with serial imaging studies to document resolution of the pseudocyst. Once the pseudocyst has resolved, the stents or drains may be removed, though long-term plastic stent placement may be considered in cases of suspected pancreatic duct disruption or recurrent pseudocyst formation.
- **Pancreatic necrosis**
  - **Acute necrotic collections (ANC)** occurs during the first 4 weeks and may involve the pancreatic parenchyma and/or the peripancreatic tissues. CT scans demonstrate heterogeneous collections with varying amounts of solid necrotic material and fluid and may or may not be associated with a disruption of the MPD.[4]
  - **Walled off necrosis (WON)** occurs >4 weeks after necrotizing pancreatitis and is a mature, encapsulated collection of pancreatic and peripancreatic necrosis. WON may involve the parenchyma, may be multiplus, and may involve sites distant from the pancreas.[4]
  - **Infected necrosis** can occur in an ANC or a WON and should be suspected if there is clinical deterioration (SIRS) and/or gas within the collection on CT. Fine needle

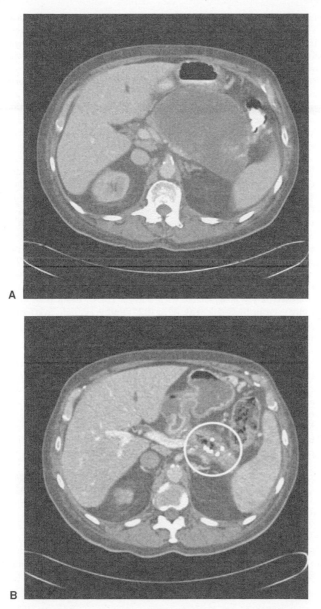

A

B

Figure 23-2. Demonstration of efficacy of endoscopic pancreatic pseudocyst drainage in a 58-year-old man with severe pancreatitis who developed a large pseudocyst as seen on computed tomography (**A**). He was symptomatic with abdominal pain, early satiety, and nausea. Therefore, multiple "pigtail" stents were endoscopically placed from the stomach into the cavity, and the cyst resolved over a period of 4 months (*white circle*) (**B**).

aspiration may be considered but the large majority of cases can be managed without FNA especially as transgastric or transcutaneous drainage are frequently part of the management algorithm. Surgical debridement has consistently been shown to be associated with high morbidity and mortality and is generally avoided whenever possible.[4,24]

Management

- *Empiric antibiotics/supportive care:* Conservative treatment with a combination of intensive care, antibiotics (in particular carbapenems, quinolones, and metronidazole), and nutritional support may delay the need for intervention, allowing for optimization of the patient and maturation of the WON. In particular, even without necrosectomy (but with percutaneous drainage) conservative management has been shown to be successful in up to 64% of patients.[42]

- *Endoscopic drainage and debridement of WOPN*
  - Utilizing EUS, the creation of an internal fistulous tract is made and direct endoscopic necrosectomy can be completed either with the fistula maintained with plastic double-pigtail stents, fully covered self-expanding metal stents (SEMS), or lumen-apposing metallic stents. This technique has been shown to have comparable clinical efficacy and may be associated with a lower rate of fistula formation, reinterventions, and length of stay.[43] A recent systematic review and meta-analysis comparing endoscopic versus percutaneous management demonstrated technical/clinical success rates in 99%/89% and had a higher success rate and lower morbidity/mortality in comparison to percutaneous and surgical therapies.[44] In a large pooled analysis, endoscopic necrosectomy was associated with a lower risk of death than open necrosectomy even in high-risk (risk ratio 0.27) and very high–risk (risk ratio 0.43) patients.[45]
  - Percutaneous drainage may have some advantages in early infected ANC that are not appropriate for the creation of a cyst-gastrostomy.
  - Specific protocols for the timing of intervention or reintervention have not been well codified, but we generally proceed with initial necrosectomy after the creation/maturation of a cyst-gastrostomy tract and repeat necrosectomy on a demand basis. Serial CT scan imaging allows for the efficient and complete resolution of necrotic debris.
  - Management should be individualized, and completed in the context of high-volume, multidisciplinary centers with hepatobiliary surgery, therapeutic endoscopic, and interventional radiology expertise.

Chronic Pancreatitis

GENERAL PRINCIPLES

Definition

Chronic pancreatitis is characterized by progressive inflammatory changes in the pancreas leading to irreversible damage of the pancreatic architecture. This leads to impairment of exocrine and endocrine function, often in conjunction with pain.[46–49]

Epidemiology

The incidence of chronic pancreatitis ranges from 4.4–11.9 per 100,000 per year, higher in men by a factor of 1.5–3 fold. The prevalence ranges from 36.9–41.8 per 100,000 persons.[49]

Etiology

The comprehensive TIGAR-O classification system for etiologic risk factors for chronic pancreatitis is shown in Table 23-2.[50]

TABLE 23-2 TIGAR-O CLASSIFICATION SYSTEM OF CHRONIC PANCREATITIS

Toxic metabolic	Alcohol, tobacco, hypercalcemia, hyperlipidemia, chronic renal failure, medications (phenacetin abuse)
Idiopathic	Early onset, late onset, tropical
Genetic	Cationic trypsinogen, CFTR mutations
Autoimmune	Sjögren syndrome, inflammatory bowel disease, primary biliary cirrhosis
Recurrent and severe acute pancreatitis	Postnecrotic, recurrent acute pancreatitis, vascular disease, postirradiation
Obstructive	Pancreas divisum, duct obstruction (tumor), posttraumatic pancreatic duct scars, preampullary duodenal wall cysts

CFTR, cystic fibrosis transmembrane conductance regulator.

Adapted from Etemad B, Whitcomb DC. Chronic pancreatitis: diagnosis, classification, and new genetic developments. *Gastroenterology.* 2001;120:682–707.

- **Alcohol**
  - Long-term ingestion of large quantities of alcohol (on average, >5 drinks per day) over 5–10 years is generally felt to be required, although only about 2–5% of heavy drinkers develop chronic pancreatitis. Smoking is a dose-dependent cofactor for causation of chronic pancreatitis—smokers are three times more likely to develop chronic pancreatitis compared with nonsmokers.[49]
  - In Western societies, alcohol consumption is the most common etiology, accounting for 70–80% of cases. Of note, however, only 5–10% of alcoholics develop chronic pancreatitis.[46]
- **Genetic syndromes**
  - Germline mutations in PRSS1, which encodes the cationic trypsinogen protein, are associated with **hereditary pancreatitis**.[51] Trypsinogen found in pancreatic acinar cells normally functions by hydrolyzing proteins at lysine and arginine residues and activating proenzymes. However, premature activation of trypsinogen can result in acute pancreatitis.
  - Clinically, patients with hereditary pancreatitis have recurrent bouts of acute pancreatitis, often in childhood, which can progressively evolve into chronic pancreatitis. The overall lifetime risk for developing pancreatic cancer is estimated at 35-fold (or more) by ages 70–75.[52] Treatment options are limited and are focused on limiting potential damage to the patient's pancreas and progression to chronic pancreatitis. Recommendations include a low-fat (low-triglyceride) diet, abstinence from cigarette smoking and alcohol, and consideration for total pancreatectomy with auto islet cell transplant.
  - In addition to mutations in PRSS1, hereditary pancreatitis has also been demonstrated due to mutations in the chymotrypsin C (CTRC) gene due to mutations that boost the effects of cationic trypsinogen.[52,53] The Kazal-type serine protease inhibitors (SPINK) are a family of genes in which SPINK1 mutations (e.g., N34S) are found to be associated in some patients with idiopathic chronic pancreatitis. Similarly, heterozygous mutations in the cystic fibrosis transmembrane receptor (CFTR) gene may be found in a subset of these patients.[54] CFTR is an ion channel

involved in the transport of chloride and thiocyanate. Traditionally CFTR gene mutations are associated with cystic fibrosis; however, they may also contribute to chronic pancreatitis.

- **Ductal obstruction:** This may result from trauma, stones, neoplasms, or sphincter of Oddi dysfunction.[46]
- **Autoimmune disease:** Includes systemic lupus erythematosus, inflammatory bowel disease, and AIP.
- **Idiopathic**

Pathophysiology

- While the specific pathogenesis is not clear, there are several theories including the oxidative stress theory (ethanol and other toxic compounds induce oxidative stress via CYP enzymes), toxic-metabolic theory (ethanol and metabolites can cause acinar cell necrosis, fatty degeneration, and ultimately fibrosis), stone/ductal obstruction theory (chronic obstruction leads to a self-reinforcing cycle of stasis, fibrosis, and stone formation), necrosis fibrosis theory (informed by patients with PRSS1 mutations or animal models of chronic pancreatitis [i.e., cerulein], recurrent bouts of acute pancreatitis lead to atrophy of the organ), and the sentinel acute pancreatitis event (SAPE) hypothesis which aims to unify the disparate theories and include more modern immune-mediated mechanisms.[55,56]
- *SAPE hypothesis*—This requires an initiating event (sentinel event) causing acute pancreatitis and acinar cell injury. Subsequently, counterregulatory profibrotic events enable the progression to chronic pancreatitis. While exposure to alcohol, nicotine, or oxidative compounds prior to the sentinel event may occur, it is this event that leads to unrestrained trypsinogen activation and protease activation that allows for cellular damage. This is followed by a late phase of acute pancreatitis with anti-inflammatory/profibrotic healing process, marked by stellate cells.
- Clinically overt malabsorption occurs when enzyme secretion is reduced by more than 90%, which usually takes 10–20 years in alcoholic pancreatitis.[57] However, steatorrhea may occur earlier in the course due to decreased lipase secretion and its lack of efficacy with impaired bicarbonate secretion.[58] In only a small minority (<5%) can pancreatic exocrine insufficiency be present without morphologic alterations.

DIAGNOSIS

Clinical Presentation

- The most common presenting symptoms are nausea, vomiting, anorexia, and a dull, constant epigastric/periumbilical abdominal pain that may radiate to the back. Pain could occur periodically, lasting several days, or occasionally be constant.
- Exacerbation of pain by eating is common in chronic pancreatitis, but other medical conditions (e.g., mesenteric ischemia and irritable bowel syndrome) can also have a similar presentation. However, in advanced stages, chronic pancreatitis can be painless (15% of patients).
- If chronic pancreatitis is complicated by exocrine insufficiency, the patient may present with weight loss (due to anorexia, malabsorption, uncontrolled diabetes mellitus), steatorrhea, malnutrition, or fat-soluble vitamin deficiencies (A, D, E, K). Stools are described as voluminous sticky/shiny/oily stools, though physical descriptions are neither sensitive nor specific.
- Less common manifestations of chronic pancreatitis include jaundice (extrinsic bile duct obstruction or stricture), ascites, pleural effusion, painful subcutaneous nodules (pancreatic panniculitis), and polyarthritis of the small joints of the hands.

Diagnostic Testing

Laboratory Testing

- **Exocrine function** can be tested directly.
  - Testing may be performed by stimulation with secretin, cholecystokinin, or both, followed by measurement of bicarbonate concentrations or enzyme activity. Subnormal measured levels are suggestive of chronic pancreatitis.[59]
  - Another method is the measurement of pancreatic polypeptide. A subnormal rise in plasma pancreatic polypeptide levels after stimulation with a protein-rich meal or secretin infusion is an indication of chronic pancreatitis.
- **Exocrine function** can also be tested indirectly.
  - Testing may be performed by measuring pancreatic enzyme levels or by assessing the absorption of a compound that requires initial digestion by pancreatic enzymes.[59]
  - The bentiromide test involves ingestion of N-benzoyl-L-tyrosyl-p-aminobenzoic acid (NBT-PABA), a tripeptide that is digested by chymotrypsin with the release of p-aminobenzoic acid (PABA). Free PABA is absorbed in the small bowel and excreted by the kidney. The quantity excreted in urine is used as a measure of pancreatic exocrine function.[59]
  - Fecal chymotrypsin activity measurement is rapid and simple, but its sensitivity is considered too low to be recommended in clinical practice.
  - Fecal elastase measurement is much more sensitive and specific in the diagnosis of moderate to severe pancreatic insufficiency.[59] However, especially in early chronic pancreatitis, it has limited sensitivity (50–93%) and specificity (62–93%) and may be falsely positive in the setting of high stool-water content.[60,61]
  - Alternatively, exocrine function can be assessed by measuring the absorption of a compound that requires initial digestion by pancreatic enzymes. However, because clinically detectable nutrient malabsorption does not occur until pancreatic enzyme secretion has diminished to <10% of normal, this approach cannot detect early chronic pancreatitis.

Imaging

- **Plain x-ray of the abdomen:** Demonstration of diffuse, speckled calcification of the pancreas on a plain x-ray film is diagnostic of chronic pancreatitis, but this is an insensitive modality.
- **CT:** The most common diagnostic findings of chronic pancreatitis on CT include duct dilation (3.5–7 mm or >7 mm), PD contour, PD stricture, parenchymal/intraductal calcifications, atrophy/decreased pancreas diameter, and cystic lesions.[62]
- **MRCP**
  - Allows for accurate delineation of the pancreatic duct (presence of dilation, stones, or strictures), evaluation of pancreatic parenchyma, and the detection of subtle solid and cystic lesions.
  - May be more desirable than CT because it avoids exposure to ionizing radiation and iodinated intravenous contrast and delineates the pancreatic duct and intraductal pathology with superior fidelity.

Diagnostic Procedures

- **Endoscopic ultrasound (EUS)**
  - Provides more detailed structural information than abdominal ultrasonography and CT, without the risk of complications of ERCP, and allows for direct tissue sampling with FNA if indicated.
  - Allows for evaluation of ductal and parenchymal changes, such as echotexture of the gland, calcifications, lobulations, and bands of fibrosis.
  - Criteria have been proposed (Rosemont criteria) (Table 23-3) that include MPD calculi, irregular MPD, dilated side branches, MPD dilation (>3.5 mm in the body, >1.5 mm in the tail), hyperechoic MPD margins, hyperechoic foci with shadowing, lobularity

TABLE 23-3 EUS ROSEMONT CRITERIA

Parenchymal Features

Major criteria	(A) hyperechoic foci with shadowing and lobularity; (B) Lobularity with honeycombing
Minor criteria	Lobularity without honeycombing, hyperechoic foci without shadowing, cysts, stranding

Ductal Features

Major criteria	Main pancreatic duct calculi
Minor criteria	Irregular main pancreatic duct contour, dilated ducts (≥3.5 mm), dilated side branches (≥1 mm), hyperechoic duct wall

Adapted from Catalano MF, Sahai A, Levy M, et al. EUS-based criteria for the diagnosis of chronic pancreatitis: the Rosemont classification. *Gastrointest Endosc.* 2009;69:1251–1261.

with/without honeycombing, hyperechoic foci without shadowing, cysts, stranding.[63] However, many of the parenchymal EUS features in noncalcific chronic pancreatitis are nonspecific and may be seen in obese or elderly populations and subsequent validations with histopathologic correlates have shown only moderate accuracy.[64]

○ EUS correlates only moderately to pancreatic exocrine insufficiency—overall sensitivity of 68% and specificity of 79% in one study.[65]

- **ERCP:** The widespread availability of EUS and MRCP has largely supplanted the use of ERCP for diagnostic pancreatography. ERCP is typically performed with intent to deliver therapy as directed by other imaging modalities rather than purely as a diagnostic procedure.

TREATMENT

- Alcohol and tobacco cessation are paramount in the treatment of chronic pancreatitis. Avoiding alcohol decreases the frequency and severity of abdominal pain in chronic alcoholic pancreatitis, especially as alcohol acts as a pancreatic secretagogue.[10]
- All patients with excessive alcohol consumption should be referred to an appropriate treatment program. Similarly, counseling for smoking cessation should be performed with appropriate pharmacologic and nonpharmacologic aids provided.

Medications

- **Analgesics**
  ○ Initially, analgesia should follow the World Health Organization (WHO) "pain relief ladder" with stepwise increase of nonopioid analgesics such as acetaminophen. The dose or frequency of these nonopioid analgesics should be titrated and maximized before adding on or switching to an opioid.[66]
  ○ Adjunctive analgesics have been heterogeneously applied including anticonvulsants, anxiolytics, and antispasmodics. A randomized controlled trial demonstrated pregabalin to have moderate pain relief in chronic pancreatitis, and thus neuromodulating agents should be utilized where possible to limit chronic narcotic use.[67]
  ○ Antidepressants are widely used for functional and visceral pain disorders that are thought to overlap with chronic pancreatitis pain and may be effective in chronic pancreatitis though high-quality evidence is lacking.

For severe or uncontrolled pain, opioid analgesics may be required; however, their use is associated with constipation, hyperalgesia, as well as addictive potential. Tramadol is often the preferred step-up analgesic as it was shown to have a similar effect as morphine in patients with chronic pancreatitis with fewer GI side effects.[68]

Because of the recurrent nature of chronic pancreatitis with the frequent use of opioid analgesics, many of these patients demonstrate opioid dependence and drug-seeking behaviors, making evaluation and treatment of pain quite complex. Consultation from a pain management specialist may be helpful.

- **Pancreatic enzyme replacement therapy**
  - Nutrients stimulate the release of cholecystokinin-releasing factor from the duodenum, which releases cholecystokinin and stimulates pancreatic secretion and may cause intraductal hypertension in patients with strictures or leakage in patients with discontinuity of their pancreatic duct.[2] Theoretically, ingestion of enzymes allow for feedback of this loop and may lessen pancreatic secretion.
  - *Pain control:* In the six trials that have examined pancreatic enzymes for pain relief, positive effects were noted in two trials and no effect was noted in four trials.[69] If utilized, enzymes should be given without enteric coating, contain large amounts of proteases, and be given up to four times a day to maximize their effect. Patients may consider a histamine-2 receptor antagonist or proton pump inhibitor to diminish enzyme degradation by gastric acid.
  - *Exocrine insufficiency*
    - This is the cornerstone of therapy for malabsorption in patients with chronic pancreatitis. It is critical that sufficient amounts of enzyme are delivered to the small bowel to reduce steatorrhea.
    - It is estimated the healthy human pancreas can produce 900,000 USP units of lipase with each meal but only 10% is required for normal fat absorption (90,000 USP units). Enteric coating allows for maximal duodenal/small bowel concentration of the enzymes. Generally, 40,000 to 50,000 USP units of lipase are recommended to start with each meal and half that amount with snacks.[48] The dosage of the pancreatic enzyme supplements can be titrated to treat the symptoms and malabsorption adequately.
    - Therapy may be ineffective due to insufficient dosing, inappropriate diet, acid inactivation of the lipase, or asynchrony in the delivery of enzymes/food (especially an issue for gastric bypass/pancreatic resection patients). If diarrhea persists despite correction of these issues, alternative etiologies like bacterial overgrowth should be considered.

Surgical/Procedural Management

- **Celiac plexus block/neurolysis**
  - In patients who have failed other medical treatments, celiac plexus blocks or neurolysis may be performed either percutaneously or with EUS guidance.
  - Celiac plexus blocks do not provide durable relief and carry risk of postural hypotension and, in the case of neurolysis, theoretical paralysis/weakness. In those patients with an initial response, repeated treatment may not be as effective.[66]
- **Pancreatic duct endotherapy during ERCP**
  - ERCP with pancreatic duct endotherapy is predicated under the premise that pain is due to an outflow obstruction of the MPD from strictures and/or intraductal stones that may be relieved with a combination of short-term stent placement and/or pancreatic stone fragmentation and extraction. The goal of ERCP in these patients is pain relief as these therapies have never been shown to clearly prolong endocrine or exocrine function of the pancreas. Therefore, these interventions should be limited to those patients symptomatic with pain with MRCP/CT/EUS demonstrating pancreatic duct strictures/stones with resultant pancreatic duct dilation who have not

responded sufficiently to medical therapy. As it is difficult to assess *a priori* which patients may have pain due to ductal hypertension, as opposed to complex neuropathic pain syndromes or opioid hyperalgesia, it is critical that patients are counseled extensively regarding the complexity and expected outcomes of these technically challenging interventions.

○ The combined effectiveness of endoscopic therapy is felt to approach approximately 50–60% with pain relief both in short- and long-term follow-up.[66] However, the quality of data is poor as most studies are observational, retrospective, and marred by selection bias and nongeneralizable endoscopic skill.

○ In the two randomized control trials that have compared endoscopic and surgical management of chronic pancreatitis, both demonstrated surgery to be superior in pain control and durability though there was a lower technical success rate of ERCP in these studies as compared to prior reports.[70,71]

○ As surgical intervention carries significant morbidity, and possible mortality, patients with multiple comorbidities and older age may be considered for endoscopic therapy. Factors that predict success include: complete clearance of stones, <5 endoscopic procedures, location of the obstruction/stones (head vs. body/tail), shorter duration of disease prior to endoscopy, tobacco cessation, and decreased MPD dilation.[66] Response to endoscopic therapy may also predict response to surgical decompression of the pancreatic duct.

- **Extracorporeal shock wave lithotripsy (ESWL)**
  ○ ESWL is indicated for patients with recurrent attacks of pain, with moderate/marked changes in the pancreatic ducal system associated with obstructing ductal stones (2–5 mm) that are ideally radiolucent.
  ○ ESWL has a high success rate in stone fragmentation (54–100%) and has been shown to decrease narcotic use in 80% of patients with 50% patients reporting pain resolution.[72]
  ○ In a prospective, randomized controlled trial of ESWL alone compared with ESWL with endoscopy, there was no evidence that the combination was superior to ESWL alone.[73] However, in certain patients, the combination may be considered as complete stone clearance, may be challenging with multiple stones especially in the setting of pancreatic duct strictures.[66]

- **Surgical management**
  ○ There are several types of surgeries available for the management of chronic pancreatitis ranging from resections (distal pancreatectomy/Whipple procedure), drainage procedures (pancreaticojejunostomy), or total pancreatectomy with auto islet cell transplant.
  ○ Surgery should only be considered in a high-volume center with multidisciplinary support and after the failure of nonsurgical options. The type of surgery should be selected according to the perceived mechanism for the pain, the severity of pain, and anatomic factors like pancreatic duct dilation >6 mm. As noted above, randomized controlled trials have established the efficacy of surgical versus endoscopic management for these patients.[70,71]

COMPLICATIONS

- **Diabetes mellitus:** Clinically evident diabetes, which occurs relatively late in the disease, is frequently seen in patients with chronic pancreatitis. Type 3 diabetes, characterized by a lack of insulin secretion and glucagon secretion is seen later in the disease process and may be noted with treatment-induced hypoglycemia and rarely ketoacidosis.[48]
- **Pseudocysts** are generally asymptomatic in chronic pancreatitis patients, but may also cause symptoms as discussed above in the section on acute pancreatitis. These symptoms may include abdominal pain, duodenal/biliary obstruction, vascular occlusion, fistula formation, pseudoaneurysm, and abscess.

- **Bile duct obstruction or duodenal obstruction**
  - Causes include inflammation and fibrosis in the head of the pancreas, or a pseudocyst.
  - Bile duct obstruction characteristically causes pain as well as elevated levels of transaminases and bilirubin.
  - Duodenal obstruction characteristically causes postprandial pain and early satiety.
  - Diagnosis is made by upper GI series, upper endoscopy, or CT.
  - ERCP with biliary stent placement has been shown to be highly effective in the management and remediation of chronic pancreatitis strictures.[74]
- **Pancreatic ascites**
  - May develop due to disruption of the pancreatic duct, which leads to fistulization to the abdomen or rupture of a pseudocyst. Pancreatic juice then tracks into the peritoneal cavity, causing ascites. Pleural effusions may develop in a similar manner as well.
  - Fluid obtained by paracentesis (or thoracentesis in the setting of pleural effusion) has a characteristically high amylase concentration, usually exceeding 1000 IU/L.
  - Treatment may be nonoperative, consisting of repeated aspiration, diuretics, or octreotide. Parenteral nutrition to decrease pancreatic secretion and endoscopic stenting of the pancreatic duct may be employed as well.
- **Splenic vein thrombosis**
  - Because of its location along the posterior pancreas, the splenic vein may thrombose due to adjacent inflammation.
  - Gastric varices may develop due to subsequent portal hypertension. Splenectomy is a curative option for patients who develop bleeding from varices.

Pancreatic Cancer

GENERAL PRINCIPLES

Definition

Pancreatic ductal adenocarcinoma (PDAC) and its variants account for >90% of all malignant exocrine pancreatic tumors.[75]

Epidemiology

- Approximately 50,000 new cases of pancreatic cancer occur every year in the United States.[75] It continues to have one of the highest mortality rates of any solid tumor type, and is projected to be the leading cause of cancer deaths by 2030.[76]
- According to SEER data, PDAC generally presents later in life (fifth to seventh decades), most frequently at a locally advanced or metastatic stage (52% metastatic, 29% regional, 10% localized). Metastatic disease continues to carry a dismal 5-year survival of 2.7%.

Risk Factors

- **Tobacco exposure** significantly contributes to the development of pancreatic cancer, with some estimates of up to 25% of cases related to smoking exposure.[77]
- **Chronic pancreatitis**
  - Older studies have noted an association between chronic pancreatitis of various etiologies and pancreatic cancer; however even at this time, there were questions of confounding effects of smoking status, degree of inflammation, and length of symptoms.[78]
  - A Swedish inpatient registry examined the incidence of PDAC in those with a single episode of pancreatitis versus recurrent pancreatitis versus chronic pancreatitis. Interestingly, these authors found that irrespective of the type of pancreatitis, there was an excess risk of being diagnosed with pancreatic cancer immediately around the time of the diagnosis of pancreatitis, but after 10 years or more this risk declined. Selection

bias, alcohol abuse, smoking, or a lack of recognition of hereditary pancreatitis cases may have contributed to previous associations of pancreatitis and pancreatic cancer.[79]

○ Recent data suggest that acute pancreatitis is associated with a small, but demonstrable risk of PDAC as well.[80]

○ Overall there is likely a small higher risk of PDAC in chronic pancreatitis patients, but this is most pronounced around the time of initial diagnosis.

- **Obesity/Diabetes**
  ○ Individuals with a BMI of 30 kg/m^2 or more had an elevated risk of pancreatic cancer compared with those with a BMI of <23kg/m^2. Similarly there was a negative correlation observed between self-reported moderate physical activity and the development of pancreatic cancer, particularly in those with a BMI of >25kg/m^2.[81]
  ○ Diabetes has been both investigated as a risk factor for as well as an early manifestation of pancreatic cancer. In a large meta-analysis examining patients with long-standing diabetes (>5 years), the relative risk for diabetics relative to nondiabetics was 2.0 for developing pancreatic cancer.[82] In addition to long-standing diabetes, new-onset (<2 years prior to diagnosis) diabetes has also been studied. In a study of U.S. Veterans, there was a 2.2-fold higher risk of developing pancreatic cancer within 2 years of a diabetes diagnosis.[83]

- **Familial pancreatic cancer**
  ○ It is estimated that 5–10% of PDAC has a hereditary basis.[84]
  ○ If we define familial pancreatic cancer to be a kindred with a pair of first-degree relatives with pancreatic cancer, an affected family member would have a sixfold increased risk of pancreatic cancer.[84] This risk rises significantly if there are three or more first-degree relatives with pancreatic cancer.[85,86]
  ○ Known genetic syndromes that increase the risk for pancreatic cancer include hereditary pancreatitis, familial atypical mole and multiple melanoma, Peutz–Jeghers syndrome, Lynch syndrome, BRCA mutations (BRCA1/2, PALB2, ATM), and Li–Fraumeni syndrome. Genetic testing should be performed in conjunction with genetic counseling, and testing of an affected family member is preferred if possible.[87]
    ○ *Pancreatic cancer screening*
      ■ The goal of pancreatic cancer screening is to identify pancreatic cancer at an early, curable stage or, ideally, to identify precancerous lesions that can be resected to prevent the development of cancer.
      ■ EUS and MRCP are generally considered to be complementary, although an advantage of EUS is that cysts or solid lesions can be sampled at the time of the procedure.
      ■ Published results of small cohorts of high-risk patients in pancreatic cancer screening programs have demonstrated that screening programs are effective and may increase survival.[88,89]

DIAGNOSIS

Clinical Presentation

- Jaundice: presenting symptom in majority of cases of pancreatic cancer in the head.[75]
- Abdominal pain
  ○ Epigastric pain or right upper quadrant pain can occur due to biliary tree obstruction.
  ○ Similar pain or discomfort in the left upper quadrant, back, or periumbilical areas could also result from pancreatic duct distention associated with pancreatic duct obstruction, or invasion of retroperitoneal or somatic nerves.
  ○ Emesis may be caused by duodenal or gastric outlet obstruction from tumor invasion.
- Weight loss
  ○ By the time of diagnosis, weight loss of >10% of ideal body weight is common.

Anorexia may be to tumor-associated pain, decreased food intake, malabsorption from pancreatic insufficiency, and proinflammatory cytokines.

- Diabetes mellitus sometimes appears as an early manifestation of pancreatic cancer, occurring many months before the tumor becomes evident.
- Other
  - Migratory thrombophlebitis (Trousseau sign) is reported in approximately 10% of patients and may be the earliest presenting sign.[75]
  - There is also a poorly understood association between pancreatic malignancy and major depressive disorder.

Diagnostic Testing

Laboratory Testing

- **Serum carbohydrate antigen 19-9 (CA 19-9) level** is a tumor-associated glycoprotein that is elevated in the serum of 85% of patients with PDAC.[48] However about 5–10% of the population is unable to produce CA 19-9 due to lack of an enzyme needed for epitope production, which does limit its use as biomarker.[51]
- CA 19-9 level may be abnormal due to other cancers (gastric, colorectal cancer) and with some benign conditions (cholangitis, biliary obstruction).
- In those that produce CA 19-9, serial assessment can be helpful in response to surgery/chemotherapy.

Imaging

- **Computed tomography**
  - Triple-phase CT is an excellent tool for diagnosis and the preoperative staging of pancreatic cancer as it delineates vascular involvement of the superior mesenteric artery (SMA)/celiac axis/PV and distant liver metastases/peritoneal involvement.
  - In terms of assessing resectability, studies range in estimates of accuracy of 70–80% with sensitivity ranging 75–84% and specificity ranging from 85–98%.[90–92] Sensitivity and specificity for assessing nodal metastasis by CT have demonstrated more limited accuracy.[93]
- **Magnetic resonance imaging**
  - MRI is not clearly superior to triple-phase multidetector CT for local staging and evaluation of pancreatic cancer, though some reports suggest it may identify smaller tumors.[94]
  - In intraductal papillary mucinous neoplasm (IPMN)- or mucinous cystic neoplasm (MCN)-associated pancreatic cancers where assessment of the association between the pancreatic duct and the tumor are critical, MRCP may have clear advantages.[95]
- **Endoscopic ultrasonography**
  - EUS has emerged as a critical component in the imaging, staging, and diagnosis of pancreatic cancer. Not only can EUS delineate a mass utilizing sonography through the wall of the stomach or duodenum, but it also can obtain diagnostic FNA of lesions.
  - Estimates of accuracy for assessing preoperative resectability have ranged in several studies from 63–93%.[96–98]
  - FNA for tissue diagnosis can be performed percutaneously under CT or ultrasound guidance or can be performed endoscopically by EUS.
  - Tissue sampling should be pursued when cytologic proof of malignancy alters management—for example, equivocal imaging, as a prerequisite for chemotherapy, radiation therapy, clinical trial inclusion, or palliative stenting with a permanent metal stent.
- **Staging laparoscopy**
  - Complements the noninvasive staging and aids the surgeon in assessing the resectability of the tumor. Laparoscopy can assist in identifying small or diffuse metastases

(such as hepatic or peritoneal implants) that may be unrecognized in the initial diagnostic evaluation.

- During laparoscopy, the abdominal cavity is inspected for frank metastases. Also, peritoneal washings are taken for cytology, peritoneal nodules or lymph nodes are sampled, and intraoperative ultrasonography of the pancreas or liver can be performed.

TREATMENT

Surgical Management

- **Tumor resection**
  - Surgery for pancreatic cancer is performed with curative intent only if no evidence of metastatic disease is seen on preoperative imaging studies and staging laparoscopy.
  - The type of surgery performed for pancreatic cancer is dependent on the location of the tumor.
  - **Pancreaticoduodenectomy** (Whipple or pylorus-sparing Whipple resection) is typically performed for tumors involving the pancreatic head. The classic Whipple resection involves a partial gastrectomy (antrectomy), cholecystectomy, and removal of the distal common bile duct, head of the pancreas, duodenum, proximal jejunum, and regional lymph nodes. Reconstruction requires pancreaticojejunostomy, hepaticojejunostomy, and gastrojejunostomy.
  - For tumors involving the body or tail of the pancreas, distal pancreatectomy and splenectomy are performed.
  - Rarely, patients are offered a total pancreatectomy for large or multifocal tumors.
- **Surgical palliation**
  - When resection of the primary tumor is not possible, palliative procedures are performed.
  - An anastomosis between the common bile duct and jejunum (choledochojejunostomy) serves to bypass the bile duct obstruction.
- **Endoscopic retrograde cholangiopancreatography**
  - At the time of ERCP, cytology brushings from the bile duct can be obtained, which have a moderate sensitivity for diagnosing pancreatic cancer and should be used in conjunction with EUS-guided FNA.
  - If there is jaundice present, ERCP should be considered with or without biliary sphincterotomy for the placement of a biliary stent which may either be plastic (if the mass is nonbiopsy proven, there is <3 month life expectancy, there is prompt expectation of surgical management) or a SEMS; please see Figure 23-3.
  - A multicenter study demonstrated a significantly increased rate of complications in patients who underwent routine preoperative biliary drainage.[99] However, the study was limited by high rates of cannulation failure (25%), post-ERCP complications (46%), and plastic stent–related early occlusion (26%). Preoperative biliary drainage may alleviate jaundice and cholestasis-associated adverse events and allow time for delivery of neoadjuvant chemoradiation which has increasingly become the standard of care.
  - Tumor ingrowth can result in stent occlusion, and a new stent can be placed within the old stent to relieve the recurrent biliary obstruction.
- **Enteral stent placement**
  - Gastric outlet obstruction can also be palliated effectively by endoscopic placement of expandable metal stents.
  - In a randomized control trial of gastrojejunostomy versus enteral stent placement, there was no difference in survival or quality of life scores, though surgical gastrojejunostomy had more durable relief with fewer reinterventions.[100] However, multiple

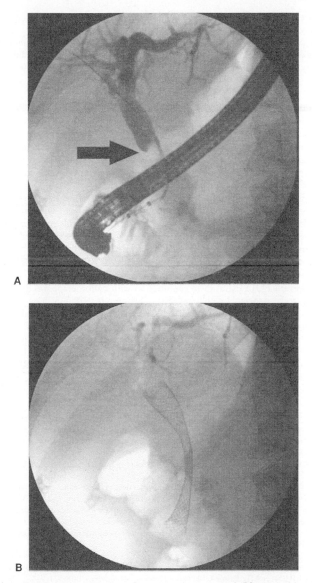

Figure 23-3. Endoscopic palliation of pancreatic cancer. A 69-year-old man developed jaundice, and a pancreatic mass was found that had metastasized to the liver. The decision was to administer palliative chemotherapy and place a metal biliary stent. The initial fluoroscopic cholangiogram demonstrates markedly dilated proximal and intrahepatic bile ducts with a "cutoff" (*arrow*) in the distal bile duct resulting from a malignant stricture (**A**). Fluoroscopic image demonstrates successful placement of a metallic self-expanding biliary stent across the malignant stricture (**B**).

studies have demonstrated a faster resolution of obstructive symptoms, shorter hospital stay, and lower costs associated with stent placement.

Stent placement is a preferable to palliative surgery in patients with a short life expectancy or those with ascites. However, stent placement may precipitate biliary obstruction or make future endoscopic access of the bile duct more challenging

Medications

- **Adjuvant chemotherapy**
  Gemcitabine has been shown to increase the quality of life in patients with advanced pancreatic cancer, but survival is only modestly improved.[101]

  In patients who can tolerate its increased side effect profile (i.e., neutropenia, diarrhea, anemia, neuropathy), FOLFIRINOX (oxaliplatin plus irinotecan with leucovorin and 5-FU) has been shown to be superior to gemcitabine alone for metastatic disease[102] and locally advanced disease.[103]

  Gemcitabine in combination with nab-paclitaxel has similarly been shown to be more modestly superior to gemcitabine alone for metastatic disease with fewer side effects than FOLFIRINOX.[104] The LAPACT trial is examining this combination in locally advance disease and preliminary results appear to mirror the metastatic data.

- **Neoadjuvant chemotherapy**
  Studies have sequentially demonstrated benefit for Mitomycin C + 5-FU,[105] 5-FU monotherapy,[106] and gemcitabine monotherapy.[107]

  Neoadjuvant FOLFIRINOX in conjunction with radiotherapy was found in a Phase 2 study to be associated with a high R0 resection rate (97%) in those that underwent resection (32/48) with median overall survival of 37.7 months.[108] Randomized control trial data are still being collected.

  Randomized data on gemcitabine plus Abraxane is lacking, though in a recent propensity-matched analysis of a surgical series comparing neoadjuvant gemcitabine/Abraxane versus FOLFIRINOX, the treatment effect of FOLFIRINOX was to increase overall survival by 4.9 months.[109]

REFERENCES

1. Dominguez-Munoz JE. *Clinical Pancreatology*. Hoboken, New Jersey: John Wiley & Sons; 2008.
2. Podolsky DK, Camilleri M, Fitz JG, et al. *Yamada's Textbook of Gastroenterology*. Hoboken, New Jersey: John Wiley & Sons; 2015.
3. Forsmark CE, Swaroop VS, Wilcox CM. Acute pancreatitis. *N Engl J Med*. 2016;375: 1972–1981.
4. Banks PA, Bollen TL, Dervenis C, et al. Classification of acute pancreatitis—2012: revision of the Atlanta classification and definitions by international consensus. *Gut*. 2013;62:102–111.
5. Ranson JH, Rifkind KM, Roses DF, et al. Prognostic signs and the role of operative management in acute pancreatitis. *Surg Gynecol Obstet*. 1974;139:69–81.
6. Wu BU, Johannes RS, Sun X, et al. The early prediction of mortality in acute pancreatitis: a large population-based study. *Gut*. 2008;57:1698–1703.
7. Crockett SD, Wani S, Gardner TB, et al. American Gastroenterological Association Institute Guideline on Initial Management of Acute Pancreatitis. *Gastroenterology*. 2018;154:1096–1101.
8. Frossard JL, Steer ML, Pastor CM. Acute pancreatitis. *Lancet*. 2008;371:143–152.
9. Forsmark CE, Baillie J; AGA Institute Clinical Practice and Economics Committee, AGA Institute Governing Board. AGA Institute technical review on acute pancreatitis. *Gastroenterology*. 2007;132:2022–2044.
10. Gorelick FS. Alcohol and zymogen activation in the pancreatic acinar cell. *Pancreas*. 2003;27: 305–310.
11. Trivedi CD, Pitchumoni CS. Drug-induced pancreatitis: an update. *J Clin Gastroenterol*. 2005;39:709–716.
12. Debi U, Kaur R, Prasad KK, et al. Pancreatic trauma: a concise review. *World J Gastroenterol*. 2013;19:9003–9011.

13. Dumonceau JM, Andriulli A, Elmunzer BJ, et al. Prophylaxis of post-ERCP pancreatitis: European Society of Gastrointestinal Endoscopy (ESGE) Guideline—updated June 2014. *Endoscopy*. 2014;46:799–815.

14. Parenti DM, Steinberg W, Kang P. Infectious causes of acute pancreatitis. *Pancreas*. 1996;13: 356–371.

15. Mosler P, Akisik F, Sandrasegaran K, et al. Accuracy of magnetic resonance cholangiopancreatography in the diagnosis of pancreas divisum. *Dig Dis Sci*. 2011;57:170–174.

16. Borak GD, Romagnuolo J, Alsolaiman M, et al. Long-term clinical outcomes after endoscopic minor papilla therapy in symptomatic patients with pancreas divisum. *Pancreas*. 2009;38:903–906.

17. Shimosegawa T, Chari ST, Frulloni L, et al. International consensus diagnostic criteria for autoimmune pancreatitis: guidelines of the International Association of Pancreatology. *Pancreas*. 2011;40:352–358.

18. Stone JH, Zen Y, Deshpande V. IgG4-related disease. *N Engl J Med*. 2012;366:539–551.

19. Hart PA, Kamisawa T, Brugge WR, et al. Long-term outcomes of autoimmune pancreatitis: a multicentre, international analysis. *Gut*. 2013;62:1771–1776.

20. Raina A, Yadav D, Krasinskas AM, et al. Evaluation and management of autoimmune pancreatitis: experience at a large US center. *Am J Gastroenterol*. 2009;104:2295–2306.

21. Sandanayake NS, Church NI, Chapman MH, et al. Presentation and management of post-treatment relapse in autoimmune pancreatitis/immunoglobulin G4-associated cholangitis. *Clin Gastroenterol Hepatol*. 2009;7:1089–1096.

22. Frank B, Gottlieb K. Amylase normal, lipase elevated: is it pancreatitis? A case series and review of the literature. *Am J Gastroenterol*. 1999;94:463–469.

23. Ben-Horin S, Farfel Z, Mouallem M. Gastroenteritis-associated hyperamylasemia: prevalence and clinical significance. *Arch Intern Med*. 2002;162:689–692.

24. Tenner S, Baillie J, Dewitt J, et al. American College of Gastroenterology guideline: management of acute pancreatitis. *Am J Gastroenterol*. 2013;108:1400–1415.

25. Koutroumpakis E, Wu BU, Bakker OJ, et al. Admission hematocrit and rise in blood urea nitrogen at 24 h outperform other laboratory markers in predicting persistent organ failure and pancreatic necrosis in acute pancreatitis: a post hoc analysis of three large prospective databases. *Am J Gastroenterol*. 2015;110:1707–1716.

26. Mao EQ, Fei J, Peng YB, et al. Rapid hemodilution is associated with increased sepsis and mortality among patients with severe acute pancreatitis. *Chin Med J*. 2010;123:1639–1644.

27. Wu BU, Johannes RS, Sun X, et al. Early changes in blood urea nitrogen predict mortality in acute pancreatitis. *Gastroenterology*. 2009;137:129–135.

28. Wu BU, Bakker OJ, Papachristou GI, et al. Blood urea nitrogen in the early assessment of acute pancreatitis: an international validation study. *Arch Intern Med*. 2011;171:669–676.

29. Wu BU, Hwang JQ, Gardner TH, et al. Lactated Ringer's solution reduces systemic inflammation compared with saline in patients with acute pancreatitis. *Clin Gastroenterol Hepatol*. 2011;9:710–717.e1.

30. Cardoso FS, Ricardo LB, Oliveira AM, et al. C-reactive protein prognostic accuracy in acute pancreatitis: timing of measurement and cutoff points. *Eur J Gastroenterol Hepatol*. 2013;25:784–789.

31. Lerch MM, Conwell DL, Mayerle J. The anti-inflammasome effect of lactate and the lactate GPR81-receptor in pancreatic and liver inflammation. *Gastroenterology*. 2014;146:1602–1605.

32. Mole DJ, Hall A, McKeown D, et al. Detailed fluid resuscitation profiles in patients with severe acute pancreatitis. *HPB (Oxford)*. 2011;13:51–58.

33. Wittau M, Mayer B, Scheele J, et al. Systematic review and meta-analysis of antibiotic prophylaxis in severe acute pancreatitis. *Scand J Gastroenterol*. 2011;46:261–270.

34. Chang YS, Fu HQ, Xiao YM, et al. Nasogastric or nasojejunal feeding in predicted severe acute pancreatitis: a meta-analysis. *Crit Care*. 2013;17:R118.

35. Li JY, Yu T, Chen GC, et al. Enteral nutrition within 48 hours of admission improves clinical outcomes of acute pancreatitis by reducing complications: a meta-analysis. *PLoS ONE*. 2013;8:e64926.

36. Bakker OJ, van Brunschot S, van Santvoort HC, et al. Early versus on-demand nasoenteric tube feeding in acute pancreatitis. *N Engl J Med*. 2014;371:1983–1993.

37. ASGE Standards of Practice Committee; Maple JT, Ben-Menachem T, Anderson MA, et al. The role of endoscopy in the evaluation of suspected choledocholithiasis. *Gastrointest Endosc*. 2010;71:1–9.

38. Choudhary A, Bechtold ML, Arif M, et al. Pancreatic stents for prophylaxis against post-ERCP pancreatitis: a meta-analysis and systematic review. *Gastrointest Endosc*. 2011;73:275–282.

39. Elmunzer BJ, Scheiman JM, Lehman GA, et al. A randomized trial of rectal indomethacin to prevent post-ERCP pancreatitis. *N Engl J Med.* 2012;366:1414–1422.

40. Yeo CJ, Bastidas JA, Lynch-Nyhan A, et al. The natural history of pancreatic pseudocysts documented by computed tomography. *Surg Gynecol Obstet.* 1990;170:411–417.

41. Shamah S, Okolo PI. Systematic review of endoscopic cyst gastrostomy. *Gastrointest Endosc Clin N Am.* 2018;28:477–492.

42. Mouli VP, Sreenivas V, Garg PK. Efficacy of conservative treatment, without necrosectomy, for infected pancreatic necrosis: a systematic review and meta-analysis. *Gastroenterology.* 2013;144:333–340.e2.

43. Akshintala VS, Saxena P, Zaheer A, et al. A comparative evaluation of outcomes of endoscopic versus percutaneous drainage for symptomatic pancreatic pseudocysts. *Gastrointest Endosc.* 2014;79:921–928; quiz 983.e2–983.e5.

44. Luigiano C, Pellicano R, Fusaroli P, et al. Pancreatic necrosectomy: an evidence-based systematic review of the levels of evidence and a comparison of endoscopic versus non-endoscopic techniques. *Minerva Chir.* 2016;71:262–269.

45. van Brunschot S, Hollemans RA, Bakker OJ, et al. Minimally invasive and endoscopic versus open necrosectomy for necrotising pancreatitis: a pooled analysis of individual data for 1980 patients. *Gut.* 2018;67:697–706.

46. Steer ML, Waxman I, Freedman S. Chronic pancreatitis. *N Engl J Med.* 1995;332:1482–1490.

47. Witt H, Apte MV, Keim V, et al. Chronic pancreatitis: challenges and advances in pathogenesis, genetics, diagnosis, and therapy. *Gastroenterology.* 2007;132:1557–1573.

48. Forsmark CE. Management of chronic pancreatitis. *Gastroenterology.* 2013;144:1282–1291.e3.

49. Conwell DL, Lee LS, Yadav D, et al. American Pancreatic Association Practice Guidelines in Chronic Pancreatitis: evidence-based report on diagnostic guidelines. *Pancreas.* 2014;43:1143–1162.

50. Etemad B, Whitcomb DC. Chronic pancreatitis: diagnosis, classification, and new genetic developments. *Gastroenterology.* 2001;120:682–707.

51. Whitcomb DC, Gorry MC, Preston RA, et al. Hereditary pancreatitis is caused by a mutation in the cationic trypsinogen gene. *Nat Genet.* 1996;14:141–145.

52. Rustgi AK. Familial pancreatic cancer: genetic advances. *Genes Dev.* 2014;28:1–7.

53. Rosendahl J, Witt H, Szmola R, et al. Chymotrypsin C (CTRC) variants that diminish activity or secretion are associated with chronic pancreatitis. *Nature Genetics.* 2008;40:78–82.

54. Cohn JA, Friedman KJ, Noone PG, et al. Relation between mutations of the cystic fibrosis gene and idiopathic pancreatitis. *N Engl J Med.* 1998;339:653–658.

55. Stevens T, Conwell DL, Zuccaro G. Pathogenesis of chronic pancreatitis: an evidence-based review of past theories and recent developments. *Am J Gastroenterol.* 2004;99:2256–2270.

56. Schneider A, Whitcomb DC. Hereditary pancreatitis: a model for inflammatory diseases of the pancreas. *Best Pract Res Clin Gastroenterol.* 2002;16:347–363.

57. DiMagno EP, Go VL, Summerskill WH. Relations between pancreatic enzyme outputs and malabsorption in severe pancreatic insufficiency. *N Engl J Med.* 1973;288:813–815.

58. Keller J, Layer P. Human pancreatic exocrine response to nutrients in health and disease. *Gut.* 2005;54(Suppl 6):1–28.

59. Lieb JG, Draganov PV. Pancreatic function testing: here to stay for the 21st century. *World J Gastroenterol.* 2008;14:3149–3158.

60. Stein J, Jung M, Sziegoleit A, et al. Immunoreactive elastase I: clinical evaluation of a new non-invasive test of pancreatic function. *Clin Chem.* 1996;42:222–226.

61. Keller J, Aghdassi AA, Lerch MM, et al. Tests of pancreatic exocrine function—clinical significance in pancreatic and non-pancreatic disorders. *Best Pract Res Clin Gastroenterol.* 2009;23:425–439.

62. Tirkes T, Shah ZK, Takahashi N, et al. Reporting standards for chronic pancreatitis by using CT, MRI, and MR cholangiopancreatography: the Consortium for the Study of Chronic Pancreatitis, Diabetes, and Pancreatic Cancer. *Radiology.* 2019;290:207–215.

63. Catalano MF, Sahai A, Levy M, et al. EUS-based criteria for the diagnosis of chronic pancreatitis: the Rosemont classification. *Gastrointest Endosc.* 2009;69:1251–1261.

64. Leblanc JK, Chen JH, Al-Haddad M, et al. Endoscopic ultrasound and histology in chronic pancreatitis. *Pancreas.* 2014;43:1–5.

65. Stevens T, Conwell DL, Zuccaro G Jr, et al. Comparison of endoscopic ultrasound and endoscopic retrograde pancreatography for the prediction of pancreatic exocrine insufficiency. *Dig Dis Sci.* 2007;53:1146–1151.

66. Drewes AM, Bouwense SAW, Campbell CM, et al. Guidelines for the understanding and management of pain in chronic pancreatitis. *Pancreatology.* 2017;17:720–731.

67. Olesen SS, Bouwense SAW, Wilder-Smith OHG, et al. Pregabalin reduces pain in patients with chronic pancreatitis in a randomized, controlled trial. *Gastroenterology.* 2011;141:536–543.

68. Wilder-Smith CH, Hill L, Osler W, et al. Effect of tramadol and morphine on pain and gastrointestinal motor function in patients with chronic pancreatitis. *Dig Dis Sci.* 1999;44:1107–1116.

69. Warshaw AL, Banks PA, Fernandez-del Castillo C. AGA technical review: treatment of pain in chronic pancreatitis. *Gastroenterology.* 1998;115:765–776.

70. Cahen DL, Gouma DJ, Nio Y, et al. Endoscopic versus surgical drainage of the pancreatic duct in chronic pancreatitis. *N Engl J Med.* 2007;356:676–684.

71. Díte P, Ruzicka M, Zboril V, et al. A prospective, randomized trial comparing endoscopic and surgical therapy for chronic pancreatitis. *Endoscopy.* 2003;35:553–558.

72. Moole H, Jaeger A, Bechtold ML, et al. Success of extracorporeal shock wave lithotripsy in chronic calcific pancreatitis management: a meta-analysis and systematic review. *Pancreas.* 2016;45:651–658.

73. Dumonceau J-M, Costamagna G, Tringali A, et al. Treatment for painful calcified chronic pancreatitis: extracorporeal shock wave lithotripsy versus endoscopic treatment: a randomised controlled trial. *Gut.* 2007;56:545–552.

74. Coté GA, Slivka A, Tarnasky P, et al. Effect of covered metallic stents compared with plastic stents on benign biliary stricture resolution. *JAMA.* 2016;315:1250–1257.

75. Ryan DP, Hong TS, Bardeesy N. Pancreatic adenocarcinoma. *N Engl J Med.* 2014;371:1039–1049.

76. Rahib L, Smith BD, Aizenberg R, et al. Projecting cancer incidence and deaths to 2030: the unexpected burden of thyroid, liver, and pancreas cancers in the United States. *Cancer Res.* 2014;74:2913–2921.

77. Lowenfels AB, Maisonneuve P. Epidemiology and risk factors for pancreatic cancer. *Best Pract Res Clin Gastroenterol.* 2006;20:197–209.

78. Lowenfels AB. Chronic pancreatitis, pancreatic cancer, alcohol, and smoking. *Gastroenterology.* 1984;87:744–745.

79. Karlson BM, Ekbom A, Josefsson S, et al. The risk of pancreatic cancer following pancreatitis: an association due to confounding? *Gastroenterology.* 1997;113:587–592.

80. Kirkegård J, Cronin-Fenton D, Heide-Jørgensen U, et al. Acute pancreatitis and pancreatic cancer risk: a nationwide matched-cohort study in Denmark. *Gastroenterology.* 2018;154:1729–1736.

81. Michaud DS, Giovannucci E, Willett WC, et al. Physical activity, obesity, height, and the risk of pancreatic cancer. *JAMA.* 2001;286:921–929.

82. Everhart J, Wright D. Diabetes mellitus as a risk factor for pancreatic cancer. A meta-analysis. *JAMA.* 1995;273:1605–1609.

83. Gupta S, Vittinghoff E, Bertenthal D, et al. New-onset diabetes and pancreatic cancer. *Clin Gastroenterol Hepatol.* 2006;4:1366–1372; quiz 1301.

84. Permuth-Wey J, Egan KM. Family history is a significant risk factor for pancreatic cancer: results from a systematic review and meta-analysis. *Fam Cancer.* 2009;8:109–117.

85. Hruban RH, Canto MI, Goggins M, et al. Update on familial pancreatic cancer. *Adv Surg.* 2010;44:293–311.

86. Klein AP. Identifying people at a high risk of developing pancreatic cancer. *Nat Rev Cancer.* 2013;13:66–74.

87. Das KK, Early D. Pancreatic cancer screening. *Curr Treat Options Gastroenterol.* 2017;15:562–575.

88. Canto MI, Harinck F, Hruban RH, et al. International Cancer of the Pancreas Screening (CAPS) Consortium summit on the management of patients with increased risk for familial pancreatic cancer. *Gut.* 2013;62:339–347.

89. Canto MI, Almario JA, Schulick RD, et al. Risk of neoplastic progression in individuals at high risk for pancreatic cancer undergoing long-term surveillance. *Gastroenterology.* 2018;155:740–751.e2.

90. Valls C, Andía E, Sanchez A, et al. Dual-phase helical CT of pancreatic adenocarcinoma: assessment of resectability before surgery. *Am J Roentgenol.* 2002;178:821–826.

91. Bronstein YL, Loyer EM, Kaur H, et al. Detection of small pancreatic tumors with multiphasic helical CT. *Am J Roentgenol.* 2004;182:619–623.

92. Lu DS, Reber HA, Krasny RM, et al. Local staging of pancreatic cancer: criteria for unresectability of major vessels as revealed by pancreatic-phase, thin-section helical CT. *Am J Roentgenol.* 1997;168:1439–1443.

93. Roche CJ, Hughes ML, Garvey CJ, et al. CT and pathologic assessment of prospective nodal staging in patients with ductal adenocarcinoma of the head of the pancreas. *Am J Roentgenol.* 2003;180:475–480.

94. Irie H, Honda H, Kaneko K, et al. Comparison of helical CT and MR imaging in detecting and staging small pancreatic adenocarcinoma. *Abdom Imaging*. 1997;22:429–433.

95. Waters JA, Schmidt CM, Pinchot JW, et al. CT vs MRCP: optimal classification of IPMN type and extent. *J Gastrointest Surg*. 2008;12:101–109.

96. Soriano A, Castells A, Ayuso C, et al. Preoperative staging and tumor resectability assessment of pancreatic cancer: prospective study comparing endoscopic ultrasonography, helical computed tomography, magnetic resonance imaging, and angiography. *Am J Gastroenterol*. 2004;99:492–501.

97. Ramsay D, Marshall M, Song S, et al. Identification and staging of pancreatic tumours using computed tomography, endoscopic ultrasound and mangafodipir trisodium-enhanced magnetic resonance imaging. *Australas Radiol*. 2004;48:154–161.

98. Gress FG, Hawes RH, Savides TJ, et al. Role of EUS in the preoperative staging of pancreatic cancer: a large single-center experience. *Gastrointest Endosc*. 1999;50:786–791.

99. van der Gaag NA, Rauws EAJ, van Eijck CHJ, et al. Preoperative biliary drainage for cancer of the head of the pancreas. *N Engl J Med*. 2010;362:129–137.

100. Jeurnink SM, Steyerberg EW, van Hooft JE, et al. Surgical gastrojejunostomy or endoscopic stent placement for the palliation of malignant gastric outlet obstruction (SUSTENT study): a multicenter randomized trial. *Gastrointest Endosc*. 2010;71:490–499.

101. Loehrer PJ, Feng Y, Cardenes H, et al. Gemcitabine alone versus gemcitabine plus radiotherapy in patients with locally advanced pancreatic cancer: an Eastern Cooperative Oncology Group trial. *J Clin Oncol*. 2011;29:4105–4112.

102. Conroy T, Desseigne F, Ychou M, et al. FOLFIRINOX versus gemcitabine for metastatic pancreatic cancer. *N Engl J Med*. 2011;364:1817–1825.

103. Conroy T, Hammel P, Hebbar M, et al. FOLFIRINOX or gemcitabine as adjuvant therapy for pancreatic cancer. *N Engl J Med*. 2018;379:2395–2406.

104. Hoff Von DD, Ervin T, Arena FP, et al. Increased survival in pancreatic cancer with nab-paclitaxel plus gemcitabine. *N Engl J Med*. 2013;369:1691–1703.

105. Hoffman JP, Lipsitz S, Pisansky T, et al. Phase II trial of preoperative radiation therapy and chemotherapy for patients with localized, resectable adenocarcinoma of the pancreas: an Eastern Cooperative Oncology Group Study. *J Clin Oncol*. 1998;16:317–323.

106. Pisters PW, Abbruzzese JL, Janjan NA, et al. Rapid-fractionation preoperative chemoradiation, pancreaticoduodenectomy, and intraoperative radiation therapy for resectable pancreatic adenocarcinoma. *J Clin Oncol*. 1998;16:3843–3850.

107. Evans DB, Varadhachary GR, Crane CH, et al. Preoperative gemcitabine-based chemoradiation for patients with resectable adenocarcinoma of the pancreatic head. *J Clin Oncol*. 2008;26:3496–3502.

108. Murphy JE, Wo JY, Ryan DP, et al. Total neoadjuvant therapy with FOLFIRINOX followed by individualized chemoradiotherapy for borderline resectable pancreatic adenocarcinoma: a phase 2 clinical trial. *JAMA Oncol*. 2018;4:963–969.

109. Dhir M, Zenati MS, Hamad A, et al. FOLFIRINOX versus gemcitabine/nab-paclitaxel for neoadjuvant treatment of resectable and borderline resectable pancreatic head adenocarcinoma. *Ann Surg Oncol*. 2018;25:1896–1903.

Biliary Tract Disorders

Bader A. Alajlan and Gabriel D. Lang

24

Introduction

Diseases of the biliary tract are frequently encountered in both primary care and specialty settings. They represent a broad spectrum of diseases, ranging from benign gallstone disease to life-threatening cholangitis and malignancies. Biliary tract disorders can be classified into three spectrums:
- Calculous biliary disease
- Acalculous biliary disease
- Neoplastic biliary disease

Calculous Biliary Disease (Gallstone Disorders)

GENERAL PRINCIPLES

Definition

- **Cholelithiasis:** The presence of concretions (gallstones) in the gallbladder or bile ducts.
- **Choledocholithiasis:** The presence of stones within the biliary system; including common bile duct, common hepatic duct, right and left hepatic ducts, and intrahepatic ducts.

Classification

- **Cholesterol stones**
  - The most common type of gallstones are cholesterol stones, representing 75–90% of all gallstones.
  - Cholesterol stones are formed when supersaturation of cholesterol occurs in bile in the presence of biliary stasis within the gallbladder and nucleation of cholesterol molecules to form crystals.
- **Brown stones**
  - These form when bacteria within the biliary tree cause bilirubin to deconjugate and combine with calcium, forming an insoluble product, calcium bilirubinate.
  - Brown stones are more commonly observed in Asia and usually present 2 years or more following cholecystectomy.
- **Black stones**
  - Black stones develop in conditions associated with chronic hemolysis, most commonly sickle cell disease and hereditary spherocytosis.
  - Black stones may also be seen in cirrhotic patients partly due to hemolysis from hypersplenism or spur cell anemia.

Epidemiology

- Gallstone disease is a common disorder, particularly in women and obese patients.
- Prevalence ranges from 10–20% in white Americans to as high as 73% in female Pima Indians.[1,2] Although cholelithiasis is common, 80% of patients with gallstones never develop symptoms or complications.[3] The risk of developing biliary colic and major complications is 2% per year.[4]

Risk Factors

- Female sex (twice as common in women than in men)
- Advanced age
- Native Americans
- Multiparity
- Pregnancy
- Obesity
- Rapid weight loss
- Crohn disease (Bile salts pool depletion due to disease or removal of terminal ileum)
- Lipid abnormalities (high triglycerides)
- Total parenteral nutrition (TPN)
- Medication (oral contraceptives, steroids, estrogens, lipid-lowering agents, octreotide, and ceftriaxone)

DIAGNOSIS

Clinical Presentation

- Patients typically present with right upper quadrant pain when gallstones occlude the cystic duct, pass into the common bile duct, or erode through the wall of the gallbladder.
- Presentations of gallstone disease depend on the location of the stone in the biliary tree and include biliary pain, acute cholecystitis, choledoholithiasis, acute cholangitis, gallstone pancreatitis, Bouveret syndrome, and gallstone ileus.
- Stones may pass from the gallbladder into the common bile duct or develop de novo in the bile ducts.

History

- The most common presentation is right upper quadrant pain or biliary colic.
- The pain is caused by transient occlusion of the neck of the cystic duct by a gallstone.
- Biliary colic consists of sudden and intense epigastric or right upper quadrant pain that may radiate to the right scapula or shoulder. It can be precipitated by fatty meals, which induce gallbladder contraction. Associated nausea or vomiting may occur.
- Biliary colic is often a misnomer, as the pain is constant rather than colicky.
- After the initial attack, the chance of symptoms recurrence is 30–50% per year for the first 2 years. The interval between attacks is variable, and weeks or months may pass between episodes.[5]
- It is important to differentiate true biliary colic from nonspecific dyspepsia as it is a major determinant of the success of cholecystectomy in relieving symptoms.

Diagnostic Testing

Laboratory Testing

- Typically, no laboratory abnormalities are noted unless a complication is present.
- Elevated levels of transaminases, alkaline phosphatase, and bilirubin can be seen with choledocholithiasis and elevations of amylase and lipase levels can be seen in those with pancreatitis.

Imaging

- **Transabdominal ultrasound (TUS)**
  - TUS has a 95% sensitivity and specificity for gallstones.[6]
  - TUS is sensitive for biliary dilation (77–87%) but less sensitive for common bile duct stones (32–90%). This is especially true for stones in the distal common bile duct as it is often obscured by bowel gas.[7]

- The yield of TUS is highest after fasting, and stones are identified by the presence of mobile echogenic objects that produce acoustic shadowing.
- Gallbladder sludge may also be seen as echogenic material that layers but does not produce acoustic shadowing.
- **Computed tomography (CT):** Cholelithiasis may also be identified by CT scanning, although the sensitivity is lower than that of ultrasonography (40% compared to 95% for TUS). CT is useful for demonstrating biliary dilatation and mass lesions. It is often the test of choice if there is a clinical suspicion of malignant biliary obstruction.

TREATMENT

- Gallstones are often found incidentally during evaluation for other conditions. Because 80% of patients remain asymptomatic, prophylactic cholecystectomy is not indicated in the majority of patients.
  - Important exceptions are patients with a calcified or "porcelain" gallbladder and Native Americans with gallstones. These patients are at high risk for gallbladder cancer, so cholecystectomy should be performed in the absence of symptoms.
  - Patients with chronic medical conditions that can be adversely affected by an episode of cholecystitis or pancreatitis (e.g., brittle type 1 diabetes mellitus) may also benefit from elective cholecystectomy.
- Patient with symptomatic gallstones should be referred for cholecystectomy given their higher risk of symptoms recurrence.
- For choledocholithiasis, management options include nonsurgical treatments via endoscopic retrograde cholangiopancreatography (ERCP) and surgical approaches including cholecystectomy with laparoscopic stone removal.[8]
- ERCP affords the ability to both diagnose and extract bile duct stones in 95% of patients.[9]
- An ERCP should be performed in high-risk patients for choledocholithiasis even if both ultrasonography and a CT do not demonstrate choledocholithiasis.[10]
- In patients in whom clinical suspicion is intermediate further imaging via magnetic resonance cholangiopancreatography (MRCP) or endoscopic ultrasound (EUS) can be used to evaluate for choledocholithiasis. MRCP and EUS have been shown to have similar sensitivity and specificity in diagnosing choledocholithiasis (sensitivity 92–97% and specificity 92–96%).[11]
- Surgical candidates with choledocholithiasis who undergo biliary sphincterotomy should then have a cholecystectomy for definitive management of gallstones. While endoscopic sphincterotomy is somewhat protective against further episodes of choledocholithiasis, patients without subsequent cholecystectomy may be at an increased risk of recurrent symptoms or complications. It must be noted that this approach may be reasonable in some patients who are considered nonoperative candidates.[12]

Medications

- Opioids can be used in patient who cannot use NSAIDs or who have severe pain.
- Anticholinergic agents do not appear to relieve biliary colic.[13]
- In patients who are poor surgical candidates, oral dissolution therapy with ursodiol or chenodiol can be attempted. However, this rarely results in complete resolution of stones, especially stones larger than 5 mm. Even after initial resolution, the recurrence rate is 45% in 5 years.[14]

Surgical Management

- Laparoscopic cholecystectomy is the treatment of choice for symptomatic gallstones. The laparoscopic approach is associated with a significantly shorter hospital stay and quicker convalescence than with open cholecystectomy.[15]

- Less than 5% of laparoscopic cholecystectomies will be converted intraoperatively to an open procedure due to technical reasons.[15]
- Complications of cholecystectomy include bile duct injuries (0.14–0.3%) and bile leaks (0.3–0.9%).[16]
  - Biliary peritonitis occurs when bile leaks into the peritoneal cavity leading to acute peritoneal inflammation and severe abdominal pain.
  - The majority of bile leaks post cholecystectomy occurs at the cystic duct stump or duct of Luschka. Occasionally, large collections of bile (bilomas) can form around the biliary tree, resulting in pain and bacterial infections.
  - Patients with bile leaks typically present shortly after surgery (2–10 days) with abdominal pain. CT scan usually reveals fluid or a biloma centered on the biliary tree. A hepatoiminodiacetic acid (HIDA) scan can confirm the diagnosis by revealing spillage of radioactive tracer into the abdominal cavity.
  - Large bilomas may require percutaneous drainage, especially if infected.
  - Endoscopic treatment of bile leaks is performed to encourage preferential flow of bile into the duodenum, which allows the leak site to heal. This is typically done by performing a biliary sphincterotomy, biliary stent placement, or both in combination.
  - Most bile leaks heal within 4 weeks. The biliary stent should be removed at a follow-up interval of 4–8 weeks. A cholangiogram is performed at the time of stent removal to confirm resolution of the bile leak. Persistent leaks are uncommon but can be treated with longer duration stenting with or without a concomitant biliary sphincterotomy or with surgery.
  - A much more uncommon form of a bile leak or biliary injury is secondary to a transected common hepatic duct. This type of injury requires surgical repair.

COMPLICATIONS

- A major complication from gallstone disease is acute cholecystitis.

Acute Choleycystitis

GENERAL PRINCIPLES

Definition

Acute calculous cholecystitis consists of inflammation or hemorrhagic necrosis, with variable infection, ulceration, and neutrophilic infiltration of the gallbladder wall, usually resulting from impaction of a stone in the cystic duct.

Epidemiology

Acute cholecystitis develops in 20% of symptomatic biliary colic patients per year.[15]

Etiology

Cystic duct occlusion results in bile stasis, gallbladder wall edema, gallbladder distention, inflammatory exudate, and bacterial infection.

DIAGNOSIS

Clinical Presentation

- Patients typically present with steady upper abdominal pain that lasts hours (>6 hours) to days, with associated nausea, vomiting, and fever.

- If bacteremic, patients may present with high fever, rigors, and severe abdominal tenderness.
- Examination often reveals right upper quadrant tenderness or a positive Murphy sign, consisting of pain with palpation of the right upper quadrant during inspiration with subsequent inhibition of inspiration. Murphy sign can also be elicited during ultrasonography, when pressure is applied directly on the gallbladder with the ultrasound probe.

Diagnostic Testing

Laboratory Testing

- Most patients have a modest leukocytosis and normal or only slightly increased transaminases and bilirubin, usually not more than twice the upper limit of normal.
- Significantly elevated transaminases or bilirubin should raise the suspicion of choledocholithiasis.

Imaging

- Patients with suspected acute cholecystitis should undergo ultrasonography. Important findings include gallstones, sonographic Murphy sign, gallbladder wall thickening (>5 mm), and pericholecystic fluid.
- If the diagnosis remains in doubt, cholescintigraphy (HIDA, para-isopropyl iminodiacetic acid, or diisopropyl iminodiacetic acid scan) should be performed. Radiolabeled iminodiacetic acid derivatives are administered, which are rapidly extracted by the liver and then excreted into bile. A normal study shows radioactivity in the gallbladder, common bile duct, and small intestine within 60 minutes. In acute cholecystitis, there is delayed filling of the gallbladder because of cystic duct obstruction.

TREATMENT

- Patients with acute cholecystitis are made NPO and given intravenous fluids.
- NSAIDs or opioids are administered to control pain.
- Broad-spectrum antibiotics are used to treat secondary bacterial infections.
- Nasogastric suction can be performed if the abdomen is distended or if the patient is vomiting.
- Prompt surgical consultation should be obtained. Definitive management is cholecystectomy.
- Most clinicians recommend waiting 24–48 hours to perform cholecystectomy until the patient has clinically stabilized, but surgery can be performed more urgently if the condition deteriorates.
- If possible, cholecystectomy should be performed during the initial hospitalization. Procedural delays have been shown to increase costs without clinical benefit.[17,18]
- Patients who are poor surgical candidates, have severe cholecystitis, or failed medical therapy may require percutaneous cholecystostomy. This approach resolves acute cholecystitis in approximately 90% of patients. Elective removal of the catheter can be considered once the tract is mature (usually 3–6 weeks) and cholecystitis has resolved. Stone extraction can then be attempted when the tract is mature. This may obviate the need for surgery.[19]
- Transmural EUS-guided gallbladder drainage using lumen apposing metal stents is a novel alternative approach to percutaneous therapy with a high clinical success rate in treating acute cholecystitis. Although long-term data regarding the use of this therapy are limited.[19]

COMPLICATIONS

Complications of acute cholecystitis include gallbladder perforation, emphysematous cholecystitis caused by gas-forming bacteria, and gallstone ileus.

Acute Cholangitis

GENERAL PRINCIPLES

Definition

Acute cholangitis consists of inflammation of the bile duct, typically from bacterial infection stemming from an obstructed duct.[20]

Etiology

- Choledocholithiasis causes most cases of cholangitis, although patients with biliary neoplasms or inflammatory biliary strictures can develop cholangitis, especially if they have undergone prior biliary interventions (e.g., ERCP).
- Gallstones can cause cholangitis even after a cholecystectomy, as stones are retained in the common bile duct with some frequency, and can be present for years before causing biliary obstruction.
- The most common bacterial pathogens are enterobacteria (68%), enterococci (14%), bacteroides (10%), and *Clostridium* species (7%).

Risk Factors

- Choledocholithiasis
- Instrumentation of the biliary tract

DIAGNOSIS

Clinical Presentation

- Patients may present with fever (90–95%), abdominal pain (90%), and/or jaundice (80%).
- Approximately 40% of patients present with all three of the above components (Charcot triad: pain, jaundice, and fever). Charcot triad has 36% sensitivity and 93% specificity[21] for the diagnosis of cholangitis.
- If suppurative cholangitis develops, patients will additionally present with mental status changes and hypotension (Reynolds pentad). Although Reynolds pentad has a low sensitivity (<10%) for acute cholangitis.[21]

Diagnostic Testing

This diagnosis must be made quickly, as patients with cholangitis are at a high risk of developing severe sepsis.

Laboratory Testing

- Most patients will have leukocytosis with a neutrophil predominance.
- Most patients will have a cholestatic pattern to their liver function tests with elevated alkaline phosphatase and bilirubin above >2 mg/dL.
- High aminotransferases to levels around or higher than 2000 IU/L can be seen, especially with acute hepatic necrosis and microabscess formation in the liver.
- Blood cultures are frequently positive if gram-negative bacteria are the cause of the infection, especially in cases of suppurative cholangitis (50–70%).
- Patients who have had recent biliary surgery, biliary instrumentation or stents are more likely to harbor *Enterococcus* or hospital-acquired organisms such as *Pseudomonas* species, methicillin-resistant *Staphylococcus aureus* or vancomycin-resistant *Enterococcus*.

Imaging

- All patients with Charcot triad and abnormal liver test should proceed directly to ERCP to both confirm the diagnosis and to provide biliary drainage.

- Patients with indeterminate findings for cholangitis should undergo TUS or abdominal CT to evaluate for ductal dilatation or common bile duct stones.
- A negative study finding, however, does not rule out cholangitis, because the common duct may not be dilated early in the course of disease and common duct stones may be missed.

Diagnostic Procedures
- ERCP should be performed urgently in suspected cases of cholangitis, especially if the patient is clinically deteriorating.[22]
- If ERCP is unsuccessful or cannot be performed, percutaneous transhepatic cholangiography (PTC) or surgical decompression should be pursued.
- Both of these procedures have higher morbidity and mortality rates than ERCP.

TREATMENT

- Broad-spectrum antibiotics and aggressive fluid resuscitation should be immediately started if cholangitis is suspected.
  - Typically, ureidopenicillins, carbapenems, or the combination of third/fourth-generation cephalosporins + metronidazole are the empiric antibiotics of choice.
  - If the patient is penicillin allergic, metronidazole with either aztreonam or ciprofloxacin can be used.
  - Eighty percent of patients will have an initial response to antibiotics and supportive therapy.
  - Antibiotics are typically given for a total of 7–14 days.
- ERCP allows for drainage of the biliary tree and may resolve biliary obstruction from choledocholithiasis. In the event that the obstruction is insurmountable, either due to a large stone or a neoplasm, a stent can be placed to maintain bile flow.
- **Mirizzi syndrome**
  - A stone impacted in the cystic duct or neck of the gallbladder that causes external compression of the common bile duct. Typically presents with pain and jaundice.
  - Surgery is the mainstay of therapy.
- **Gallstone pancreatitis** is discussed in detail in Chapter 23.
- **Porcelain gallbladder**
  - Characterized by calcification of the gallbladder due to chronic inflammation of the gallbladder secondary to gallstones.
  - Carries a 2–3% risk of adenocarcinoma of gallbladder.[23]
  - Patients with porcelain gallbladder should be referred for prophylactic cholecystectomy.
- **Gallstone ileus**
  - Consists of mechanical intestinal obstruction resulting from the passage of a large gallstone (typically 25 mm or larger) into the bowel lumen.[24]
  - The process starts with a gallstone eroding through the gallbladder wall into the small intestine. The stone can then cause obstruction, usually at the terminal ileum. Patients typically present with acute partial small bowel obstruction.
  - Rarely, the stone can become impacted within the pyloric channel or duodenum, causing gastric outlet obstruction (Bouveret syndrome).
  - Gallstone ileus is responsible for 0.1–4% of all cases of intestinal obstruction and develops in 0.3–3% of all cholelithiasis patients. It is associated with high mortality (6.7–18%). It is seen more commonly in the elderly (eighth decade) and in women.[24]
  - The diagnosis is suggested by air in the biliary tree with dilated loops of bowel and air fluid levels on an x-ray study, with or without an ectopic gallstone.

Abdominal ultrasonography is useful in detecting biliary stones, and barium upper gastrointestinal series may be needed to detect a duodenal-biliary fistula.

Treatment is surgical enterotomy with removal of the stones. In addition, cholecystectomy with surgical closure of the duodenal fistula may be performed. However, this procedure is associated with high morbidity and mortality and should be pursued only in patients in excellent general health.

- **Hemobilia**
  - This manifestation can range from a microscopic bleed due to stone-induced biliary mucosal injury to major bleed due to gallstone-induced pseudoaneurysm.
  - 10% of major hemobilia cases are secondary to gallstone disease. These cases are treated with angiography using selective embolization.[25]

Acalculous Biliary Disease

ACUTE ACALCULOUS CHOLECYSTITIS

- An acute inflammatory disease of the gallbladder not associated with gallstones but associated with biliary stasis due to impaired gallbladder motility from ischemia. This condition is usually encountered in the setting of other significant comorbid illnesses.
- Acute acalculous cholecystitis should be excluded in critically ill patients who develop sepsis of unclear origin.
- Complications can occur rapidly in these patients. Therefore, early antibiotics followed by cholecystectomy or cholecystostomy tube placement is paramount.

SPHINCTER OF ODDI DYSFUNCTION (SOD)

- A benign and acalculous obstructive disorder that occurs at the level of the sphincter of Oddi.
- Classification of biliary SOD has recently changed based in Rome IV criteria to two types instead of three.
- Sphincter of Oddi stenosis (formally type I biliary SOD) is defined as biliary type pain, abnormal liver test, and biliary duct dilation. This is typically treated with endoscopic biliary sphincterotomy.
- Functional biliary sphincter of Oddi disorder (formally type II biliary SOD) is defined as biliary type pain and abnormal liver test or biliary duct dilation. This is also treated with endoscopic biliary sphincterotomy.
- The previously named type III SOD is no longer recognized as a clinical entity and should not be treated with biliary sphincterotomy.

GALLBLADDER POLYPS

- Occur in 1–10% of the general population.
- Most (>95%) of these polyps are benign and non-neoplastic. Cholesterol polyps are the most common type, followed by inflammatory polyps and gallbladder adenomyomas.
- Patients with gallbladder polyps larger than 10 mm or patient with any size gallbladder polyp and gallstones or primary sclerosing cholangitis (PSC) should undergo cholecystectomy given the high risk for gallbladder malignancy.[26]
- Patients with gallbladder polyps less than 10 mm in size need TUS assessment every 6–12 months to exclude rapid growth. If the polyp remains stable in size after 2 years, no further follow-up is recommended.[26]

BILIARY CYSTS

- Choledochal cysts are congenital anomalies of the biliary tract. They are more common in females and Asia. The majority of cases are diagnosed before age 30.
- Symptoms vary from abdominal pain, intermittent jaundice, abdominal masses, and recurrent cholangitis. Complications include recurrent cholangitis, cyst rapture, acute pancreatitis, and malignancy.
- Some biliary cysts are a result of pancreaticobiliary maljunction. These patients are at an increased risk for gallbladder adenocarcinoma and should have a cholecystectomy.
- Biliary cysts are classified based on anatomical features and are all treated surgically except for type III choledochal cysts which can be treated endoscopically.

BENIGN BILIARY STRICTURES

- These can result from multiple etiologies: postsurgical, chronic pancreatitis, infection, HIV cholangiopathy, ischemia, autoimmune cholangiopathy, or PSC.
- Chronic pancreatitis–induced biliary strictures have a variable presentation ranging from incidental to abdominal pain, overt jaundice, and cholangitis. Patients with persistent symptoms and CBD >12 mm or alkaline phosphatase >3 times normal should be considered for therapy. Endoscopic therapy with remediation of the stricture (dilation and serial stenting) can be attempted, although several treatment sessions are often required and long-term success is suboptimal (10–40%) especially in patient with calcific chronic pancreatitis. Recent reports describe improved results with the use of fully covered metal stents left in place for 6–12 months. Surgical management should be considered in operative candidates.
- Postcholecystectomy biliary strictures can be a result of an injury to the right hepatic duct during cholecystectomy and typically present years later with segmental cholangitis and right hepatic atrophy. This is treated surgically. Postcholecystectomy biliary strictures can also be a result of injuries to the CHD or CBD. Patients with this type of injury present with pain, abnormal liver function tests, and biliary dilation. These patients can be treated with biliary stenting.
- Postliver transplant strictures commonly occur at the ductal anastomosis and have a favorable response to multiple sessions of biliary stenting, especially if treated within 6 months of liver transplantation. Nonanastomotic strictures usually present with multiple intra- and extrahepatic strictures and usually due to hepatic artery thrombosis. Nonanastomotic strictures are difficult to treat and less responsive to stenting. As such, many patients with diffuse strictures may require retransplantation.
- HIV cholangiopathy is an infectious phenomenon (commonly from *Cryptosporidium parvum*) that occurs when the CD4 count is less than 100/μL. Patients usually present with abdominal pain and diarrhea. Imaging findings are consistent with sclerosing cholangitis with papillary stenosis. Treatment is primarily endoscopic, although the approach varies with the anatomic abnormality identified.
- IgG4 cholangiopathy is the biliary manifestation of IgG4-related system disease and associated with autoimmune pancreatitis. It is characterized by increased serum levels of IgG4 and intra- and extrahepatic biliary strictures. Multifocal infiltrate of IgG4-containing lymphoplasmacytic infiltrates are seen in the liver and bile ducts. Patients typically have good response to steroids.

MALIGNANT BILIARY STRICTURES

- Malignant biliary strictures are secondary to ampullary cancer, pancreatic cancer, cholangiocarcinoma, lymphoma, gallbladder cancer, metastatic disease, and external compression from large lymph nodes.

- Cross-sectional imaging followed by EUS for tissue sampling is typical for most of these malignancies.
- Treatment of malignant biliary obstruction often requires a multidisciplinary approach including oncology, surgery, and gastroenterology.

Primary Sclerosing Cholangitis (PSC)

GENERAL PRINCIPLES

Definition

- PSC consists of inflammation and fibrosis of the intra- and extrahepatic bile ducts secondary to an autoimmune or idiopathic mechanism.[27] The disease, as discussed here, is from a biliary perspective. Please see Chapter 19 for further details on PSC.
- PSC is insidious in onset. It typically presents with fatigue, jaundice, and cholestasis. It progresses irreversibly to end-stage liver disease (ESLD).[28]

Epidemiology

- Seventy-five percent of patients are male.
- The average age at diagnosis is 40 years, although the disease can often be diagnosed in childhood.

Etiology

- The etiology of PSC is unknown.
- Animal and *in vitro* models have identified infections, autoimmunity, cytokines, and bile acid transporter or ion channel abnormalities as underlying causes for PSC.

Pathophysiology

- Both intra- and extrahepatic bile ducts can become strictured.
- The disease process is usually diffuse, with obliterative fibrosis distributed throughout the biliary system.
- Tight strictures predispose the patient to intermittent obstruction of biliary flow with subsequent bacterial cholangitis.

Risk Factors

- Up to 70% of PSC occurs in the setting of inflammatory bowel disease (IBD), with ulcerative colitis accounting for 90% of those cases.[29]
- No relationship exists between the duration and severity of IBD and the development of PSC.
- Although colectomy is curative for colonic disease in ulcerative colitis, it does not eliminate the risk of PSC.

Associated Conditions

- Metabolic bone disease, most commonly osteoporosis, occurs frequently in PSC.
- Patients with PSC have a 10–30% chance of developing cholangiocarcinoma, which is often difficult to diagnose in the setting of PSC.
- Despite knowing that patients with PSC are at high risk for cholangiocarcinoma, no effective screening method has been identified.
- Patients with PSC with concomitant IBD have an increased risk of colon cancer, this risk is increased three- to fivefold in patients with PSC and IBD as compared with those with IBD alone.[30]

DIAGNOSIS

Clinical Presentation

- The onset of disease is often insidious, with the gradual onset of fatigue, pruritus, and jaundice.
- Pruritus can be particularly severe in PSC and difficult to manage.
- The exact mechanism remains unknown but may involve the accumulation of pruritogenic substances secondary to decreased bile excretion or increased opioidergic tone.
- If advanced liver disease has developed, patients can present with variceal bleeding, encephalopathy, or ascites.
- Steatorrhea and malabsorption of fat-soluble vitamins may develop late in disease because of decreased secretion of bile acids.

Diagnostic Testing

Laboratory Testing

- Approximately 25% of patients are diagnosed from abnormal laboratory tests before symptoms have developed.
- Most have significantly elevated alkaline phosphatase, γ-glutamyltransferase, and bilirubin.
- Transaminases are elevated to a lesser degree.
- In addition, many patients will have positive antinuclear antibodies and antineutrophil cytoplasmic antibodies (p-ANCA) levels, suggesting that PSC is immune mediated.
- Patients with IBD who present with elevated alkaline phosphatase levels should have an aggressive evaluation for PSC.

Imaging

- Definitive diagnosis is made by imaging of the biliary tree. MRCP is a noninvasive option with similar diagnostic accuracy and should be used instead of ERCP whenever possible.
- The classic finding is multifocal stricturing of the intra- and extrahepatic bile ducts with intervening normal or dilated segments. This is often described as a "string of beads" appearance.
- Secondary causes of strictures, including trauma, ischemia, tumors, IgG4-related disease, and certain infections (Cytomegalovirus, *Cryptosporidium*), need to be excluded.
- A minority of patients who do not have the classic cholangiographic findings demonstrate small duct cholangitis on liver biopsy.

TREATMENT

- Various medical therapies, such as immunosuppressants, corticosteroids, and antibiotics, have not been proved successful in slowing progression of disease or improve survival, although ursodeoxycholic acid (15 mg/kg/day) improves biochemical abnormalities.
- Management is therefore primarily supportive until ESLD develops, at which point liver transplantation is offered.
- Referral for transplantation should be made when MELD exceeds 14. Although additional MELD points may be offered in specific clinical situation like intractable pruritus, those with cholangiocarcinoma <3 cm in size, and those with recurrent episodes of bacterial cholangitis.

- The survival rate 10 years after transplantation is 70%, although patients with PSC have a higher retransplantation rate than all other patients with ESLD caused by recurrent disease.
- Medications:
  - Pruritus often respond to bile acid–binding resins, such as cholestyramine at a dose of 4 g PO BID to QID.[31]
  - Antihistamines seem to have no effect on pruritus beyond possible sedation effects.[32]
  - Nonpharmacologic therapies of pruritus that have shown a promise include photodynamic therapy and, in extreme cases, liver transplantation.

COMPLICATIONS

- **Dominant stricture**
  - Approximately 40–60% of patients develop a dominant stricture.
  - If cholangiography demonstrates a dominant stricture in a patient with elevated liver function tests, treatment via balloon dilatation is often successful. Stent placement can be performed, although a long-term endoscopic stenting to prevent recurrent stricture formation is not supported by controlled data.
  - It can be difficult to differentiate a dominant stricture from cholangiocarcinoma.
  - Tumor markers, such as carbohydrate antigen 19-9 (CA 19-9), carcinoembryonic antigen, and cytologic brushings or forceps biopsies with fluorescence in situ hybridization (FISH) may be of some value in identifying patients with cholangiocarcinoma. Although the sensitivity of these tests are modest.
  - Cholangioscopy allows direct visualization of the bile duct during ERCP and affords the ability to directly sample the stricture, potentially improving the detection of early cholangiocarcinoma.
- **Bacterial cholangitis**
  - Bacterial cholangitis is more frequent in patients who have had manipulation of the biliary tract or have developed a dominant stricture.
  - Patients typically present with fever and worsening jaundice, and they often have recurrent episodes.
  - After empiric antibiotics are started, treatment is directed at relieving the obstruction, usually endoscopically.
  - ERCP allows dilation of large strictures, biliary decompression, and removal of stones.
  - Prospective studies have not shown any benefit in placing endoprostheses across PSC strictures.
  - Long-term prophylactic antibiotics have not been shown to have any benefit in preventing cholangitis.

OUTCOME/PROGNOSIS

PSC follows a slowly progressive course, with a median survival of 10 years from diagnosis.

Neoplastic Biliary Disease

Most neoplastic biliary diseases are asymptomatic early in the disease course. Symptoms are vague and may include prolonged abdominal pain, which may be difficult to differentiate from biliary pain, or acute cholecystitis. Other common symptoms include nausea, vomiting, weight loss, and jaundice. These vague symptoms make early diagnosis of these malignancies extremely difficult. Tumor markers such as carcinoembryonic antigen and CA 19-9 can be elevated, as are liver function tests. Cross-sectional imaging, either CT or MRI, remains the best ways to identify these neoplastic processes.

Gallbladder Carcinoma

GENERAL PRINCIPLES

Definition

This consists of neoplasia involving the gallbladder, typically adenocarcinoma.

Epidemiology

- Gallbladder cancer is the most common biliary tract malignancy.[33]
- It is predominantly seen in elderly women. It is the most common gastrointestinal malignancy in Native Americans.
- Up to 80% of patients have a history of gallstones.
- Approximately 90% of patients are diagnosed after the neoplasm has spread beyond the gallbladder.
- Patients who have a calcified or "porcelain" gallbladder are at high risk of gallbladder cancer and should undergo cholecystectomy even if asymptomatic.
- Other risk factor also includes gallstones >3 cm, adenomatous gallbladder polyps >1 cm, abnormal pancreaticobiliary junction, segmental adenomyomatosis, chronic *Salmonella typhi* carriers, PSC, and xanthogranulomatous cholecystitis.[34]

DIAGNOSIS

- Imaging
  - Ultrasonography often detects masses within the gallbladder lumen or irregular gallbladder wall thickening. A normal ultrasound does not rule out gallbladder cancer, however.
  - CT demonstrates masses and gallbladder thickening and provides additional evidence for extent of disease.
- Diagnostic procedures
  - Fine-needle aspiration during EUS has also been used to evaluate peripancreatic and periportal lymphadenopathy in patients with gallbladder cancer.[35]
  - ERCP or PTC is indicated in patients with evidence of biliary obstruction.
  - Histologic diagnosis for tumors that appear unresectable can be accomplished with percutaneous biopsy or ERCP.

TREATMENT

- Most patients present with advanced unresectable disease.
- The overall 5-year survival rate is <5%, and patients with advanced cancer have a median survival of only 45–127 days.

Surgical Management

- Patients stage I–III cancer may be surgically resectable.
- Depending on the extent of diseases spread, surgery may require a cholecystectomy or an extensive resection.

Palliative Management

- Patients with unresectable disease may be given chemotherapy with agents such as 5-fluorouracil, Adriamycin, gemcitabine, and nitrosoureas, but results are not encouraging.
- Most patients with unresectable disease will require palliative treatments such as endoscopic stent placement or percutaneous biliary drainage.

Cholangiocarcinoma

GENERAL PRINCIPLES

Definition

Neoplasia developing within the bile ducts.

Epidemiology

- The reported incidence of cholangiocarcinoma in the United States is 2 cases per 100,000 population. This malignancy is increasing in incidence.
- Cholangiocarcinoma is classified by anatomical location: intrahepatic cholangiocarcinoma (10%), hilar cholangiocarcinoma (60%), and distal extrahepatic bile duct cancers (30%).[36]
- The increase in incidence is mainly seen in intrahepatic cholangiocarcinoma.[37,38]

Etiology

Unknown.

Pathophysiology

Chronic biliary inflammation is thought to contribute to cancer formation.

Associated Conditions

- The strongest association is with PSC.
- Also seen with chronic liver disease, ulcerative colitis, parasitic biliary disease, choledochal cysts, pancreaticobiliary maljunction, viral hepatitis (HBV and HCV), toxic exposures, and smoking.

DIAGNOSIS

Clinical Presentation

- Patients typically present with anorexia, weight loss, acholic stool, abdominal pain, pruritus, and jaundice when the tumor causes significant obstruction.
- Some bile duct tumors spread diffusely throughout the liver, making it difficult to distinguish from PSC.
- Most tumors are locally invasive and do not metastasize.
- Prognosis is grim, with rare patient survival of >1 year.

Diagnostic Testing

Laboratory Testing

- Most patients have elevated alkaline phosphatase and bilirubin levels.
- Aminotransferases may be moderately increased.
- Elevated CA 19-9 levels have a wide variation in sensitivity (50–90%) and specificity (50–90%) as tumor marker in cholangiocarcinoma.
- CA 19-9 has been used to help in the diagnosis of cholangiocarcinoma, follow treatment effect, assess recurrence of disease, and for cholangiocarcinoma surveillance in PSC patients. This marker can also be also elevated in benign biliary disease such as cholangitis and benign biliary obstruction, although CA 19-9 concentrations >1000 unit/mL are typically consistent with advanced metastatic disease.

Imaging

- Ultrasonography and abdominal CT scan are useful in identifying intrahepatic or extrahepatic ductal dilation, but the primary tumors are often difficult to visualize.

- Magnetic resonance imaging (MRI) or MRCP may be more sensitive in identifying the primary tumor.

Diagnostic Procedures
- ERCP or PTC provides direct imaging of the biliary system and can define the extent of tumor spread.
- During ERCP, a tissue diagnosis can be made using cytology brushes or cholangioscopic biopsies.
- Biopsies obtained through percutaneous or transluminal means are not recommended because of the danger of tumor seeding and are relative contraindication for liver transplantation in some institutes.
- Regional lymph node sampling can be performed via EUS in early-stage disease to evaluate for surgical resectability or liver transplantation.
- The histologic diagnosis of cholangiocarcinoma may be challenging, because many tumors are well differentiated and occur in the setting of PSC.

TREATMENT

- Surgical resection or liver transplantation represents the only options for long-term survival.
- Chemotherapy and radiation therapy are uniformly ineffective in prolonging survival.

Surgical Management
- Distal extrahepatic and intrahepatic tumors are more likely to be resectable than proximal extrahepatic tumors.
- A high recurrence rate is seen after resection. Adjuvant chemoradiation has not been shown to improve survival.
- Liver transplantation combined with neoadjuvant chemoradiation has led to increased survival rates in patients with locally unresectable cancer with otherwise normal hepatic and biliary function and patients with a history of PSC.

Palliative Management
- Patients with unresectable tumors are usually offered ERCP with stent placement versus percutaneous biliary drainage.
- Recent preliminary reports of other palliative treatments (e.g., photodynamic therapy) have been encouraging, but more studies are needed before this treatment becomes widely adopted.

OUTCOME/PROGNOSIS

- Median survival for resectable tumors is 3 years, but falls to 1 year if the tumor is unresectable.
- Death usually results from recurrent biliary sepsis or liver abscess formation.

Ampullary Carcinoma

GENERAL PRINCIPLES

Definition
This consists of neoplasia developing within the ampulla of Vater.

Epidemiology

- Reported incidence in United States is six cases per million population and it is increasing.[39]
- The incidence is dramatically increased with hereditary polyposis syndromes, such as familial adenomatous polyposis (FAP) and hereditary nonpolyposis colorectal cancer (HNPCC), compared with the general population.

DIAGNOSIS

Clinical Presentation

Patients usually present with jaundice. Other manifestations include pruritus, abdominal pain, bleeding, and acholic stools. Cholangitis or pancreatitis from malignant obstruction are uncommon.

Diagnostic Testing

- Liver function test usually show a cholestatic pattern.
- Imaging studies with CT typically reveal intra- and extrahepatic bile duct dilatation as well as pancreatic ductal dilatation.
- ERCP is the singlemost useful endoscopic study for diagnostic confirmation with direct visualization of the ampulla and ability to biopsy, as well as decompress the biliary tract.
- EUS is helpful for the preoperative staging of these patients.

TREATMENT

- Ampullary adenomas and early carcinomas may be amenable to endoscopic or local surgical resection (ampullectomy).
- Patients with invasive carcinoma should be referred to surgery.
- Patients who have unresectable tumors are usually offered ERCP with stent placement for palliative decompression.

OUTCOME/PROGNOSIS

- Five-year overall survival based on stages range from 0% in advanced disease to 84% in early-stage disease.
- The outcome of resected tumors depends upon the extent of local invasion, surgical margins, and the presence or absence of nodal metastases. The five-year survival rates can range from 60–80% in patients without nodal involvement to 20–50% in patients with nodal involvement.[40]

REFERENCES

1. Diehl AK. Epidemiology and natural history of gallstone disease. *Gastroenterol Clin North Am.* 1991;20(1):1–19.
2. Stinton LM, Myers RP, Shaffer EA. Epidemiology of gallstones. *Gastroenterol Clin North Am.* 2010;39(2):157–169, vii.
3. Sakorafas GH, Milingos D, Peros G. Asymptomatic cholelithiasis: is cholecystectomy really needed? A critical reappraisal 15 years after the introduction of laparoscopic cholecystectomy. *Dig Dis Sci.* 2007;52(5):1313–1325.
4. Stinton LM, Shaffer EA. Epidemiology of gallbladder disease: cholelithiasis and cancer. *Gut Liver.* 2012;6(2):172–187.
5. Festi D, Reggiani ML, Attili AF, et al. Natural history of gallstone disease: expectant management or active treatment? Results from a population-based cohort study. *J Gastroenterol Hepatol.* 2010;25(4):719–724.

6. Bortoff GA, Chen MY, Ott DJ, et al. Gallbladder stones: imaging and intervention. *Radiographics.* 2000;20(3):751–766.

7. Gurusamy KS, Giljaca V, Takwoingi Y, et al. Ultrasound versus liver function tests for diagnosis of common bile duct stones. *Cochrane Database Syst Rev.* 2015;(2):CD011548.

8. Hungness ES, Soper NJ. Management of common bile duct stones. *J Gastrointest Surg.* 2006;10(4):612–619.

9. Fogel EL, McHenry L, Sherman S, et al. Therapeutic biliary endoscopy. *Endoscopy.* 2005;37(2):139–145.

10. ASGE Standards of Practice Committee; Maple JT, Ben-Menachem T, Anderson MA, et al. The role of endoscopy in the evaluation of suspected choledocholithiasis. *Gastrointest Endosc.* 2010;71(1):1–9.

11. Verma D, Kapadia A, Eisen GM, et al. EUS vs MRCP for detection of choledocholithiasis. *Gastrointest Endosc.* 2006;64(2):248–254.

12. Boerma D, Rauws EA, Keulemans YC, et al. Wait-and-see policy or laparoscopic cholecystectomy after endoscopic sphincterotomy for bile-duct stones: a randomised trial. *Lancet.* 2002;360(9335):761–765.

13. Tytgat GN. Hyoscine butylbromide—a review on its parenteral use in acute abdominal spasm and as an aid in abdominal diagnostic and therapeutic procedures. *Curr Med Res Opin.* 2008;24(11):3159–3173.

14. Petroni ML, Jazrawi RP, Pazzi P, et al. Risk factors for the development of gallstone recurrence following medical dissolution. The British-Italian Gallstone Study Group. *Eur J Gastroenterol Hepatol.* 2000;12(6):695–700.

15. Strasberg SM. Clinical practice. Acute calculous cholecystitis. *N Engl J Med.* 2008;358(26):2804–2811.

16. Strasberg SM, Hertl M, Soper NJ. An analysis of the problem of biliary injury during laparoscopic cholecystectomy. *J Am Coll Surg.* 1995;180(1):101–125.

17. Wilson E, Gurusamy K, Gluud C, et al. Cost-utility and value-of-information analysis of early versus delayed laparoscopic cholecystectomy for acute cholecystitis. *Br J Surg.* 2010;97(2):210–219.

18. Gurusamy K, Samraj K, Gluud C, et al. Meta-analysis of randomized controlled trials on the safety and effectiveness of early versus delayed laparoscopic cholecystectomy for acute cholecystitis. *Br J Surg.* 2010;97(2):141–150.

19. Baron TH, Grimm IS, Swanstrom LL. Interventional approaches to gallbladder disease. *N Engl J Med.* 2015;373(4):357–365.

20. Qureshi WA. Approach to the patient who has suspected acute bacterial cholangitis. *Gastroenterol Clin North Am.* 2006;35(2):409–423.

21. Rumsey S, Winders J, MacCormick AD. Diagnostic accuracy of Charcot's triad: a systematic review. *ANZ J Surg.* 2017;87(4):232–238.

22. Lai EC, Mok FP, Tan ES, et al. Endoscopic biliary drainage for severe acute cholangitis. *N Engl J Med.* 1992;326(24):1582–1586.

23. Khan ZS, Livingston EH, Huerta S. Reassessing the need for prophylactic surgery in patients with porcelain gallbladder: case series and systematic review of the literature. *Arch Surg.* 2011;146(10):1143–1147.

24. Halabi WJ, Kang CY, Ketana N, et al. Surgery for gallstone ileus: a nationwide comparison of trends and outcomes. *Ann Surg.* 2014;259(2):329–335.

25. Luu MB, Deziel DJ. Unusual complications of gallstones. *Surg Clin North Am.* 2014;94(2):377–394.

26. American Society for Gastrointestinal Endoscopy Standards of Practice Committee; Anderson MA, Appalaneni V, Ben-Menachem T, et al. The role of endoscopy in the evaluation and treatment of patients with biliary neoplasia. *Gastrointest Endosc.* 2013;77(2):167–174.

27. LaRusso NF, Shneider BL, Black D, et al. Primary sclerosing cholangitis: summary of a workshop. *Hepatology.* 2006;44(3):746–764.

28. Lee YM, Kaplan MM. Primary sclerosing cholangitis. *N Engl J Med.* 1995;332(14):924–933.

29. Chapman R, Fevery J, Kalloo A, et al. Diagnosis and management of primary sclerosing cholangitis. *Hepatology.* 2010;51(2):660–678.

30. Zheng HH, Jiang XL. Increased risk of colorectal neoplasia in patients with primary sclerosing cholangitis and inflammatory bowel disease: a meta-analysis of 16 observational studies. *Eur J Gastroenterol Hepatol.* 2016;28(4):383–390.

31. Mela M, Mancuso A, Burroughs AK. Review article: pruritus in cholestatic and other liver diseases. *Aliment Pharmacol Ther.* 2003;17(7):857–870.

32. Holtmeier J, Leuschner U. Medical treatment of primary biliary cirrhosis and primary sclerosing cholangitis. *Digestion.* 2001;64(3):137–150.

33. Jones RS. Carcinoma of the gallbladder. *Surg Clin North Am.* 1990;70(6):1419–1428.

34. Cariati A, Piromalli E, Cetta F. Gallbladder cancers: associated conditions, histological types, prognosis, and prevention. *Eur J Gastroenterol Hepatol.* 2014;26(5):562–569.

35. Chang KJ. State of the art lecture: endoscopic ultrasound (EUS) and FNA in pancreatico-biliary tumors. *Endoscopy.* 2006;38(Suppl 1):S56–S60.

36. Rizvi S, Gores GJ. Pathogenesis, diagnosis, and management of cholangiocarcinoma. *Gastroenterology.* 2013;145(6):1215–1229.

37. Shaib YH, Davila JA, McGlynn K, et al. Rising incidence of intrahepatic cholangiocarcinoma in the United States: a true increase? *J Hepatol.* 2004;40(3):472–477.

38. Khan SA, Thomas HC, Davidson BR, et al. Cholangiocarcinoma. *Lancet.* 2005;366(9493):1303–1314.

39. Castro FA, Koshiol J, Hsing AW, et al. Biliary tract cancer incidence in the United States—demographic and temporal variations by anatomic site. *Int J Cancer.* 2013;133(7):1664–1671.

40. Beger HG, Treitschke F, Gansauge F, et al. Tumor of the ampulla of Vater: experience with local or radical resection in 171 consecutively treated patients. *Arch Surg.* 1999;134(5):526–532.

Genetic Testing in Gastrointestinal Disease

25

Motaz H. Ashkar and Elizabeth J. Blaney

Introduction

- About 5–10% of cancers are linked to a hereditary cancer predisposition syndrome.[1]
- The diagnosis of a hereditary cancer syndrome guides the index patient surveillance and management strategy, as well as risk assessment and screening intervals for immediate and extended family members.[1]
- A familial form of cancer is suspected in the following setting:
  - Early age of diagnosis
  - Synchronous or metachronous tumors
  - Multiple primary tumor types
  - Family history of the same cancer type in one or more first-degree relatives
  - High rate of cancer occurrence in a family
  - Associated congenital anomalies or known phenotypic syndromes
- Many gastrointestinal diseases have known causative mutations and testing is available for clinical use (Table 25-1).
- In addition to determining risk for heritable diseases, genetic testing is also used to determine polymorphisms that can guide pharmacotherapy.
- Genetic counseling should be offered to all patients before testing due to potential psychological impact and possibility of insurance or employment discrimination in the event of a positive test result.

Lynch Syndrome

GENERAL PRINCIPLES

- Lynch syndrome is also known as **hereditary nonpolyposis colorectal cancer** (HNPCC). This is an autosomal dominant (AD) condition, representing the most common cause of inherited colorectal cancer (CRC) syndromes and accounts for 3% of all CRC.[2]
- Lynch syndrome is the result of germline mutation in DNA **mismatch repair** (MMR) genes causing changes in tumor DNA nucleotide length (termed microsatellites instability [MSI]) and subsequently, loss of expression in *MLH1, MSH2, MSH6,* and *PMS2* proteins.
- Deletion in the *EPCAM* gene causing loss of *MSH2* protein expression.
- Several regulatory genes for cell growth and cellular apoptosis are affected by *MMR* gene mutations and accumulation of MSI abnormalities, promoting cells vulnerability and the carcinogenesis process in HNPCC.
- Germline mutations of *MLH1* or *MSH2* account for 90% of Lynch syndrome cases.

DIAGNOSIS

Clinical Presentation

- Colorectal cancer:
  - The lifetime risk of CRC in Lynch syndrome patients reaches 70% by age 70 and it depends on the gender (males > females) and the (MMR) gene mutation (*MLH1* > *MSH2* > *MSH6*).

TABLE 25-1 SUMMARY OF GENETICS AND GASTROINTESTINAL DISEASES

Disease	Inheritance	Gene	Test	Testing Indication	Test Result Follow-Up
FAP AFAP	AD	APC	Gene sequence analysis on blood sample	Patients with polyposis phenotype	Screen at-risk family members if mutation is identified
MAP	AR	MUTYH		Patients with polyposis lacking APC mutation or apparent (AR) inheritance	
HDGC	AD	CDH1		Diffuse gastric cancer at age <50, family history, characteristic pathology on tumor specimen	
PJS	AD	LKB1 (STK11)		PJS phenotype by diagnostic criteria	
JPS		SMAD4 (MADH4), BMPR1A		JPS phenotype by diagnostic criteria	
CS		PTEN, SDH, KLLN		CS phenotype by diagnostic criteria	
SPS	Unknown	Unknown, MUTYH-18%		MUTYH testing if colon adenomas present	
Hereditary pancreatitis (HD)	AD or AR	PRSS, CFTR, SPINK1		Patients with unexplained pancreatitis as child, unexplained recurrent acute or chronic pancreatitis as adult, suggestive family history	Identifies the etiology of pancreatitis

				High-risk individuals	
Hereditary pancreatic cancer	AD	BRCA1/2, CDKN2A, ATM, HD/PJS/LS genes			MRI and EUS screening
Lynch syndrome (HNPCC)	AD	MMR genes—MLH1, MSH2, MSH6, PMS2	IHC of tissue specimen to determine loss of expression of MMR genes; MSI testing of tumor or polypectomy specimen	Patients with suspected Lynch syndrome undergoing resection of tumors or polyps	Once IHC determines which gene is likely mutated or MSI-H is found in the tumor, gene sequencing and mutational analysis is performed; at-risk family members may then be screened.
HH	Variable genetics penetrance	HFE—C282Y, H63D	HFE gene mutation testing on blood sample	Patients with clinical iron-overload state	Screen first-degree relatives of patients with symptomatic HH
Celiac disease	HLA associated	HLA DQ2/DQ8	HLA typing	Negative celiac disease serology in patients on gluten-free diet	Rules out celiac disease in absence of DQ2 or DQ8
IBD	Pharmacokinetic genetic polymorphisms	TPMT	TPMT genotype by gene sequence analysis; TPMT phenotype by enzyme activity RBC assay	Prior to initiation of thiopurine-based IBD treatment	Patients with homozygous mutant alleles are not candidates for thiopurine therapy; those with low enzyme activity require decreased drug dosage

AD, autosomal dominant; AFAP, attenuated familial adenomatous polyposis; APC, adenomatous polyposis coli; AR, autosomal recessive; CS, Cowden syndrome; EUS, endoscopic ultrasound; FAP, familial adenomatous polyposis; HDGC, hereditary diffuse gastric cancer; HH, hereditary hemochromatosis; HLA, human leukocyte antigen; HNPCC, hereditary nonpolyposis colon cancer; IBD, inflammatory bowel disease; IHC, immunohistochemistry; JPS, juvenile polyposis syndrome; MAP, MUTYH-associated polyposis; MMR, mismatch repair; MRI, magnetic resonance imaging; MSI, microsatellite instability; MSI-H, high level of microsatellite instability; MUTYH, MUTY homolog; PJS, Peutz-Jeghers syndrome; SPS, serrated polyposis syndrome; TPMT, thiopurine methyl transferase.

This risk is 66% in males with an average diagnosis age of 42 years and 43% in females with an average age of 47 years.[3]

○ Cancerous lesions in Lynch syndrome are commonly right sided evolving from **flat high-risk adenomas** (larger in size with dysplasia or villous histology) compared to sporadic adenomas.

○ Smoking and obesity increase the risk of colorectal adenomas in Lynch syndrome.

- Extracolonic cancers: Lynch syndrome is associated with extracolonic cancers, including endometrial (most common), ovarian, stomach, small bowel, pancreatic, hepatobiliary, renal pelvis, ureteral, brain gliomas, and Muir–Torre syndrome (sebaceous tumors, cutaneous keratoacanthomas and Lynch syndrome cancers).

Diagnostic Criteria

- It is important to identify individuals with Lynch syndrome, which lack an easy to identify phenotype, as surveillance decreases the incidence of CRC and associated mortality.
- There are several proposed diagnostic criteria to identify individuals with Lynch syndrome including (Amsterdam I, Amsterdam II, and Bethesda guidelines) (Table 25-2).
- Genetic testing
  ○ Direct sequencing of MMR gene to look for germline mutation is expensive and may lead to discovery of variants of uncertain significance.

TABLE 25-2   DIAGNOSTIC CRITERIA FOR LYNCH SYNDROME

Amsterdam I criteria

At least three relatives with histologically verified CRC

1. One is a first-degree relative of the other two
2. At least two successive generations affected
3. At least one of the relatives was diagnosed with CRC at age <50
4. FAP is excluded

Amsterdam II criteria

At least three relatives with an HNPCC-associated cancer (CRC, endometrial, stomach, ovary, ureter/renal pelvis, brain, small bowel, hepatobiliary tract, and sebaceous tumors of skin)

1. One is a first-degree relative of other two
2. At least two successive generations affected
3. At least one HNPCC-associated cancer diagnosed at age <50
4. FAP is excluded

Bethesda guidelines

1. CRC diagnosed in a patient aged <50
2. Presence of synchronous or metachronous CRC or other HNPCC-associated cancers, regardless of age
3. CRC with MSI-high histology in a patient aged <60
4. CRC or HNPCC-associated tumor diagnosed at age <50 in at least one first-degree relative
5. CRC or HNPCC-associated tumor diagnosed at any age in two first- or second-degree relatives

---

CRC, colorectal cancer; FAP, familial adenomatous polyposis; HNPCC, hereditary nonpolyposis colon cancer; MSI, microsatellite instability.

When Lynch syndrome is suspected, **genetic analysis** can be performed on tumor or polypectomy specimen to identify loss of expression of *MLH1, MSH2, MSH6,* or *PMS2* by immunohistochemistry (IHC) testing and/or MSI testing.

- **IHC testing** regardless of the *MMR* gene involved, it has test sensitivity of 83% and specificity of 89%.
- **MSI** is another useful test to identify patients with Lynch syndrome. It is measured by PCR of tumor tissue.
  - (MSI) testing sensitivity reaches 91% depending on the gene mutation (*MLH1* or *MSH2* > *MSH6*, or *PMS2*); the specificity of MSI testing is 90%.
  - Greater than 90% of HNPCC-associated tumors have high level of microsatellite instability (MSI-H), whereas sporadic CRC usually have low level of MSI.
  - IHC and MSI analysis have comparable test sensitivity and prove complementary to maximize it in identifying Lynch syndrome. Choice of testing may depend on the expertise of the pathology department.
- *BRAF* **mutation** or **promoter hypermethylation** studies is an adjunct screening test to identify the mechanism of *MLH1* protein loss observed on IHC testing.
  - About 68% of sporadic (non-Lynch syndrome) CRC cases carry *BRAF* mutation, whereas tumors of Lynch syndrome do not.
  - Up to 15% of sporadic CRC can have MSI-H, which is associated with epigenetic inactivation of *MLH1* by methylation or *BRAF* mutation. This aids in excluding Lynch syndrome in MSI-H tumors.
- **Germline mutation analysis** is performed on the proband by gene sequencing and deletion analysis for the (*MLH1, MSH2, MSH6,* and *PMS2*) and/or *EPCAM* genes, or other mutated genes on IHC testing.
  - Germline should be offered, if Lynch syndrome is suspected (tumors with MMR deficiency and high level of MSI with no *BRAF* mutation, history that fulfills Amsterdam criteria or Bethesda guidelines).
  - Positive test confirms the diagnosis, but in some families a specific mutation is not identified.

SURVEILLANCE AND TREATMENT

- **Colorectal cancer (CRC):**
  - CRC surveillance in suspected Lynch syndrome cases reduces cancer related death by 65%.
  - **Screening colonoscopy** at least every 2 years starting at age 20–25 or 2–5 years prior to the earliest age of CRC diagnosis in the family, whichever comes first.
  - **Enhanced cancer surveillance with annual colonoscopy** is recommended for those who carry MMR germline mutation.
  - **Total colectomy with ileorectal anastomosis (IRA)** is the treatment of choice. If not suitable (i.e., elderly individuals), then subtotal colectomy with continued annual surveillance of the remaining colon/rectum is an option given the high rate of metachronous lesions.
  - Primary prophylactic surgery is generally not recommended.
- **Extracolonic cancers**
  - Endometrial and ovarian cancer: Annual screening starting at age 30–35 by pelvic examination with **endometrial biopsies** and **transvaginal ultrasound**. Prophylactic hysterectomy and bilateral salpingo-oophorectomy should be offered to Lynch syndrome mutation carriers when finished child bearing (40–45 years of age).
  - Gastric cancer: Baseline screening **esophagogastroduodenoscopy (EGD)** with random gastric biopsies starting at age 30–35 and treatment for *Helicobacter pylori*

infection if positive. Limited data for surveillance, but repeating EGD every 3–5 years can be considered in cases with family history of gastric or duodenal cancer.

○ Small bowel tumors: Routine surveillance is not cost effective. Majority of the lesions are duodenal and ileal within reach of EGD and colonoscopy examinations. **Video capsule endoscopy** has also been suggested.

○ Urinary tract and pancreatic cancer: Annual screening starting at age 30–35 with urinalysis and cytological examination. Screening for pancreatic cancer with endoscopic ultrasound (EUS) or pancreas protocol cross-sectional imaging is only recommended if there is family history.

Adenomatous Polyposis Syndromes

GENERAL PRINCIPLES

- This includes familial adenomatous polyposis (FAP), attenuated familial polyposis, and *MUTYH*-associated polyposis (MAP), and other variants.
- Inherited syndromes characterized by early development of CRC secondary to germline mutations that amplify carcinogenesis.

Familial Adenomatous Polyposis (FAP)

GENERAL PRINCIPLES

- An **autosomal dominant** disease characterized by 100 or more synchronous colorectal adenomas.
- It is distributed equally between men and women. Considered the most common inherited polyposis syndrome with prevalence of 3 cases per 100,000.
- Patients with FAP usually develop symptoms after puberty, and polyposis is diagnosed by an average age of 36, with death from cancer at age 42.
- Average age of colon cancer diagnosis is 39 years. The risk of colon cancer in classic FAP approaches 100% by age 35–40.
- Left-sided adenomas are common. Their malignant potential is directly proportional to their high numbers as they share similar histologic features compared to sporadic adenomas.
- Genetics
  - The genetic basis for the disease is germline mutation with **inactivation and loss of tumor suppressor function in the *adenomatous polyposis coli (APC)* gene on chromosome 5q21–22**, which leads to cellular resistance to apoptosis and chromosomal instability, predisposing the cell to tumorigenesis.
  - Carcinogenesis in FAP requires *APC* gene mutation on both alleles, one is inherently mutated while the second is affected by somatic factors.
  - More than 800 mutations in the *APC* gene have been associated with FAP, with almost all mutations resulting in protein truncation.
  - One-third of patients have no family history of the disease, many representing sporadic "*de novo*" germline mutations. Colon cancer incidence at diagnosis in those patients reaches 25%.
  - The disease pathogenicity (i.e., number of adenomas, presence of desmoid tumors, risk of colon cancer) is linked to the mutations location in the *APC* gene. FAP is usually due to *APC* gene mid-portion mutations.

Attenuated Familial Adenomatous Polyposis (AFAP)

GENERAL PRINCIPLES

Definition

- A variant of FAP, with autosomal dominant inheritance pattern characterized by <100 synchronous colorectal adenomas. Average number of adenomas is 25 and tend to be proximal (75%) and flat rather than polypoid with infrequent rectal involvement.
- Onset of polyp development is delayed up to 20 years compared to FAP. The average of CRC diagnosis is 58 years.
- Genetics: AFAP is secondary to *APC* gene mutation, with overall high pathogenicity but less compared to FAP. Mutations are common at the far or proximal ends of the *APC* gene.

MUTYH-Associated Polyposis (MAP)

GENERAL PRINCIPLES

Definition

- A variant of FAP or AFAP, with autosomal recessive inheritance pattern. The average age of CRC diagnosis is 48 years.
- Genetics
  - MAP results from homozygous *MUTYH* mutations in two alleles.
  - *MUTYH* is a base excision repair gene to prevent DNA oxidative damage. *MUTYH* mutations cause *APC* and *KRAS* changes that initiate the cascade of tumorigenesis.

DIAGNOSIS

Clinical Presentation

- Patients with adenomatous polyposis syndromes are at risk for **extracolonic neoplasia** including small intestinal adenomas, gastric carcinomas, desmoid tumors, follicular and papillary thyroid cancer, childhood hepatoblastoma, CNS tumors (mostly medulloblastomas), congenital hypertrophy of the retinal pigmented epithelium (CHRPE), epidermoid cysts, and sebaceous gland adenomas.
- **Gastric polyps** occur in 30–50% of cases, but most are non-neoplastic, characterized by hyperplasia of fundic glands without epithelial dysplasia. Gastric cancer risk in FAP is <1%.
- The lifetime risk of **duodenal adenoma** approaches 100%, and duodenal and ampullary adenocarcinoma has become the leading cause of death in FAP patients who have undergone prophylactic colectomy with a lifetime risk of 5%.
- The second and third portion of the duodenum and especially the periampullary region are the most commonly affected areas. Polyps may cause biliary obstruction.
  - **Thyroid cancer** is present in 12% of FAP patients with female predominance and mean age of 28 years. Papillary histology is more common, while benign thyroid nodularity is observed up to 80%.
  - 1.6% of FAP will develop childhood **hepatoblastoma** with male predominance.

Diagnostic Testing

- Direct commercial blood tests are available for *APC* mutations, although they do not detect all mutations that cause FAP.

- *APC* gene sequencing should be performed on an affected family member with polyposis phenotype to determine if a mutation is found.
  - If mutation is present, other at-risk family members may be screened for the same mutation.
  - Genetic screening for children should start at age 10–12.
- Testing is available for *MUTYH* mutations in those with polyposis but lacking *APC* mutation and those with apparent autosomal recessive pattern inheritance.

SURVEILLANCE AND TREATMENT

- Colorectal cancer (CRC)
  - Gene carriers, at-risk family members who did not undergo genetic testing, or whose genetic testing is uninformative should be offered annual screening starting age 10–12.
  - Classic FAP may be screened with sigmoidoscopy or colonoscopy, while AFAP requires colonoscopy given predominance of right-sided tumors at a later starting age of 25.
  - **Colectomy** should be performed when polyposis is diagnosed with documented CRC or high-grade dysplasia.
  - Early colectomy is indicated in patients with symptoms or high-risk polyposis (i.e., large polyps >1 cm diameter, increase in polyps number in repeated examinations) or in cases of inadequate colon surveillance.
  - Colectomy options are determined by the disease distribution and the patient comorbidities:
    - **Colectomy with IRA** is preferred in polyposis with less rectal involvement (<20 rectal) and (<1000 colonic).
    - **Proctocolectomy with ileal pouch anal anastomosis (IPAA)** is preferred in severe polyposis with (>20 rectal) and (1000> colonic adenomas).
  - Because adenomas or cancers can still arise from the ileal pouch, continued annual surveillance of the ileal pouch, rectal cuff, and anastomosis by endoscopy is required.
- Extracolonic cancers
  - Gastric and duodenal polyps:
    - Surveillance for duodenal polyps should include baseline examination with both forward and side-viewing upper endoscopy at the time of colectomy or early in the third decade of life (25–30 years).
    - Patients with a history of duodenal polyps should undergo surveillance endoscopy on the basis of the Spigelman stage of duodenal polyps (Table 25-3).
    - Surveillance can be performed every 4 years for stage 0, every 2–3 years for stage I, every 1–3 years for stage II, and every 6–12 months for stage III. Stage IV polyps need duodenectomy.
    - Gastric fundic gland polyps must be randomly sampled. Surgery is considered for high-grade dysplasia or gastric cancer.
  - Thyroid cancer screening is recommended to all adenomatous polyposis syndromes types by annual ultrasound, while biannual ultrasound and AFP to screen for hepatoblastoma screening up to the age of 7 is controversial.
  - Desmoid tumors screening with abdominal computed tomography (CT) is indicated in high-risk patients (mid-portion *APC* gene mutation) before colectomy, or symptomatic patients with palpable masses or bowel obstruction.

OTHER FAP VARIANTS

Gardner Syndrome

- Gardner syndrome includes the same genetic lesions (*APC* gene) and gastrointestinal manifestations as FAP and is distinguished by **prominence of extraintestinal lesions**

TABLE 25-3 SPIGELMAN STAGE OF DUODENAL POLYPS

Score	1	2	3
No. of polyps	1–4	5–20	>20
Size (mm)	0–4	5–10	>10
Histologic type	Tubular	Tubulovillous	Villous
Dysplasia	Mild	Moderate	Severe

- Stage 0: score 0
- Stage I: score 1–4
- Stage II: score 5–6
- Stage III: score 7–8
- Stage IV: score 9–12

including desmoid tumors, sebaceous or epidermoid cysts, lipomas, osteomas (particularly of the mandible), supernumerary teeth, gastric polyps, and juvenile nasopharyngeal angiofibromas.
- More than 90% of patients with Gardner syndrome have **CHRPE**. Consisting of pigmented ocular fundic lesions, CHRPE is present in only 5% of controls; therefore, this examination finding is highly suggestive of gene carriage of adenomatous polyposis, especially when present bilaterally in patients with a positive family history.
- **Desmoid tumors or diffuse mesenteric fibromatosis** is found in 4–20% of FAP patients and can lead to intestinal obstruction or constriction of the mesenteric vasculature or uterus.
- Desmoid tumors frequently develop in areas of previous surgical procedures such as colectomy or cesarian section. Desmoid tumors can prove a lethal complication, ranking second behind metastatic disease in patients with FAP. There is no proven treatment or prevention strategy.

Turcot Syndrome
- Turcot syndrome refers to the **association between brain tumors and FAP or HNPCC**. There is no directly established mechanism for the development of brain tumors with the mutations that lead to CRC.
- Mutations to *APC* tend to be associated with medulloblastomas.
- Mutations in MMR genes are typically associated with glioblastoma.

Hamartomatous Polyposis Syndromes

GENERAL PRINCIPLES
- Autosomal dominant genetic syndromes known with hamartomatous polyp development in the GI tract and extragastrointestinal manifestations.
- These syndromes include: **Peutz–Jeghers syndrome** (PJS), **juvenile polyposis syndrome** (JPS), **Cowden syndrome** (*PTEN* hamartoma tumor syndrome), and **serrated/hyperplastic polyposis syndrome**.
- Hamartomatous polyps are frequent in other syndromes including neurofibromatosis type-1 (NF-1), multiple endocrine neoplasia type 2B (MEN-2B), Gorlin syndrome, and Birt-Hogg-Dubé.

Peutz–Jeghers Syndrome

GENERAL PRINCIPLES

Definition

- Peutz–Jeghers syndrome (PJS) is an **autosomal dominant** disease of multiple hamartomatous polyps in the gastrointestinal tract associated with mucocutaneous pigmentation.
- PJS incidence is about 1 in 50,000 to 1 in 200,000 births with equal distribution between males and females.
- Genetics
  - The genetic defect is in a gene encoding serine threonine kinase (*LKB1* or *STK11*) on chromosome 19p, which is proposed to function as a tumor suppressor.
  - *STK11* mutations are present in up to 90% of PJS families while 25% of cases arise from *de novo* mutations.

DIAGNOSIS

Clinical Presentation

- **Mucocutaneous pigmentation** (>95%): These are **melanin pigment spots**, appearing as flat 1–5-mm blue-gray to brown lesions on the lips (usually cross the vermilion border and darker than common freckles) and perioral region (94%), hands (74%), buccal mucosa (66%), and feet (62%). Pigmentations appear in infancy and regress after puberty, with exception of buccal lesions.
- **Hamartomatous polyps** (88–100%) are most commonly in small intestine (up to 90% and likely jejunal), but can also be found in the colon (up to 60%), stomach (up to 30%), and rectum (24%). They have **nondysplastic** unique histology. Usually multilobulated and contain **proliferation of smooth muscle** with branching bands extending into the lamina propria in a treelike fashion **with normal overlying mucosa.** Polyps may lead to obstruction, intussusception, infarction, and bleeding by the second to third decade of life.
- **Gastrointestinal malignancy** (38–66%) increased risk in PJS patients. Most commonly colorectal (39%), followed by pancreas (11–36%), stomach (29%), and small bowel (13%).
- **Extragastrointestinal malignancy** (9–54%): Women are at increased risk for **gynecologic cancers** such as breast (30–54%), ovary (21%), and cervical cancers (10%) such as "sex-cord tumors with annular tubules (SCTAT)." Young men are at increased risk for **Sertoli cell testicular tumors** (9%). **Lung cancer** risk is (7–17%).

Diagnostic Testing

- Genetic testing must be offered to high-risk family members and to confirm the diagnosis in those with at minimum one diagnostic criteria (≥2 histologically proven PJS polyps, one or more PJ polyps with family history of PJS, typical mucocutaneous pigmentation and family history of PJS, one or more PJ polyps with typical mucocutaneous pigmentation).
- Genetic testing on blood samples is commercially available through several laboratories and *LKB1* mutations can be identified in about 80% of families with PJS.[3]
- Genetic testing is offered starting at age 8, as up to 30–40% of patients may start to develop complications such as bowel obstruction by age 10.

SURVEILLANCE AND TREATMENT

- **Regular surveillance** of affected individuals aims to detect cancers of the breast, colon, pancreas, stomach, small bowel, ovaries, uterus, cervix, and testicles.
- **Gastrointestinal malignancy**
  - Annual CBC to early detect symptomatic PJS polyps with iron deficiency anemia secondary to bleeding GI polyps.
  - Upper endoscopy, colonoscopy, small bowel video capsule endoscopy at age 8 years every 2–3 years starting age 8. Subsequent surveillance depends on baseline screening findings:
    - If polyps found, repeat all three examinations (EGD, colonoscopy, and VCE) every 3 years.
    - If no polyps found, repeat all three examinations at age 18 years then every 3 years.
    - MRE/CTE can be performed if VCE is contraindicated.
  - Polypectomy of lesions >0.5–1.0 cm to decrease the complications risk (i.e., bleeding, intussusception, obstruction, transition to neoplasia).
  - PJS polyps express COX-2 receptors and hyperactivation of mammalian target of rapamycin (mTOR). Chemoprevention with COX-2 inhibitors or (mTOR) inhibitors (i.e. Everolimus) to control the polyps burden is not recommended due to lack of supportive evidence.
  - EUS or MRCP every 1–2 years starting at age 30 to screen for pancreatic cancer.
- **Extragastrointestinal malignancy**
  - Men require annual **testicular examination** starting at birth, followed by testicular ultrasound when abnormalities are palpated or feminization occurs (i.e., gynecomastia).
  - Women require annual pelvic examination with Papanicolaou (Pap) smear, transvaginal ultrasound, starting at age 21 years. While annul mammography and/or breast MRI is recommended starting at age 25 years.
  - No evidence for lung cancer screening but counseling about symptoms and smoking cessation is essential.
- Annual screening and clinical examination for at-risk first-degree relatives should start at birth.

Juvenile Polyposis Syndrome

GENERAL PRINCIPLES

- Juvenile polyposis syndrome (JPS) is an **autosomal dominant** disease of multiple hamartomatous polyps in the gastrointestinal tract.
- JPS is rare with incidence between 1 in 100,000 and 1 in 160,000 births.
- JPS polyps can be sessile or large pedunculated and multilobulated with white exudate on their surface. Histologically, abundance of lamina propria with mucin-filled cystically dilated gland and absence of a smooth muscle core with epithelial lining reflecting the GI tract surface lining.
- Genetics
  - JPS results from germline mutations in the *SMAD4* gene (known as *MADH4*) on chromosome 18q21.1 or *BMPR1A* gene on chromosome 10q22–23. Both genes function as tumor suppressors of tumor growth and apoptosis by transforming growth factor (TGF-β).
  - Gene mutations are present in up to 75% of JPS families while 25% of cases arise from *de novo* mutations.

DIAGNOSIS

Clinical Presentation

- **Hamartomatous polyps** are most commonly in the colorectum (98%), stomach (14%), and small intestine (7%).
- Symptomatic polyps more commonly present with rectal bleeding and anemia by the first to second decade of life. Abdominal pain, diarrhea, and intussusception are less common.
- **Gastrointestinal malignancy** increased lifetime risk in JPS patients. Most commonly colorectal (17–22%) and gastric (2–30%) with a mean diagnosis age of 34 and 58 years, respectively. Small intestinal and pancreatic cancer occurrence in JPS patients is rare.
- **Hereditary hemorrhagic telangiectasia (HHT)** mainly in JPS with *SMAD4* gene mutations. Symptomatic presentation usually with epistaxis, occult GI bleeding, or cardiopulmonary complications (i.e., pulmonary AV malformations, mitral valve prolapse).

Diagnostic Testing

- Genetic evaluation should include testing for mutations in both *SMAD4* and *BMPR1A* genes.
- Genetic testing must be offered to family members of known JPS patients, to distinguish JPS from other conditions with juvenile polyps and to confirm the diagnosis in those with at minimum one diagnostic criteria (>5 histologically proven JPS polyps in the colorectum, one or more JPS polyps in other areas of the GI tract, one or more JPS polyps with known family history of JPS).

SURVEILLANCE AND TREATMENT

- There is no international consensus for cancer screening, surveillance, and treatment in JPS. However, the 2015 American College of Gastroenterology (ACG) guidelines recommend:
  - Annual screening for both colorectal and gastric cancer with colonoscopy and EGD starting at 12 years of age or earlier if symptomatic.
  - Surveillance for both colorectal and gastric cancer with colonoscopy and EGD should be repeated every 1–3 years. All polyps ≥5 mm must be resected.
  - No screening for small bowel disease but periodic surveillance is indicated depending on prior small bowel polyp findings with enteroscopy, VCE, or CTE.
  - Prophylactic gastrectomy, proctocolectomy, and IPAA are indicated for polyp-related symptoms or if it cannot be managed endoscopically.
- Periodic cardiovascular examination is recommended for HHT evaluation in *SMAD4 gene* mutation carriers.

Cowden Syndrome

GENERAL PRINCIPLES

Definition

- Cowden syndrome (CS) is an inherited **autosomal dominant** disease featured by multiple hamartomas in various organs. CS incidence is 1 in 200,000.
- It's a phenotypic variant of (*PTEN* hamartoma tumor syndrome). Other variants are Bannayan–Riley–Ruvalcaba (BRRS), *PTEN*-related Proteus syndrome (PS), and Proteus-like syndrome.

- Genetics
  - CS genetic defect and carcinogenesis are secondary to point mutations of the phosphatase and tensin homolog (*PTEN*) gene on chromosome 10q23.
  - *PTEN* mutations result in loss of tumor suppression capacity to negatively regulate both phosphoinositide-3-kinase (*PI3K-AKT*) and mTOR signaling pathways.[4]
  - With normal *PTEN* gene, CS can still arise from mutations in the succinate dehydrogenase (*SDH*) gene or mutations in the DNA synthesis inhibition regulatory (*KLLN*) gene.[5–7]
  - Gene mutations are found in only 20–34% of subjects with CS clinical diagnostic criteria.[8]

DIAGNOSIS

Clinical Presentation

- CS has a wide range of clinical features, including mucocutaneous and extramucocutaneous hamartomatous lesions, benign thyroid diseases including multinodular goiter, adenomas, and Hashimoto thyroiditis in (>50%), adult Lhermitte–Duclos disease (dysplastic gangliocytoma of the cerebellum), macrocephaly (84%), gastrointestinal polyps, and mental retardation.
- **Malignancy risk:** Individuals with CS have lifetime cumulative cancer risk of 85% by the age of 70 years. Cancers are most commonly breast (85%), nonmedullary thyroid (35.2%), renal cell carcinoma (33.6%), endometrial (28.2%), colorectal (9%), and melanoma (6%).[9,10]
- **Gastrointestinal manifestations:**
  - Polyps are the most common gastrointestinal pathology in CS patients and found up to 95% in the colon. The incidence of gastric and duodenal polyps is over 66%.[1,11,12]
  - Hamartomatous polyps constitute the majority of CS polyps (35–85%), while other histologic types (ganglioneuromatous, hyperplastic, adenomas, inflammatory and lipomas) are less frequent.[12]
  - Colorectal adenocarcinoma lifetime risk in CS is 9% with an average diagnosis age of 44 years.[12] Gastric and duodenal cancer are rare.
  - **Esophageal glycogen acanthosis (80%):** Usually an incidental finding in CS on routine endoscopy. Grossly, appears as numerous gray-white nodularity in the upper and middle thirds of the esophagus with normal background mucosa.
- The revised diagnostic criteria for CS or other *PTEN*-hamartoma tumor syndrome phenotypes adopted by the National Comprehensive Cancer Network (NCCN) are summarized in (Table 25-4).[13]

Diagnostic Testing

- Genetic evaluation should include testing for *PTEN* gene mutations. Testing for other genes including *SDH and KLLN* mutations are also commercially available.
- Family members should undergo mutation-specific testing to aid in cancer-specific surveillance protocols.

SURVEILLANCE AND TREATMENT

System-based cancer surveillance in individuals with or at risk for CS must include:
- GI: Baseline colonoscopy every 2 years starting at the 15 years, and EGD every 2–3 years. Surveillance frequency can be increased according to the degree of polyposis.

TABLE 25-4 REVISED *PTEN* HAMARTOMA TUMOR SYNDROME DIAGNOSTIC CRITERIA[13]

Major Criteria	Minor Criteria
Breast cancer	Autism spectrum disorder
Endometrial cancer	Colon cancer
Thyroid cancer (follicular)	Esophageal glycogenic acanthosis ($\geq$3)
Adult Lhermitte–Duclos disease	Thyroid structural lesions (i.e., adenoma, multinodular goiter)
GI hamartomas (including ganglioneuromatous, excluding hyperplastic polyps; $\geq$3)	Thyroid cancer (papillary or follicular variant of papillary)
Macrocephaly ($\geq$97 percentile: 58 cm for women and 60 cm for men)	Renal cell carcinoma
Macular pigmentation of the glans penis	Testicular lipomatosis
Mucocutaneous lesions (any of the following)	Mental retardation (i.e., IQ $\leq$75)
1. Multiple trichilemmomas ($\geq$3, at least one biopsy proven)	Lipomas ($\geq$3)
2. Acral keratoses ($\geq$3 palmoplantar keratotic pits and/or acral hyperkeratotic papules)	Vascular anomalies (including multiple intracranial developmental venous anomalies)
3. Mucocutaneous neuromas ($\geq$3)	
4. Oral papillomas (particularly on tongue and gingiva), multiple ($\geq$3) OR biopsy proven OR dermatologist diagnosed	
Operational diagnosis in an individual (one the following):	**Operational diagnosis in family members of an individual who meets the diagnostic criteria or has *PTEN* gene mutation (one of the following):**
1. Three or more major criteria, but one must include macrocephaly, Lhermitte–Duclos disease, or gastrointestinal hamartomas.	1. Any two major criteria with or without minor criteria.
2. Two major and three minor criteria.	2. One major and two minor criteria.
	3. Three minor criteria.

- Endocrine: Annual thyroid examination with baseline ultrasound in adolescence or at time of diagnosis. All females must have monthly self-breast examination at 25years of age and annual mammogram and breast MRI at the age of 30–35 years.
- Genitourinary: Uterine cancer surveillance must start at age 30–35 years with annual transvaginal ultrasound and random endometrial sampling. Annual urine cytology and baseline renal ultrasound is recommended to screen for renal cell cancer.
- Annual detailed dermatologic examination for melanoma by the age of 18 years.

Serrated Polyposis Syndrome (Hyperplastic Polyposis Syndrome)

GENERAL PRINCIPLES

Definition

- Serrated polyposis syndrome (SPS) is a rare condition manifested by predisposition to **serrated colon polyps and increased risk of CRC**. SPS prevalence is not known but estimated to be 1:100,000.
- Polyps pathology ranges from hyperplastic, to sessile serrated and serrated adenomas.
- Genetics
  - No clear genetic defect is defined to predispose to SPS. However, hereditary etiology is suggested based on increase family history of CRC in patients with SPS.[14]
  - *MUTYH* mutations were observed in 18% of patients with SPS which indicate overlap between MAP and SPS.[15]
  - Smoking is strongly associated with SPS; the mechanism is unknown but it appears to potentiate the undefined genetic predisposition.[16]

DIAGNOSIS

Clinical Presentation

- The diagnosis of SPS requires at least one the following criteria to be present:
  - At least 5 serrated polyps proximal to the sigmoid colon with ≥2 of these polyps >10 mm in size.
  - Any number of serrated polyps proximal to the sigmoid colon and history of SPS in a first-degree relative.
  - >20 serrated polyps of any size with various colonic distribution.
- **Malignancy risk:** The lifetime risk for CRC in SPS is estimated at (>50%) and the mean age of diagnosis is 48 years.[17]

Diagnostic Testing

Genetic testing is not recommended in patients with SPS but testing for *MUTYH* mutations is optional in patients with SPS and self or family history of colonic adenomas.

SURVEILLANCE AND TREATMENT

- SPS patients undergo surveillance colonoscopy every 1–3 years with complete polypectomies. It is suggested that first-degree relatives should start screening colonoscopies by the age of 40 years or 10 years earlier than the age of diagnosis in SPS individuals (whichever comes first).[18]
- Total colectomy with IRA is indicated if polyps cannot be managed endoscopically, presence of high-grade dysplasia or CRC.

HEREDITARY PANCREATITIS

- Hereditary pancreatitis typically presents as acute pancreatitis in childhood or early adolescence, chronic pancreatitis in late adolescence or early adulthood, and patients are at risk for pancreatic cancer later in life.
- Autosomal dominant hereditary pancreatitis is usually caused by mutations in the serine protease 1 gene (*PRSS1*) on chromosome 7q35, which encodes cationic trypsin.[19]

- One-third of patients with *PRSS1*-associated hereditary pancreatitis develop pancreatic insufficiency and/or diabetes mellitus.
- Autosomal recessive pancreatitis is most commonly associated with cystic fibrosis (*CFTR* gene mutation).
- Mutations in the serine protease inhibitor Kazal type 1 gene (*SPINK1*) also result in autosomal recessive or complex genetic pattern of inherited pancreatitis.
- Both *CFTR* and *SPINK1* code for molecules that protect the pancreas from active trypsin.
- Genetic testing can be performed on those with a suggestive family history, unexplained pancreatitis in a child, or unexplained recurrent acute or chronic pancreatitis in older patients.

HEREDITARY PANCREATIC CANCER

- Genetic predisposition causes 10–15% of pancreatic cancer cases, while positive family history is present in 5–10% of all pancreatic cancer subjects.[20,21]
- The diagnosis of familial pancreatic cancer requires ≥2 first-degree relatives with history of pancreatic cancer who do not meet criteria for a known pancreatic cancer–associated hereditary syndrome.
- It follows an autosomal dominant inheritance pattern with a (35%) life risk of developing cancer by the age of 85 years, with incremental risk in relation to the number of first-degree relatives with pancreatic cancer in the kindred.
- Testing for hereditary pancreatic adenocarcinoma must be considered in high-risk individuals with:
  - Diagnosed genetic syndrome associated with pancreatic cancer, including hereditary pancreatitis (53-fold risk), PJS (132-fold risk), Lynch syndrome, familial atypical multiple melanoma and mole syndrome (FAMMM), and hereditary breast–ovarian cancer syndrome with *BRCA1/2* mutations (about 2-fold risk), ataxia–telangiectasia syndrome (*ATM* gene mutation).
  - Two relatives with pancreatic cancer (one being a first-degree relative).
  - Three or more relatives with pancreatic cancer.
  - History of hereditary pancreatitis.
- Genetic testing must include testing for mutations in *BRCA1/2*, *CDKN2A*, *ATM*. Also analysis for known gene mutations associated with PJS, Lynch syndrome and hereditary pancreatitis must be considered.
- Annual MRI and/or EUS starting at the age of 50 or 10 years younger than the earliest age of pancreatic cancer in the family (whichever first) is recommended for surveillance.

Hereditary Diffuse Gastric Cancer (HDGC)

GENERAL PRINCIPLES

Definition

- HDGC is an **autosomal dominant** inherited form of diffuse-type gastric cancer with prevalence of (1–3%).
- Genetics
- HDGC is associated with germline truncating **mutations in the gene E-cadherin (*CDH1*) on chromosome 16q22.1**, resulting in defective intercellular adhesion.

DIAGNOSIS

Clinical Presentation

- Lifetime cumulative risk for advanced gastric cancer is 40–70% in men and 60–80% in women, with 38 years as the average age of onset.[22]

- Women with HDGC are also at high risk for lobular breast cancer (60% by age 80); so enhanced breast cancer screening is recommended.

Diagnostic Testing

- Genetic testing is commercially available and consists of direct gene sequencing of peripheral blood to identify a specific mutation in an affected individual. Subsequently mutation-specific assays may be performed on at-risk family members. Mutations are identified in 25–50% of families.
- *CDH1* gene mutation is suspected in the following settings:
  - ≥2 cases of diffuse gastric cancer with at least one diagnosed at age <50.
  - Any diffuse gastric cancer at age <40.
  - ≥3 cases of diffuse gastric cancer in first- or second-degree relatives regardless of age of onset.
  - Personal or family history of diffuse gastric cancer and lobular breast cancer (one <50 years).
  - Suggestive pathology on biopsy—in situ signet ring cells or pagetoid spread of signet ring cells adjacent to diffuse-type gastric cancer.

SURVEILLANCE AND TREATMENT

- There are no reliable screening tests for carriers of germline mutation of *CDH1* to allow early diagnosis of diffuse gastric cancer, as endoscopic visualization fails to identify early-stage disease and random biopsies may miss focal advanced lesions.
- **Prophylactic total gastrectomy** is often recommended in early twenties or 5 years earlier than the youngest family member who developed gastric cancer.
- **Annual** surveillance endoscopy with random gastric biopsies in patients with established *CDH1* gene mutation before the age of 20 years or for those who refused gastrectomy.
- Enhanced breast cancer screening in women in HDGC families, starting by the age of 35 years with annual mammography/breast MRI and biannual clinical breast examination.
- CRC screening with colonoscopy at intervals of 3–5 years must start at the age of 40 years or 10 years younger than the earliest age of CRC cancer in the family.

Other Conditions to Consider Genetic Testing

HEREDITARY HEMOCHROMATOSIS (HH)

- Caused by missense mutations (*C282Y*) in the *HFE* gene on chromosome 6. It is rarely caused by other genes mutations (hemojuvelin, hepcidin, ferroportin, transferring receptor 2).
- Homozygosity for *C282Y* gene mutations is the most common disease phenotype, but patients may also be homozygous for the *H63D* mutation, heterozygous for *C282Y* or *H63D* or compound heterozygotes.[23]
- HH genetic testing is utilized to allow for early treatment, and to prevent late consequences of iron overload including cirrhosis, hepatocellular carcinoma, diabetes mellitus, and cardiomyopathy.
- Testing for *HFE* gene mutation should be performed on patients with a clinical iron overload state (transferrin saturation ≥60% in men or ≥50% in women and/or elevated ferritin).
- Optimal screening timing is between 18 and 30 years of age, when HH is evident by iron tests, but prior to onset of end-organ damage.

CELIAC DISEASE

- Celiac disease is characterized by a chronic inflammatory response to gluten in small bowel mucosa in genetically susceptible individuals. It is highly associated with *HLA DR3-DQ2* and/or *DR4-DQ8* gene locus in about 99% of patients, which are necessary but not sufficient to produce the celiac phenotype.[24]
- *HLA* typing for DQ2/DQ8, a commercially available blood test, can be useful in the diagnosis of celiac disease when patients are already on a gluten-free diet without a confirmed diagnosis (negative celiac serology). The absence of *HLA DQ2/DQ8* essentially rules out celiac disease.[25]

INFLAMMATORY BOWEL DISEASE (IBD) AND THIOPURINE METHYLTRANSFERASE (TPMT)

- Azathioprine (AZA) and 6-mercaptopurine (6-MP) are successfully used in patients IBD for inducing and maintaining remission, and as steroid-sparing agents.
- AZA is metabolized to 6-MP, which is then metabolized to 6-thioguanine (6-TG) and 6-methylmercaptopurine (6-MMP) through the enzyme thiopurine methyltransferase (TPMT). 6-TG and 6-MMP are related to the bone marrow and liver toxicities, respectively.
- TPMT enzyme activity is a major determining factor of 6-MP metabolism and its toxicity.
- Approximately 89% of population has wild-type TPMT genotype, which is associated with normal TPMT enzyme activity. Eleven percent of population is heterozygous for TPMT and has intermediate TPMT enzyme activity. About 0.3% of population is homozygous for TPMT mutant alleles, and has almost no TPMT enzyme activity, which leads to high 6-TG levels and bone marrow toxicity in patients taking AZA or 6-MP.
- Testing for genetic polymorphisms to determine the TPMT genotype before initiating therapy with thiopurines can identify patients with low or absent TPMT activity.
- Patients with homozygous mutant alleles are not candidates for therapy with AZA or 6-MP.
- TPMT genotypes correlate with enzyme activity or phenotype, which may be determined directly by RBC assay. Testing of TPMT enzyme activity can be confounded by recent blood transfusion or concomitant medications.
- Empiric dosing of thiopurines may be initiated on the basis of TPMT enzyme activity level.
- It is important to note that regardless of TPMT genotype or phenotype, monitoring of blood cell counts and liver function tests are still required, as normal TPMT screening testing does not preclude development of adverse drug reactions.

REFERENCES

1. Syngal S, Brand RE, Church JM, et al. ACG clinical guideline: genetic testing and management of hereditary gastrointestinal cancer syndromes. *Am J Gastroenterol.* 2015;110(2):223–262.
2. Moreira L, Balaguer F, Lindor N, et al. Identification of Lynch syndrome among patients with colorectal cancer. *JAMA.* 2012;308(15):1555–1565.
3. Stoffel E, Mukherjee B, Raymond VM, et al. Calculation of risk of colorectal and endometrial cancer among patients with Lynch syndrome. *Gastroenterology.* 2009;137(5):1621–1627.
4. Stambolic V, Suzuki A, De La Pompa JL, et al. Negative regulation of PKB/Akt-dependent cell survival by the tumor suppressor PTEN. *Cell.* 1998;95(1):29–39.
5. Bennett KL, Mester J, Eng C. Germline epigenetic regulation of KILLIN in Cowden and Cowden-like syndrome. *JAMA.* 2010;304(24):2724–2731.
6. Cho YJ, Liang P. Killin is a p53-regulated nuclear inhibitor of DNA synthesis. *Proc Natl Acad Sci USA.* 200;105(14):5396–5401.

7. Ni Y, Zbuk KM, Sadler T, et al. Germline mutations and variants in the succinate dehydrogenase genes in Cowden and Cowden-like syndromes. *Am J Hum Genet*. 2008;83(2):261–268.

8. Pilarski R, Stephens JA, Noss R, et al. Predicting PTEN mutations: an evaluation of Cowden syndrome and Bannayan-Riley-Ruvalcaba syndrome clinical features. *J Med Genet*. 2011;48(8):505–512.

9. Bubien V, Bonnet F, Brouste V, et al. High cumulative risks of cancer in patients with PTEN hamartoma tumour syndrome. *J Med Genet*. 2013;50(4):255–263.

10. Tan MH, Mester JL, Ngeow J, et al. Lifetime cancer risks in individuals with germline PTEN mutations. *Clin Cancer Res*. 2012;18(2):400–407.

11. Levi Z, Baris HN, Kedar I, et al. Upper and lower gastrointestinal findings in PTEN mutation-positive cowden syndrome patients participating in an active surveillance program. *Clin Transl Gastroenterol*. 2011;2:e5.

12. Heald B, Mester J, Rybicki L, et al. Frequent gastrointestinal polyps and colorectal adenocarcinomas in a prospective series of PTEN mutation carriers. *Gastroenterology*. 2010;139(6):1927–1933.

13. Pilarski R, Burt R, Kohlman W, et al. Cowden syndrome and the PTEN hamartoma tumor syndrome: systematic review and revised diagnostic criteria. *J Natl Cancer Inst*. 2013;105(21):1607–1616.

14. Kalady MF, Jarrar A, Leach B, et al. Defining phenotypes and cancer risk in hyperplastic polyposis syndrome. *Dis Colon Rectum*. 2011;54(2):164–170.

15. Boparai KS, Dekker E, van Eeden S, et al. Hyperplastic polyps and sessile serrated adenomas as a phenotypic expression of MYH-associated polyposis. *Gastroenterology*. 2008;135(6):2014–2018.

16. Walker GR, Landmann JK, Hewett DG, et al. Hyperplastic polyposis syndrome is associated with cigarette smoking, which may be a modifiable risk factor. *Am J Gastroenterol*. 2010;105(7):1642–1647.

17. Win AK, Walters RJ, Buchanan DD, et al. Cancer risks for relatives of patients with serrated polyposis. *Am J Gastroenterol*. 2012;107(5):770–778.

18. Rex DK, Ahnen DJ, Baron JA, et al. Serrated lesions of the colorectum: review and recommendations from an expert panel. *Am J Gastroenterol*. 2012;107(9):1315–1329.

19. Rosendahl J, Bödeker H, Mössner J, et al. Hereditary chronic pancreatitis. *Orphanet J Rare Dis*. 2007;2:1.

20. Klein AP, Brune KA, Petersen GM, et al. Prospective risk of pancreatic cancer in familial pancreatic cancer kindreds. *Cancer Res*. 2004;64(7):2634–2638.

21. Klein AP. Genetic susceptibility to pancreatic cancer. *Mol Carcinog*. 2012;51(1):14–24.

22. Fitzgerald RC, Hardwick R, Huntsman D, et al. Hereditary diffuse gastric cancer: updated consensus guidelines for clinical management and directions for future research. *J Med Genet*. 2010;47(7):436–444.

23. Neghina AM, Anghel A. Hemochromatosis genotypes and risk of iron overload—a meta-analysis. *Ann Epidemiol*. 2011;21(1):1–14.

24. Hadithi M, von Blomberg BM, Crusius JB, et al. Accuracy of serologic tests and HLA-DQ typing for diagnosing celiac disease. *Ann Intern Med*. 2007;147(5):294–302.

25. American Gastroenterological Association medical position statement: celiac sprue. *Gastroenterology*. 2001;120(6):1522–1525.

Gastrointestinal Procedures

Zachary L. Smith and Daniel K. Mullady

26

Introduction

- The ability to perform endoscopic procedures has radically changed the practice of gastroenterology.
- Endoscopy allows for direct visual inspection, tissue sampling, and minimally invasive therapeutic intervention. An endoscopic procedure is worth performing if the benefit for the patient exceeds the risks by a sufficiently wide margin.
- Preparation for endoscopy involves addressing important issues specific to each patient before, during and after the procedure. These include:
  - Preprocedure
    - Assessing indications, absolute and relative contraindications
    - Medication allergies
    - Patient medications and any potential drug–drug interactions with anesthetics or antibiotics
    - Presence of coagulopathy, comorbid factors, and conditions potentially requiring antibiotic prophylaxis
    - Detailed informed consent with complete understanding of the benefits and risks associated with the procedure.
  - During the procedure: continuous monitoring of vital signs including noninvasive blood pressure, telemetry, pulse oximetry, and respiratory rate.
  - Postprocedure
    - Adequate recovery from sedation using objective criteria (e.g., Aldrete score)
    - Monitoring for signs of immediate and delayed adverse events
    - Arranging and documenting the appropriate follow-up
- General indications for endoscopic procedures are listed in Table 26-1.

Upper Gastrointestinal Endoscopy

GENERAL PRINCIPLES

- Esophagogastroduodenoscopy (EGD) allows high-resolution visual inspection of the upper gastrointestinal (GI) tract from the esophagus to the second or third portion of the duodenum.
- EGD is performed for various indications, such as:
  - **Diagnosis** and **management** of abdominal pain or upper GI bleeding;
  - **Screening** and diagnosis of esophageal or gastric malignancies;
  - **Surveillance** of premalignant conditions such as Barrett esophagus;
  - Application of endoscopic **eradication therapies** for management of Barrett's esophagus–associated dysplasia and early esophageal adenocarcinoma; and
  - **Palliation** of dysphagia resulting from both malignant and benign causes.
- Procedure
  - At some institutions, examinations are performed using **topical anesthetics** applied to the oropharynx in combination with **intravenous (IV) conscious sedation**.

TABLE 26-1 GENERAL INDICATIONS FOR ENDOSCOPIC PROCEDURES

Gastrointestinal endoscopy is generally indicated:

If a change in management is probable based on results of endoscopy

After an empiric trial of therapy for a suspected benign digestive disorder has been unsuccessful

As the initial method of evaluation as an alternative to radiographic studies

When a primary therapeutic procedure is contemplated

Gastrointestinal endoscopy is generally not indicated:

When the results are not expected to contribute to a management choice

For periodic follow-up of healed benign disease unless surveillance of a premalignant condition is warranted

Gastrointestinal endoscopy is generally contraindicated:

When the risks to patient health or life are judged to outweigh the most favorable benefits of the procedure

When adequate patient cooperation or consent cannot be obtained

When a perforated viscus is known or suspected

Monitored anesthesia care can be used with assistance from an anesthesiologist when conscious sedation is anticipated to be unsuccessful.

The only patient preparation required is to **avoid oral intake of clear liquids for 2 hours and solid food for ≥6 hours before the procedure**.

- Various instruments may be passed through the working channel of the endoscope for use in tissue biopsy, cauterization, clip application, medication injection, enteral stenting, and application of endoscopic eradication therapies.

COMPLICATIONS

- Endoscopy has a small risk of complications, overall estimated to occur in 0.1% having the procedure.[1]
- Significant **bleeding** has been reported in 0.025–0.15%.
- **Perforation** has been reported in 0.02–0.2%.
- **Cardiorespiratory complications**, mostly attributed to premedication or sedation, can occur in 0.05–0.73% of patients.
- The risk of **mortality** as a result of upper endoscopy has been estimated 1 in 10,000 from large database analyses.

Colonoscopy

GENERAL PRINCIPLES

- Colonoscopy is performed to examine the colonic and terminal ileal mucosa.
- Colonoscopy is performed for various indications, including:
  - **Evaluation** and **treatment** of overt lower GI bleeding;
  - **Evaluation** of iron-deficiency anemia;
  - **Screening** and **surveillance** of colorectal cancer and polyps;
  - **Diagnosis** and cancer surveillance in inflammatory bowel disease;

- **Palliative treatment of** stenosing or bleeding neoplasms; and
- **Evaluation** of clinically significant diarrhea of unexplained origin.
- Procedure
  - As is true for upper endoscopy, colonoscopy typically involves the administration of moderate or deep sedation.
  - **Colon preparation** is required before the procedure. This usually involves the ingestion of a bowel purgative on the day or evening before the patient's colonoscopy. **Please see** Table 26-2 **for a comprehensive list of bowel purgatives**.[2]
- Various instruments may be passed through the working channel of the colonoscope for use in tissue biopsy, treatment of bleeding, polypectomy, and colonic stent placement.

COMPLICATIONS

- Colonoscopy has a small risk of complications.[3] In patients undergoing colonoscopy for average risk colon cancer screening, this risk is estimated to occur in 2.8 per 1000 procedures.
- Significant **bleeding** can be seen in up to 1.9% of patients. The rate of bleeding complications seen with therapeutic colonoscopy is roughly double than that seen with diagnostic colonoscopy.
- **Perforation** can occur in up to 0.4% of patients. Surgical consultation should be obtained in the event of suspected perforation; however, if possible, attempts to close the defect with endoscopic clips or other means should be made if the endoscopist is immediately aware of the perforation.
- **Cardiorespiratory complications** are typically attributable to the sedation used during the procedure.
- **Mortality** has been reported in up to 0.06% of patients.

Flexible Sigmoidoscopy

GENERAL PRINCIPLES

- Flexible sigmoidoscopy involves a shorter examination compared with colonoscopy and is used to examine the distal colon up to the splenic flexure.
- Flexible sigmoidoscopy is generally used for evaluation of:
  - Suspected distal colonic disease when colonoscopy is not indicated;
  - Anastomotic recurrence in rectosigmoid carcinoma; and
  - Exclusion of infection or immune-mediated processes (e.g., graft-versus-host disease) in certain patient subsets, including those with inflammatory bowel disease or following bone marrow transplantation.
- Procedure
  - This examination can be performed **without sedation**, which adds the advantages of decreased cost; fewer complications associated with sedation; and decreased lost work time for the patient. This practice varies by institution.
  - This procedure also eliminates the need for a complete colon preparation. Commonly, two enemas can be given a few hours before the procedure.

COMPLICATIONS

- Complications of flexible sigmoidoscopy are similar to those listed above under colonoscopy.
- The overall risk of perforation during flexible sigmoidoscopy is low (0.01%).

Small Bowel Enteroscopy

GENERAL PRINCIPLES

- Since standard upper GI endoscopy is limited to the proximal duodenum, longer endoscopes are needed to examine the upper GI tract beyond the ligament of Treitz.
- Various endoscopes can be used including colonoscopes (termed **push enteroscopy**) as well as longer enteroscopes with balloon overtubes (**single- and double-balloon enteroscopy**).
- **Intraoperative enteroscopy**, a technique where the small intestine is plicated over the enteroscope with the assistance of a surgeon. This is typically done laparoscopically.
- **Video capsule enteroscopy** is currently being used in many settings as a means to visualize segments of the bowel previously inaccessible to endoscopy.
- Small bowel enteroscopy is performed **for evaluation of obscure (occult or overt) GI bleeding**.
- It is also indicated for **diagnosis and treatment of small bowel polyps and masses**.
- Procedure
    - **Endoscopes which can be used for enteroscopy** are 160–240 cm in length and can be used for therapeutic intervention. They allow for controlled insertion and withdrawal.
        - Push enteroscopy is traditionally used after a negative upper endoscopy and colonoscopy.
        - The yield of push enteroscopy in this setting is approximately 60%.
    - **Balloon enteroscopy** utilizes single or double inflatable balloons on an overtube through which the enteroscope is advanced. The overtube and inflated balloons are used to grip the intestinal wall and allow deep cannulation of the small bowel.
        - Both transoral and transanal approaches can be used.
        - This form of enteroscopy allows biopsy or treatment of lesions noted beyond the reach of push enteroscopy and is replacing intraoperative enteroscopy in some centers.
    - **Video capsule enteroscopy** visualizes segments of the bowel previously inaccessible to endoscopy.
        - The patient swallows a capsule that contains a camera, light source, battery, and transmitter.
        - As the capsule traverses the GI tract, it takes pictures and transmits these images to a receiver that the patient wears on the belt. The capsule takes 8–12 hours of images, usually sufficient time to traverse the ileocecal valve.
        - The images are then loaded onto a computer where they can be viewed in a movie format.
        - The current indications for capsule endoscopy include evaluation of obscure GI bleeding and persistent occult GI bleeding.
        - The major contraindication is the presence of intestinal strictures which can obstruct passage of the capsule.[4,5]
- While capsule enteroscopy is only a diagnostic procedure, small bowel flexible enteroscopes not only provide diagnosis but also allow tissue acquisition, resection of polyps, and ablation or mechanical clipping of bleeding lesions.

COMPLICATIONS

- Complications rates are higher in balloon-assisted enteroscopy compared with standard endoscopy including higher rates of bowel perforation.
- The **main complication associated with capsule endoscopy is capsule retention**, rates of which are dependent on the indication of the procedure. Capsule retention frequently occurs in the area of pathology in the small bowel. Intestinal obstruction from a retained capsule can occur, and may require surgical intervention.

TABLE 26-2 COMMERCIALLY AVAILABLE BOWEL PREPARATIONS

	PEG-ELS	SF-PEG-ELS	Low-Volume PEG-ELS With Ascorbic Acid	Low-Volume PEG-3350-SD
Brand name	GoLYTELY	NuLYTELY; TriLyte	MoviPrep	MiraLAX
Company (location)	Braintree Laboratories (Braintree, MA)	Braintree Laboratories	Salix Pharmaceuticals (Raleigh, NC)	Merck (Boston, MA)
Composition	PEG, sodium sulfate, sodium, bicarbonate, sodium chloride, potassium chloride	PEG, sodium bicarbonate, sodium chloride, potassium chloride	PEG-3350, sodium sulfate, sodium chloride, ascorbic acid	PEG-3350
Purgative volume/amount; recommended minimum additional fluid[a]	4 L; none	4 L; none	2 L; 1 L clear liquid	238 g PEG-3350 in 2-L SD; regimens vary
FDA approval	Yes	Yes	Yes	No
Average wholesale price, US$	24.56	26.89 (NuLYTELY); 27.98 (TriLyte)	81.17	10.08
Dosing regimens[b]	Split dose: 2–3 L day before and 1–2 L day of procedure; Single dose: 4 L day before	Split dose: 2–3 L day before and 1–2 L day of procedure; Single dose: 4 L day before	Split dose: 1 L day before and 1 L day of procedure; Single dose: 2 L day before	Split dose: 1 L day before and 1 L day of procedure; Single dose: 2 L day before
Specific comments	Criterion standard; least palatable preparation	More palatable than PEG-ELS	Avoid in patients with glucose-6-phosphate dehydrogenase deficiency	Not balanced ELS; unclear whether electrolyte shifts may occur

[a]Split dose recommended whenever possible.
[b]The authors suggest an additional 1–2 L of clear fluid intake beyond that recommended in prescribing information.
From Saltzman JR, Cash BD, Pasha SF, et al. Bowel preparation before colonoscopy. *Gastrointest Endosc.* 2015;81(4):781–794.
FDA, U.S. Food and Drug Administration; NaP, sodium phosphate; OSS, oral sodium sulfate; PEG-ELS, polyethylene glycol electrolyte solution; SD, sports drink; SF, sulfate free.

Oral Sodium Sulfate	Oral Sodium Sulfate With PEG-ELS	Sodium Picosulfate/ Magnesium oxide/ Anhydrous Citric Acid	Magnesium Citrate	NaP Tablets
Suprep	Suclear	Prepopik	Generic	OsmoPrep
Braintree Laboratories	Braintree Laboratories	Ferring Pharmaceuticals Inc. (Parsippany, NJ)	Over-the-counter (OTC)	Salix Pharmaceuticals
Sodium sulfate, potassium sulfate, magnesium sulfate	Sodium sulfate, potassium sulfate, magnesium sulfate, PEG-3350	Sodium picosulfate, magnesium sulfate, anhydrous citric acid	Magnesium citrate	Monobasic and dibasic NaP
12 oz; 2.5-L water	6-oz OSS/2 L PEG-ELS; 1.25-L water	10 oz; 2-L water	20–30 oz; 2-L water	32 tablets; 2-L water[b]
Yes	Yes	Yes	No	Yes
91.96	77.94	95.34	2.48	150.84
Split dose: 6 oz OSS with 10 oz of water + 32-oz water day before and 6-oz OSS with 10 oz of water + 32-oz water day of procedure	Split dose: 6-oz OSS with 10 oz of water + 32-oz water day before and 2 L PEG-ELS day of procedure; Single dose: Evening before 6-oz OSS with 10 oz of water + 16-oz water followed by 2 L PEG-ELS + 16-oz water 2 hrs after OSS	Split dose: 5 oz Prepopik day before + 40 oz clear liquids and 5 oz Prepopik + 24 oz clear liquids day of procedure; Single dose: 5 oz + 40 oz clear liquids the afternoon or early evening before the procedure and 5 oz + 24 oz clear liquids 6 hrs later	Split dose: 1–1.5 10-oz bottles day before and 1–1.5 10-oz bottles day of procedure	Split dose: 20 tablets day before and 12 tablets day of procedure
Avoid in patients with renal insufficiency	Avoid in patients with renal insufficiency, elderly; not recommended for routine use	Avoid in patients with renal insufficiency or risk factors for acute phosphate nephropathy; not recommended for routine use		

Endoscopic Retrograde Cholangiopancreatography

GENERAL PRINCIPLES

- Endoscopic retrograde cholangiopancreatography (ERCP) is performed using a specially designed endoscope called a duodenoscope that involves a side-viewing imaging system as well as an elevator that can manipulate the angle of accessories exiting the working channel of the endoscope.
- This system allows direct visualization of the major and minor papillae and facilitates insertion of devices into the desired ductal structure.
- Iodinated contrast is injected to delineate intraductal anatomy, typically to localize stones or strictures.
- With the advent of improved noninvasive cross-sectional imaging technology including computed tomography (CT) and magnetic resonance cholangiopancreatography (MRCP), the role of ERCP as a diagnostic modality has diminished considerably.
- The most common diagnostic indications for ERCP include:
  - Primary sclerosing cholangitis where cross-sectional imaging is inconclusive in the setting of high clinical suspicion.
  - Biliary and pancreatic sphincter of Oddi manometry to assess for Type II sphincter of Oddi dysfunction
  - Assessment of postoperative bile leak
- Procedure
  - An ERCP can be used effectively in **detecting and treating choledocholithiasis**. **Biliary** sphincterotomy is usually performed to facilitate stone extraction. Biliary sphincterotomy can protect against recurrent symptomatic choledocholithiasis in patients not undergoing cholecystectomy. ERCP may also be used therapeutically to **dilate benign and malignant strictures** in the biliary tree with or without subsequent stent placement.
  - **Brushings for cytology or intraductal biopsies** may also be obtained during ERCP to assist in the diagnosis of cholangiocarcinoma and pancreatic neoplasms.
  - **Palliation of jaundice** in patients with pancreatic and biliary malignancies can be achieved by placement of self-expanding metallic stents.
- ERCP is used predominantly for the treatment or palliation of:
  - Choledocholithiasis, especially in the setting of biliary obstruction or cholangitis;
  - Benign and malignant biliary strictures;
  - Bile leak;
  - Suspected Type 1 or Type 2 sphincter of Oddi dysfunction;
  - Pancreatic duct leak;
  - Complications of acute and chronic pancreatitis such as pancreatic duct disruption, strictures, and stones; and
  - Resection of ampullary neoplasms.
- Various devices can be passed through the working channel of the duodenoscope to achieve access and cannulation of the common bile duct and pancreatic duct, and to perform maneuvers such as sphincterotomy, balloon dilation, tissue biopsies and brushings, biliary and pancreatic stenting, stone extraction, and cholangioscopy.

COMPLICATIONS

The ERCP procedure is associated with **all the risks of upper endoscopy**.[5] Additional risks include the following:

- Approximately 3–15% of patients develop **post-ERCP pancreatitis (PEP)**. This is usually mild and self-limited; however, in a small percentage of cases, this can be life threatening.

- The incidence of PEP is higher in patients with suspected sphincter of Oddi dysfunction and females less than 40 years of age.
- Rectal indomethacin has been shown in a large randomized controlled trial to reduce the risk of PEP.[6]
- Additionally, both the placement of pancreatic duct stents, and the administration of high volumes of crystalloids in the postprocedure setting, have been suggested to reduce the risk of PEP.
- Additional adverse events of ERCP include retroperitoneal or guidewire perforations, cholangitis and postsphincterotomy hemorrhage.

Endoscopic Ultrasonography

GENERAL PRINCIPLES

- Endoscopic ultrasonography (EUS) allows for imaging the luminal wall and surrounding structures.
- EUS is an effective modality for tissue acquisition and local staging of pancreaticobiliary malignancies.
- EUS-guided fine-needle aspiration (FNA) has supplanted CT-guided biopsy and ERCP in the diagnosis of pancreatic neoplasms.
- EUS is an effective modality in evaluating lesions in the GI tract, mediastinum, and other organs such as the left adrenal gland and the liver.[7]
- **EUS-guided FNA** provides clinically important diagnostic and prognostic information including cytologic confirmation of the presence (or absence) of malignancy and metastasis to secondary sites.
- The **most common indications of EUS-guided FNA** include evaluation of:
  - Pancreatic masses;
  - Mediastinal and intra-abdominal lymphadenopathy;
  - Liver masses;
  - Left adrenal masses; and
  - GI subepithelial lesions.
- EUS is the most sensitive imaging study for the diagnosis of chronic pancreatitis and choledocholithiasis and external anal sphincter defects.
- EUS is also an adjunctive tool in the evaluation of patients with fecal incontinence to assess integrity of the internal and external anal sphincters.
- Procedure
  - EUS is performed using a specially designed endoscope that involves an oblique-viewing endoscope with a sonographic imaging system.
  - Two types of echoendoscopes are commonly employed.
    - **Curvilinear array imaging:** This echoendoscope is utilized for the performance of FNA and FNB.
    - **Radial imaging:** This echoendoscope is commonly used for luminal GI tract indications (e.g., subepithelial lesions, local staging of esophageal cancer).
  - The endoscope is passed to different areas in the upper and lower GI tract allowing for targeted inspection of intra- and extraluminal structures.
  - The FNA needle can be passed through the working channel of the endoscope to perform FNA of solid lesions or aspiration of fluid from pancreatic cysts.

COMPLICATIONS

- EUS is associated with all the risks associated with upper endoscopy and with sedation.
- **Bacteremia** is a rare occurrence after EUS-guided FNA, with an incidence of approximately 0.4–1%.

- There is a small risk of **pancreatitis** (1–2%) associated with EUS-guided FNA of pancreatic masses.
- **Bleeding and bile peritonitis** as complications of EUS-guided FNA are rare and described anecdotally in the literature.

Liver Biopsy

GENERAL PRINCIPLES

- Liver biopsy can be achieved by two different techniques:
  - **Percutaneous liver biopsy**, performed at the bedside, sometimes with ultrasound guidance; rarely, it is performed under computed tomographic guidance.
  - **Transjugular liver biopsy** under fluoroscopic guidance.
- **Common indications** for liver biopsy include evaluation of abnormal liver chemistries, assessment of degree of inflammation and fibrosis in chronic liver disease (e.g., hepatitis C), and diagnosis of liver masses.[8]
- Procedure
  - Bedside percutaneous liver biopsy is commonly performed by gastroenterologists or hepatologists.
  - The patient is placed supine with the right arm behind the head.
  - With ultrasound guidance or percussion, an appropriate biopsy location is chosen in the right lateral chest wall, usually near the eighth intercostal space.
  - The area is prepared and draped in sterile fashion, and lidocaine is used to infiltrate the skin, subcutaneous fat, intercostal muscles, and liver capsule.
  - A small incision is made, and the liver biopsy needle is advanced to the liver capsule.
  - With the patient held in full expiration, the biopsy needle is advanced into the liver parenchyma, and a core of tissue is obtained.
  - The patient is then observed closely for at least 4 hours for complications.
- **Contraindications to percutaneous liver biopsy** include severe coagulopathy, thrombocytopenia, or ascites.[8]
- If percutaneous liver biopsy cannot be safely performed or if portal pressure measurements are needed, transjugular liver biopsy under radiologic guidance may be performed.
- Directed biopsy with ultrasound or CT guidance may be necessary for sampling of liver masses.

COMPLICATIONS

Complications of liver biopsy are rare but can be severe.
- The most common complication is **pain at the biopsy site or in the right shoulder**.
- Less common complications are **bleeding (including hemobilia), pneumothorax, gallbladder perforation, inadvertent kidney biopsy, or death**.
- Most complications are apparent within the first 4–6 hours, but they can occur up to 48 hours after biopsy.

Percutaneous Endoscopic Gastrostomy/Jejunostomy

GENERAL PRINCIPLES

- Percutaneous endoscopic gastrostomy/jejunostomy (PEG/PEJ) and jejunal extension through PEG (PEG-J) tubes are indicated in patients requiring long-term nutritional support.

- **Common indications** include oropharyngeal dysphagia secondary to neurologic conditions, oropharyngeal and laryngeal cancer, esophageal cancer, and head and facial trauma.[9]
- **Procedure**
  - Enteral feeding through a gastrostomy or jejunostomy has several advantages over parenteral nutrition such as lower risks of infection, preservation of gut integrity, and costs.
  - Percutaneous enterostomies should not be performed in individuals with rapidly progressive diseases with a short life expectancy or when oral feeds are expected to resume within 30 days.
  - Other contraindications include coagulopathy, pharyngeal or esophageal obstruction, inability to achieve apposition of stomach with the abdominal wall, lack of adequate gastric transillumination due to prior gastric surgery, ascites, hepatomegaly, and obesity and bowel obstruction.
  - The two common techniques of PEG and PEJ include the "pull" and "push" technique.
  - PEJ is a modification of PEG and more difficult to perform.
  - Feeding via the PEG/PEJ is typically initiated the next day or 24 hours postprocedure.

COMPLICATIONS

- Complications include wound infections, bleeding, perforation, ileus, injury to internal organs, tumor seeding, buried bumper syndrome, and death.
- Antibiotic prophylaxis is recommended to reduce the risk of peristomal wound infection.

SPECIAL CONSIDERATIONS

Conscious Sedation

- Conscious sedation provides adequate analgesia and sedation for most GI procedures while allowing the patient to cooperate with verbal commands.
- Conscious sedation for endoscopic procedures usually involves a **benzodiazepine** (e.g., midazolam) **and an opiate** (e.g., meperidine or fentanyl).
- In patients not adequately sedated with this combination, addition of other IV agents such as promethazine or diphenhydramine can be considered.
- **Propofol** is an ultra–short-acting sedative, and its use **requires the presence of an anesthesiologist** for both the administration of the drug and airway control. The use of propofol is typically reserved for providing deep sedation.[10]
- The American Society of Anesthesiologists (ASA) assessment (categories I–V) is useful in evaluating the sedation risk for a patient.
  - ASA category I represents the lowest risk.
  - Advanced age, obesity, pregnancy, sleep apnea, a history of substance abuse, or severe cardiac, respiratory, hepatic, renal, or central nervous system disease places patients at higher risk for sedation.
  - Anesthesia assistance should be considered for patients with ASA class III and above, for those who have had adverse reaction or inadequate response to moderate sedation, for patients who take opiates chronically, and for lengthy or complex endoscopic procedures.
  - The ASA guidelines state that patients should fast a minimum of 2 hours after consumption of clear liquids and 6 hours after consuming light meals before the administration of sedation.
- The most common sedation complications include airway obstruction and respiratory depression, oversedation, hypoxia, and hypotension. Patients are monitored during the procedure using continuous pulse oximetry, heart monitoring, intermittent blood

pressure recordings, and in some situations, end-tidal CO_2. These parameters are supplemental to vigilant clinical observation of the patient.

Antibiotic Prophylaxis for Endoscopy

- Mucosal trauma during GI endoscopy can result in bacterial translocation of microbial flora into the bloodstream. Bacteremia as a result of this carries a risk of localization of infection in remote tissues (e.g., infective endocarditis). Endoscopy can also contaminate a sterile space or tissue by an endoscopic accessory or by contrast injection.
- **Bacterial endocarditis** is a potentially life-threatening infection.
  - Approximately 4% of patients develop bacteremia associated with endoscopy, but this varies depending on the specific procedure performed.
  - Although infective endocarditis is a potentially life-threatening infection, this has rarely been reported post-GI endoscopy. There are no data demonstrating a causal link between endoscopic procedures and infective endocarditis.
  - Similarly, there are no data that demonstrate that antibiotic prophylaxis before endoscopic procedures protect against infective endocarditis.
  - The guidelines for antibiotic prophylaxis for GI endoscopy are outlined by the American Society for Gastrointestinal Endoscopy and have been highlighted in Table 26-3.[11] These recommendations are in accordance with the recommendations of the American Heart Association.
  - Antibiotic prophylaxis solely to prevent infective endocarditis is no longer recommended before endoscopic procedures.

Anticoagulation and Antiplatelet Agents

- Patients on chronic anticoagulation (warfarin, heparin, and low–molecular-weight heparin), antiplatelet agents (aspirin, nonsteroidal anti-inflammatory drugs [NSAIDs]), thienopyridines (clopidogrel), and glycoprotein IIb/IIIa receptor inhibitors requiring GI procedures pose a challenging problem.
- Ideally, the **platelet count should be >50,000** and **INR should be <1.5 prior to endoscopic procedures**.
- The three issues that should be considered include:
  - Risk of bleeding from antithrombotic therapy;
  - Risk of bleeding from an endoscopic intervention in the setting of antithrombotic medication use; and
  - Risk of thromboembolic event from interruption of antithrombotic therapy.
- Management of antithrombotic agents is **based on the risk of the GI procedure** (low vs. high risk), **indication for use of antithrombotic agent** (low vs. high risk for thromboembolic event), and **indication of procedure** (elective vs. emergent).
- **Low-risk GI procedures** include all diagnostic procedures including ERCP without sphincterotomy and EUS without FNA.
- **High-risk procedures** include polypectomy (especially in the small bowel and proximal colon), sphincterotomy, stricture dilation, PEG, and EUS-guided FNA.
- The guidelines for management of anticoagulation and antiplatelet therapy for GI endoscopy were recently updated by the American Society for Gastrointestinal Endoscopy.[12] These guidelines provide a comprehensive list of most individual antithrombotic agents and their specific management recommendations prior to endoscopy including duration of action and reversal agents. Please refer to these guidelines for all-inclusive recommendations. Some important updated recommendations from this guideline are as follows:
  - Elective endoscopic procedures
  - Low doses of aspirin and NSAIDs may be continued safely during the periprocedural period

TABLE 26-3 AMERICAN SOCIETY FOR GASTROINTESTINAL ENDOSCOPY RECOMMENDATIONS FOR ANTIBIOTIC PROPHYLAXIS

Antibiotic Prophylaxis and/or Treatment to Prevent Local Infections

Patient Condition	Procedure Contemplated	Goal of Prophylaxis	Periprocedural Antibiotic Prophylaxis
Bile duct obstruction in absence of cholangitis	ERCP with complete drainage	Prevention of cholangitis	Not recommended[a]
Bile duct obstruction in absence of cholangitis	ERCP with incomplete drainage	Prevention of cholangitis	Recommended; continue antibiotics after procedure[b]
Solid lesion in upper GI tract	EUS-FNA	Prevention of local infection	Not recommended[a]
Solid lesion in lower GI tract	EUS-FNA	Prevention of local infection	Not recommended[b]
Mediastinal cysts	EUS-FNA	Prevention of cyst infection	Suggested[c]
Pancreatic cysts	EUS-FNA	Prevention of cyst infection	Suggested[c]
All patients	Percutaneous endoscopic feeding tube placement	Prevention of peristomal infection	Recommended[a]
Cirrhosis with acute GI bleeding	Required for all patients regardless of endoscopic procedures	Prevention of infectious adverse events and reduction of mortality	On admission[a]
Synthetic vascular graft and other nonvalvular cardiovascular devices	Any endoscopic procedure	Prevention of graft and device infection	Not recommended[a]
Prosthetic joints	Any endoscopic procedure	Prevention of septic arthritis	Not recommended[b]
Peritoneal dialysis	Lower GI endoscopy	Prevention of peritonitis	Suggested[c]

[a]High, Further research is very unlikely to change our confidence in the estimate of effect.
[b]Moderate, Further research is likely to have an important impact on our confidence in the estimate of effect and may change the estimate.
[c]Low, Further research is very likely to have an important impact on our confidence in the estimate of effect and is likely to change the estimate.

- Continue thienopyridines for low-risk endoscopic procedures
- Discontinue thienopyridines 5 to 7 days before high-risk endoscopic procedures. Alternatively, can switch to ASA monotherapy and continue until the thienopyridine can be safely resumed
- Discontinue anticoagulation for the appropriate interval in if high-risk endoscopic procedures are planned in a patient at low risk for thromboembolic events
- Continue warfarin and novel anticoagulants in patients undergoing low-risk endoscopic procedures
- Urgent or emergent endoscopic procedures
- Recommend either 4-factor PCC and vitamin K or fresh frozen plasma be given for life-threatening GI bleeding in patients on warfarin anticoagulant therapy
- Do not delay endoscopic therapy in patients with serious GI bleeding and an INR <2.5

REFERENCES

1. Ben-Menachem T, Decker GA, Early DS, et al. Adverse events of upper GI endoscopy. *Gastrointest Endosc.* 2012;76(4):707–718.
2. Saltzman JR, Cash BD, Pasha SF, et al. Bowel preparation before colonoscopy. *Gastrointest Endosc.* 2015;81(4):781–794.
3. Fisher DA, Maple JT, Ben-menachem T, et al. Complications of colonoscopy. *Gastrointest Endosc.* 2011;74(4):745–752.
4. Laine L, Sahota A, Shah A. Does capsule endoscopy improve outcomes in obscure gastrointestinal bleeding? Randomized trial versus dedicated small bowel radiography. *Gastroenterology.* 2010;138(5):1673–1680.
5. Dumonceau JM, Andriulli A, Deviere J, et al; European Society of Gastrointestinal Endoscopy. European Society of Gastrointestinal Endoscopy (ESGE) guideline: prophylaxis of post-ERCP pancreatitis. *Endoscopy.* 2010;42(6):503–515.
6. Elmunzer BJ, Scheiman JM, Lehman GA, et al. A randomized trial of rectal indomethacin to prevent post-ERCP pancreatitis. *N Engl J Med.* 2012;366(15):1414–1422.
7. Hawes RH. The evolution of endoscopic ultrasound: improved imaging, higher accuracy for fine needle aspiration and the reality of endoscopic ultrasound-guided interventions. *Curr Opin Gastroenterol.* 2010;26(5):436–444.
8. Rockey DC, Caldwell SH, Goodman ZD, et al; American Association for the Study of Liver Diseases. Liver biopsy. *Hepatology.* 2009;49(3):1017–1044.
9. ASGE Technology Committee; Kwon RS, Banerjee S, Desilets D, et al. Enteral nutrition access devices. *Gastrointest Endosc.* 2010;72(2):236–248.
10. Cohen LB, Ladas SD, Vargo JJ, et al. Sedation in digestive endoscopy: the Athens international position statements. *Aliment Pharmacol Ther.* 2010;32(3):425–442.
11. ASGE Standards of Practice Committee; Khashab MA, Chithadi KV, Acosta RD, et al. Antibiotic prophylaxis for GI endoscopy. *Gastrointest Endosc.* 2015;81(1):81–89.
12. ASGE Standards of Practice Committee; Acosta RD, Abraham NS, Chandrasekhara V, et al. The management of antithrombotic agents for patients undergoing GI endoscopy. *Gastrointest Endosc.* 2016;83(1):3–16.

Index

Note: Page number followed by f and t indicates figure and table respectively.